Fitness and Lifestyle Management for Law Enforcement

REVISED FOURTH EDITION

Nancy Wagner Wisotzki

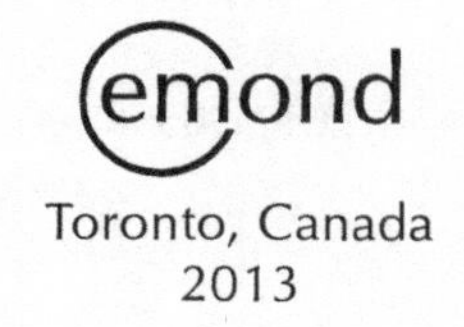

Toronto, Canada
2013

Emond Montgomery Publications Limited
60 Shaftesbury Avenue
Toronto ON M4T 1A3
http://www.emond.ca/highered

Printed in Canada.
Revised and reprinted December 2015.

We acknowledge the financial support of the Government of Canada.
Nous reconnaissons l'appui financier du gouvernement du Canada.

Canadä

Publisher, higher education: Mike Thompson
Senior developmental editor, higher education: Sarah Gleadow
Director, editorial and production: Jim Lyons
Developmental and copy editor: Francine Geraci
Proofreader: Cindy Fujimoto
Permissions editor: Maria DeCambra
Text designer and typesetter: Shani Sohn
Indexer: Paula Pike
Cover designer: Tara Wells
Cover image: epicurean / iStockphoto.com

Library and Archives Canada Cataloguing in Publication

Wagner Wisotzki, Nancy, 1959-
Fitness and lifestyle management for law enforcement / Nancy Wagner Wisotzki. — 4th ed.

Includes index.
ISBN 978-1-55239-473-1

1. Police—Health and hygiene. 2. Police—Physical training. I. Title.

HV7936.H4W33 2012 613.02'43632 C2012-905588-3

To The Kissin Cousins,
Dan, Amy, Alex, Aaron, Christine, Matt, and Kate:
For your love, laughter, and your dreams that you have yet to realize.

To the graduates and police officers who continue to touch my life and heart:
Thank you for your inspiration and zest for living well and enjoying life.

Contents

CHAPTER 12 Stress

CHAPTER 13 Shiftwork

CHAPTER 14 Common Injuries

PART 5
Fitness Standards for Law Enforcement

CHAPTER 15 Preparing to Meet Law Enforcement Fitness Standards

Appendix: Assignments

Preface

Over the course of several editions, the aim of this book has expanded beyond providing a general understanding of the importance of physical activity and how to meet the basic fitness requirements for a career in law enforcement. Although these continue to serve as its foundation, it has come to mean so much more, encompassing the importance of living a wellness *lifestyle*. This knowledge will carry you throughout your career. It will help you determine your goals and, through a personal commitment and the use of effective time- and self-management skills, to work toward living a healthy lifestyle as you learn more about general health and wellness concepts, and maintain the fitness level you need to do your job.

Entrance requirements have evolved over the years to reflect the physical demands of law enforcement jobs, particularly with the adoption of Bona Fide Occupational Requirements (BFOR) testing, which assesses the minimum physical requirements for police officers. For most of you, this challenge will not be difficult to meet. However, as your career evolves, it will become more important for you to maintain wellness in *all* areas of your life by staying healthy not only physically, but emotionally and mentally as well.

This textbook has been prepared with these goals in mind. Just as your instructors will tell you that learning is a life-long commitment, the same applies to physical activity. In the following pages and in the new companion volume, the *Fit for Duty, Fit for Life Training Guide*, you will be introduced to issues and concepts of crucial importance to law enforcement personnel, including wellness and physical fitness, time management, nutrition, hypokinetic diseases (such as obesity, diabetes, and cardiovascular disease), back pain, stress, shiftwork, and common injuries.

Meeting the minimum requirements of the job and getting hired is most likely your first goal, but it should not be your *ultimate* goal. Police work requires a lifetime commitment to yourself and to your family, and you will need to ensure that you find the balance that allows you to maintain a high quality of life both on the job and off. Having the knowledge and coping skills to deal with demands in *all* areas of your life will be key to your success in policing. Quality of life—both on the job and off, through awareness, positive choices, and physical fitness—will be your choice to make.

This fourth edition of *Fitness and Lifestyle Management for Law Enforcement* includes expanded coverage of the basics of physical activity, nutrition, updated BFOR and Ontario Police Fitness standards, and illustrations to help explain some of the topics. The companion text, *Fit for Duty, Fit for Life Training Guide*, contains photographs and descriptions of recommended stretching and weight-training exercises, as well as logs to help you track your progress as you work toward meeting your goals.

I hope you stay happy, healthy, and fit. Good luck on your journey.

Nancy Wagner Wisotzki
Georgian College

Acknowledgments

It has been an interesting journey updating this edition of this book. I want to thank the executive members of the Police Fitness Personnel of Ontario and the Faculty at Georgian College, especially Janice Pepe, who gave me continual feedback and support through this process. Your commitment to police officers' fitness and well-being in Ontario is reflected in your devotion not only to your individual services but to all officers in the province. I want to thank Francine Geraci and Sarah Gleadow for their editorial guidance, patience, and positive input throughout this process. Special thanks to the students in the School of Public Safety and Emergency Services, who inspire me always to challenge my knowledge and who inspire me to love what I do. Finally to Larry, Alexandra, and Christine—for pushing me to value our family and the goals that help us lead a healthy and active lifestyle.

PART 1

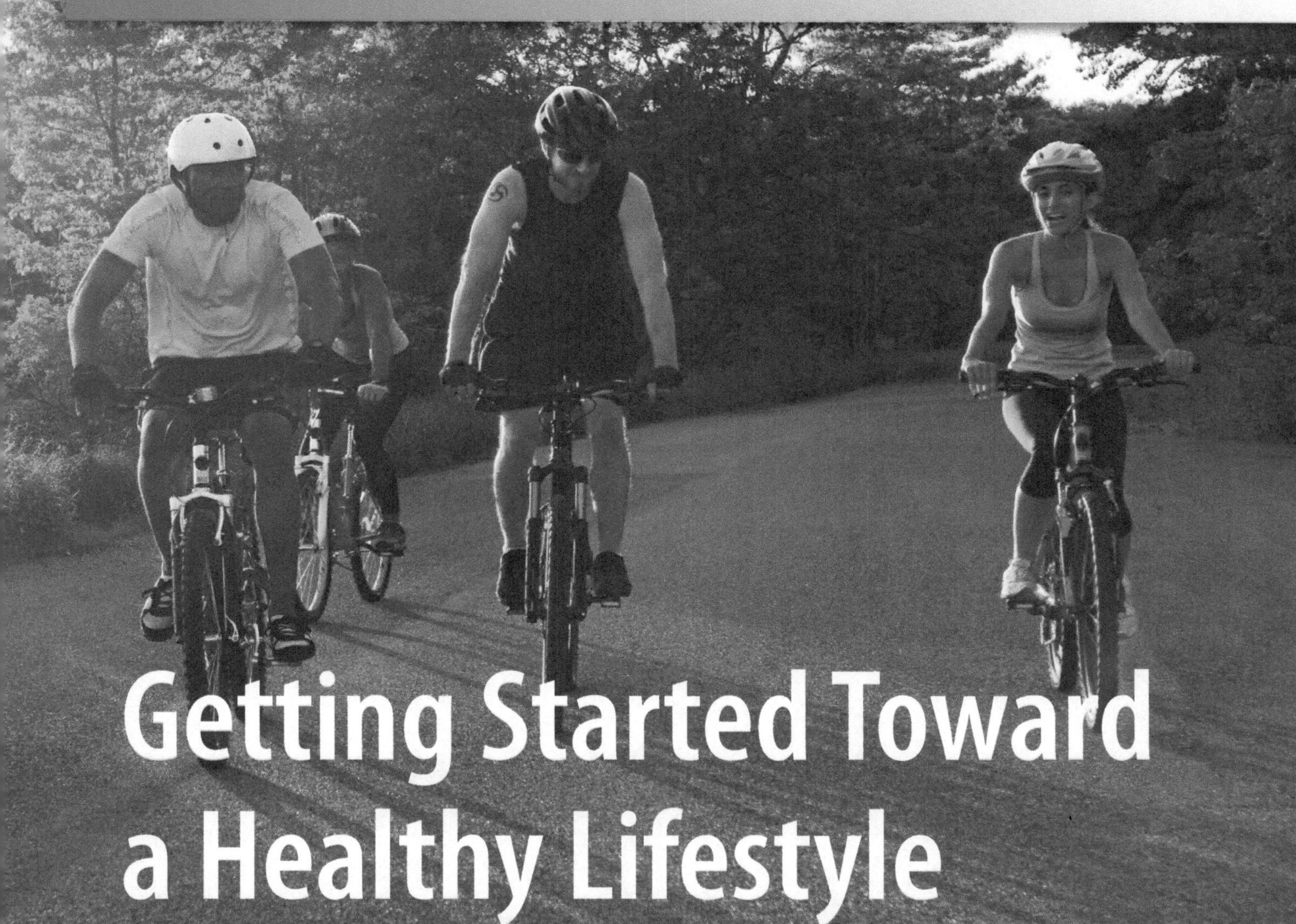

Getting Started Toward a Healthy Lifestyle

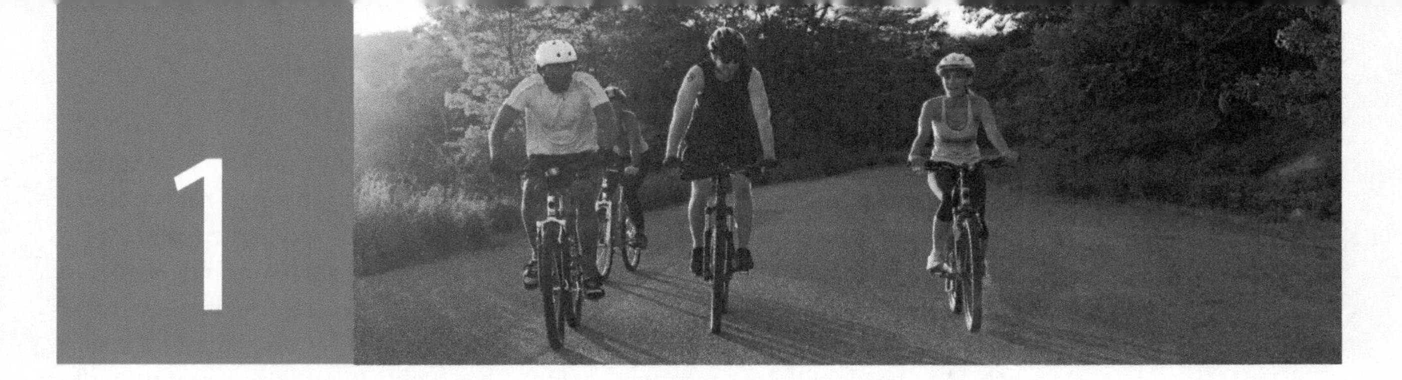

1

Wellness and Active Living: A Healthy Lifestyle

LEARNING OBJECTIVES

After completing this chapter, you should be able to:

- Explain the concepts of fitness, active living, health, and wellness.
- Describe the health benefits of physical activity.
- Describe some of the steps you can take to achieve a healthy lifestyle.
- Evaluate the physical and psychological competencies you need to meet the requirements of a law enforcement career.

OVERVIEW

During the 1970s and 1980s, Canadians embraced physical activity with enthusiasm and vigour. But by the 1990s, participation rates had dropped alarmingly. Physical inactivity in the 21st century has now reached epidemic proportions. Most of us recognize the benefits of physical activity to our independence and quality of life, yet our health and wellness are today in crisis. Ours may be the first generation whose children will have a shorter life expectancy than their parents. As a result of these concerns, "wellness" has grown to mean different things to different people. For some people, wellness equates with a certain level of fitness, while others perceive it as freedom from illness. For still others, wellness is resiliency to physical and psychological stresses that affect daily life.

This chapter discusses the concepts of fitness, active living, health, and wellness. As you prepare for a career in law enforcement, you will be required to scrutinize your health and physical fitness levels to determine your readiness to meet the occupational demands of the job. The goal of this chapter is to enable you to assess your wellness and commitment to lifelong fitness and make some decisions on how you may achieve your optimal levels.

A Wellness Profile

health
the ability of an individual to function independently in a constantly changing environment

wellness
a way of life in which you make decisions and choices to enjoy the highest level of health and well-being possible

Health and wellness are related concepts. Good **health** means being able to function independently in a constantly changing environment. **Wellness** can be defined as a way of life in which you make decisions and choices to enjoy the highest level of health and well-being possible. Wellness includes the idea that life is a journey that must be enjoyed and continually fine-tuned in order to benefit as much as possible from all aspects of your life. This means taking the appropriate steps to prevent illness and to lead a richer, more balanced, and satisfying life. By embracing small, positive changes in your lifestyle habits, you empower yourself through self-esteem and self-worth to ensure you have a healthy attitude and lifestyle.

An individual's lifestyle and behaviour clearly affect his or her health. Here is a list of behaviours and habits necessary for wellness:

- taking responsibility for your own health (including research on health issues, regular checkups, and asking questions) and taking an active role in the decisions you make about your life
- learning to manage stress effectively
- maintaining high self-esteem and being able to interact successfully with others
- understanding your sexuality and having satisfying intimate relationships
- developing healthy relationships with spouses, partners, family, friends, and colleagues
- avoiding tobacco and other drugs; using alcohol wisely, if at all
- eating well, exercising, and maintaining a healthy weight
- understanding the Ontario health-care system and the health benefits to which your employment entitles you
- knowing the facts about cardiovascular (heart and blood vessel) disease, diabetes, cancer, sexually transmitted diseases and other infections, and injuries, and using your knowledge to protect yourself against them

- understanding how the environment affects your health and taking appropriate action to protect yourself against environmental hazards
- having a sense of satisfaction with life and appreciating life's different stages
- developing a sense of humour, the ability to express yourself and share feelings, empathy with others, and a tolerance of others' opinions
- achieving a balance in all dimensions of health

The Relationship Between Wellness and Fitness

Healthy living, physical activity, exercise, physical fitness, and active living all have a relationship to overall wellness. As you pursue your career in law enforcement, it is important that you aim for balance in all aspects of your life. Understanding that wellness is a spectrum will help you appreciate the importance of physical activity and fitness throughout your career.

Healthy Living

At a population level, **healthy living** refers to the practices of population groups that are consistent with supporting, improving, maintaining, and enhancing health. As it applies to individuals, healthy living is the practice of health-enhancing behaviours, or put simply, living in healthy ways. It implies the physical, mental, and spiritual capacity to make healthy choices, including healthy eating and physical activity, and to understand their relationship to healthy weights (PHAC, 2005a).

healthy living
the practice of health-enhancing behaviours; the physical, mental, and spiritual capacity to make healthy choices including healthy eating and physical activity, and an understanding of their relationship to maintaining a healthy weight

In 2002, the federal government developed an Integrated Pan-Canadian Healthy Living Strategy (PHAC, 2005b). Under the Public Health Agency of Canada, goals were set to improve health and reduce health disparities across the country. The aim was to focus on children and youth to address physical inactivity and unhealthy eating. The Healthy Living Network was set up in 2003 for communication and health information to provide support for communities and educators in improving health quality in Canada. Healthy living incorporates appropriate choices that include healthy eating, refraining from smoking, having a support system in place, and staying physically active whether at home, school, or work. The emphasis is on the reduction of diseases and prevention of injuries. Through *Healthy Living* e-bulletins, the network promotes physical activity, healthy eating, and healthy weights across the country (for more information, see PHAC, 2012).

Physical Activity

Physical activity is all leisure and non-leisure body movement that reduces the risk of disease, helps control weight, and strengthens muscles, bones, and joints. Over the past few decades, the physical activity and fitness levels of Canadians have decreased, and overweight and obesity and their associated co-morbidity rates have steadily increased (Colley et al., 2011a, 2011b; Shields et al., 2010; Tremblay, Colley, Saunders, Healey, & Owen, 2010).

physical activity
all leisure and non-leisure body movement that results in an expenditure of energy

Sedentary behaviour is emerging as a negative contributor to health. "Sedentary" is increasingly being defined as a distinct subset of activities, rather than as simply a lack of volitional physical activity of moderate or vigorous intensity (Tremblay, Wolfson, & Connor Gorber, 2007). Sedentary behaviour encompasses a broad range of activities (for instance, occupational sitting, TV watching, eating) that occur intermittently throughout the day (Tremblay, Esliger, Tremblay, & Colley, 2007; PHAC, 2012).

For children and youth, physical activity is integral in preventing high blood pressure, overweight and obesity, **metabolic syndrome**, depression, and injury. For adults, it is important for reducing premature mortality relating to cardiovascular disease, certain types of cancer (breast and colon), and diabetes. For older adults, it has become important for functional independence: bodily movement produced by skeletal muscles results in an expenditure of energy that has a positive impact on bone density and muscle mass.

metabolic syndrome a cluster of risk factors including abdominal obesity, hypertension, high blood triglycerides, insulin resistance, low HDL (good) and high LDL (bad) cholesterol, and vascular inflammatory markers

moderate-intensity physical activity on an absolute scale, moderate intensity refers to activity that is performed 3.0–5.9 times the intensity of rest; on a scale relative to an individual's personal capacity, moderate-intensity physical activity is usually about 10–12 on the Borg scale of 0–20

vigorous-intensity physical activity on an absolute scale, vigorous intensity refers to activity that is performed at 6.0 or more times the intensity of rest for adults and typically 7.0 or more times for children and youth; on a scale relative to an individual's personal capacity, vigorous-intensity physical activity is usually about 14–16 on the Borg scale of 0–20

We know that people's health and well-being improve with daily moderate levels of activity. Moderate activities can include walking briskly, mowing the lawn, dancing, swimming, or bicycling. Occupational physical activity can include walking, hauling, lifting, pushing, carpentry, shovelling, and packing boxes. In order to continue to do your job well, it is important that physical activity become an integral component of your daily life.

In 2010, the Canadian Society for Exercise Physiology (CSEP) recommended that adults should engage in at least 150 minutes per week of **moderate to vigorous physical activity** (MVPA), accumulating in bouts lasting at least 10 minutes (Warburton, Charlesworth, Ivey, Nettlefold, & Bredin, 2010). The percentage of Canadians meeting that level by accumulating at least 30 minutes of MVPA on at least 5 days per week is about 5 percent, and approximately 63 percent accumulate 15 minutes of MVPA at least one day a week. This means that more than a third of the Canadian population (37 percent) do not reach even this modest level of activity (Colley et al., 2011a). In other words, the findings indicate that 85 percent of adults are not active enough to meet Canada's most recent physical activity recommendations (Tremblay et al., 2011).

FACTS ABOUT . . .

Physical Inactivity

- Physical inactivity has been identified as the fourth leading risk factor for global mortality (6 percent of deaths globally), behind high blood pressure (13 percent), tobacco use (9 percent), and high blood glucose (6 percent). It contributes to over 3 million preventable deaths annually.
- Overweight and obesity are responsible for 5 percent of global mortality.
- As much as 50 percent of mortality from the 10 leading causes of death in Canada can be traced to lifestyle.
- A survey of the physical activity levels of Canadians aged 20 to 79 years found that only 15 percent of adults are meeting the current physical activity recommendations. The majority—69 percent—of Canadian adults spend their waking hours in sedentary pursuits.
- It is estimated that physical inactivity costs the Canadian economy approximately $7.1 billion per year (2006 dollars).

SOURCES: WHO, 2009; Anis et al., 2009; Statistics Canada, 2008, 2011.

Exercise

Exercise is a form of leisure-time physical activity that is planned, structured, and repetitive. Its main objective is to improve or maintain physical fitness. The benefits of exercise are improved health, resistance to diseases caused by inactivity, and the capacity to perform daily activities with vigour. People who make exercise a part of their everyday activities will likely be fitter than those who do not exercise, and will, therefore, enjoy better health and more energy to perform daily tasks more effectively and skillfully. Exercise can also improve your mood by stimulating various brain chemicals that may leave you feeling more relaxed after your workout. By delivering more oxygen and nutrients to your tissues, exercise can help you breathe easier, have more efficient cardiac output, and have more energy to do the things you enjoy.

exercise
a form of leisure-time physical activity that is planned, structured, and repetitive, with the goal of improving or maintaining physical fitness

For those who suffer from arthritis or osteoporosis (a reduction in bone mass), exercise increases range of motion and bone density, which in turn improve the quality of daily life, allowing simple tasks to be done without risk of injury or pain. This is important in law enforcement, with its physical demands, whether it means being able to comfortably wear your duty belt (which can weigh 5–10 kilograms) or performing capably when intervening in an altercation.

DID YOU KNOW?

Those in the low-fitness category experience non-vehicular back injuries and vehicular back injuries at a greater proportion than those who are more fit.

SOURCES: Cady, 1985; Constance, Sullivan, & Shimizu, 1988.

Physical Fitness

Physical fitness refers to a person's health and performance, specifically in the areas of cardiorespiratory (heart and lung) fitness, body composition, muscular strength and endurance, and flexibility. A physiologic state of well-being allows one to meet the demands of daily life, provides the basis for sport performance, or both. A physically fit individual has enough energy to enjoy life and avoid fatigue.

physical fitness
a person's health and performance, specifically in the areas of cardiorespiratory fitness, body composition, muscular strength and endurance, and flexibility

Physical fitness is divided into four health-related components (cardiorespiratory, muscular strength and endurance, flexibility, body composition) and six skill-related components (agility, balance, power, speed, coordination, reaction time). Further, we can distinguish the following types of physical fitness:

- **Health-related fitness** involves aspects of fitness that are linked to a person's health. For example, people who perform weight-bearing exercises in their middle years are less likely to lose bone density when they are older. In law enforcement, this may help in a situation where you must physically respond to the demands of a chase or an altercation.

health-related fitness
the components of physical fitness that are related to health status, including cardiovascular fitness, musculoskeletal fitness, body composition, and metabolism

- **Performance/skill-related fitness** is the degree of fitness required to perform a particular job or sport. A person who exercises regularly will likely develop good motor skills (including coordination, agility, speed, and reaction time) and the endurance, muscular strength, and cardiorespiratory power and capacity necessary for peak performance. Law enforcement officers must respond to emergency situations all the time. Impaired speed and reaction time can cost them their lives or the lives of others who depend on them.

performance/skill-related fitness
the degree of fitness required to perform a particular job or sport

- **Musculoskeletal fitness** consists of three measures: muscular strength, flexibility, and muscular endurance (Statistics Canada, 2009) to provide a measure of health. Musculoskeletal fitness has been positively associated with functional independence, mobility, maintaining healthy blood sugar

musculoskeletal fitness
a combined measure of muscular strength, flexibility, and muscular endurance to provide a measure of health

levels, bone health, psychological well-being, and overall quality of life. It is negatively associated with the risk of fall, illness, disability, and premature death (Warburton, Gledhill, & Quinney, 2001a, 2001b).

It is important for law enforcement officers to maintain both the cardiorespiratory and musculoskeletal components of training so that they can deal with the various situations they will face. It is recommended that eight to ten exercises that use the major muscles of the body be performed on two or more non-consecutive days each week. Such activities include lifting weights, weight-bearing calisthenics, or similar **resistance training** exercises that use the major muscle groups of the body. Canada's newest recommendations on physical activity specify that muscle- and bone-strengthening activities should be done *in addition to* the recommended 150 minutes per week (Tremblay et al., 2011).

resistance training
an exercise program that uses repeated, progressive contractions of specific muscle groups to increase muscle strength, endurance, or power

In accordance with the most recent *Canadian Physical Activity Guidelines* (CSEP, 2011a), regular physical activity should include activity most days of the week, preferably each day. Five or more days of the week should include at least 30 minutes (which can be done in 10-minute increments) of moderate- to vigorous-intensity activities (Tremblay et al., 2011). Research has shown a direct relationship between metabolic and cardiorespiratory health and participating in at least 150 minutes of moderate-intensity activities per week (Warburton et al., 2010). However, if you want to be fitter and excel at the demands of your job, you need to ensure that you are engaging in enough activities at an intensity that enables you to see improvements.

Active Living

While physical inactivity is the fourth leading cause of death globally, it is also related, directly and indirectly, to other risk factors such as high blood pressure, high cholesterol, and high glucose levels, and to the recent striking increases in childhood and adult obesity (WHO, 2009). In the early 1990s, the Canadian government implemented an "active living" approach to dealing with this situation.

According to Fitness Canada (1991), **active living** is a way of life in which people make meaningful and satisfying physical activities an integral part of daily living.

active living
a way of life in which individuals make meaningful and satisfying physical activities an integral part of daily living

PERSONAL PERSPECTIVE

Intrinsic Motivation

Some years ago, I had the privilege to meet a grad whom I had not seen in a number of years. He had returned to Barrie to work, and connected with me through a student that he had hired. The student confided that this grad was avoiding coming to see me not because he did not want to come and talk, but because he was embarrassed by his physical condition. As I thought about this justification, I realized that I had given him only an extrinsic motivation for his success in class (passing the course and being physically fit). Apparently, I had missed the boat in terms of helping him, and perhaps other students, develop the intrinsic motivational skills necessary to maintaining or returning to fitness after graduation. I ultimately reconnected with that grad, and over the years have supported him in realizing those intrinsic reasons to be physically active again.

When you read Chapter 2, you will discover both the intrinsic and extrinsic motivational skills needed to succeed throughout your chosen career.

Because physical activity is influenced by policies and practices in education, transportation, parks and recreation, media, and business, multiple sectors of society need to be involved in the solutions. There is a clear need to inform, motivate, and support individuals and communities to be active in ways that are safe. As a result of this push, towns and cities have created Charters for Physical Activity to encourage regular exercise (Global Advocacy for Physical Activity, 2010).

Although Health Canada has intensively promoted healthy eating and physical activity, obesity continues to increase. We know that poor nutrition and lack of physical activity are primary contributors to weight gain. Lack of fruits and vegetables in the diet, as well as inactivity due to watching TV, playing video games, or using a computer, contribute to weight gain and obesity (Garriguet, 2004). We also know that socio-economic factors may play a role in obesity rates, particularly for women. Obesity is an especially important health issue among First Nations, Inuit, and Métis populations.

An interesting note regarding causes of mortality: Although cardiovascular disease has been the main cause of death in Canada over the last 25 years, it has declined (from 47 percent in 1979 to 32 percent in 2004 to 21.5 percent in 2007), making it the second leading cause of death. Cancer's mortality rate has been growing (from 23 percent in 1979 to 30 percent in 2004 to 29.6 percent in 2007), making it the leading cause of death in Canada (see Figure 1.1) (Statistics Canada, 2008).

Active living is one strategy that can combat overweight and obesity. It is essential to improved health, well-being, and quality of life. There are three types of activities you need to take part in to keep your body healthy: endurance activities, flexibility activities, and strength activities (PHAC, 2004). These activities will be covered in other chapters of this book. An active lifestyle helps increase bone density, energy

TOP TEN ...

Ways to Get Started with Active Living

1. **Walk** whenever you can—get off the bus early; use the stairs instead of the elevator.
2. **Reduce long periods of inactivity**, like watching TV—get up and move during each commercial.
3. **Get up from the couch** and stretch out.
4. **Play actively** with your kids.
5. **Choose to walk, cycle, or skateboard** for short trips.
6. **Start with a 10-minute walk**—gradually increase the time to 30 minutes.
7. **Find nearby walking and cycling paths** and use them.
8. **Observe a physical activity class** to see if you want to try it.
9. **Try one class to start**—you don't have to make a long-term commitment. Try something new, like yoga or Pilates.
10. **Do the activities you do now, more often!** Bring a friend along to help keep you motivated.

FACTS ABOUT . . .

Obesity in Canada

- Over half the Canadian population is overweight, and 1 in 4 adults aged 18 or older are obese.
- Since 1988, the prevalence of obesity has risen over 10 percentage points, with the highest percentage for men in the 60–74 age group and for women in the 20–29 age group.
- Between 1994 and 2005, rates of high blood pressure among Canadians skyrocketed by 77 percent, diabetes by 45 percent, and obesity by 18 percent—affecting both younger and older Canadians.
- Among Canadians 35–49 years of age, the prevalence of high blood pressure increased 127 percent, diabetes by 64 percent, and obesity by 20 percent—all major risk factors for heart disease.
- Some 26 percent of Canadian children and adolescents aged 2–17 are overweight or obese (a figure that has doubled since 1978–79), and 8.6 percent are obese (triple that of 1978–79).
- Beyond its adverse effects on physical health, childhood obesity can also affect mental health. There is a link with low self-esteem, body-image issues, depression, and unhealthy eating behaviours.
- Among Aboriginal Canadians, 31.8 percent of adult men, 41.1 percent of adult women, 14.0 percent of youth, and 36.2 percent of children are considered obese.
- Obesity is associated with higher risk for non-insulin-dependent (type 2) diabetes, cardiovascular disease, psycho-social difficulties, osteoarthritis, some cancers (endometrial, breast, and colon), dyslipidemia (high levels of cholesterol or fat in the blood), liver and gallbladder disease, sleep apnea, gynecological problems (abnormal menses, infertility), and premature mortality.

SOURCES: Garriguet, 2007; First Nations Regional Longitudinal Health Survey, 2002/03, 2007; Heart and Stroke, 2010; Shields et al., 2010; Shields, Carroll, & Ogden, 2011.

FIGURE 1.1 Leading Causes of Death, Canada, 2008

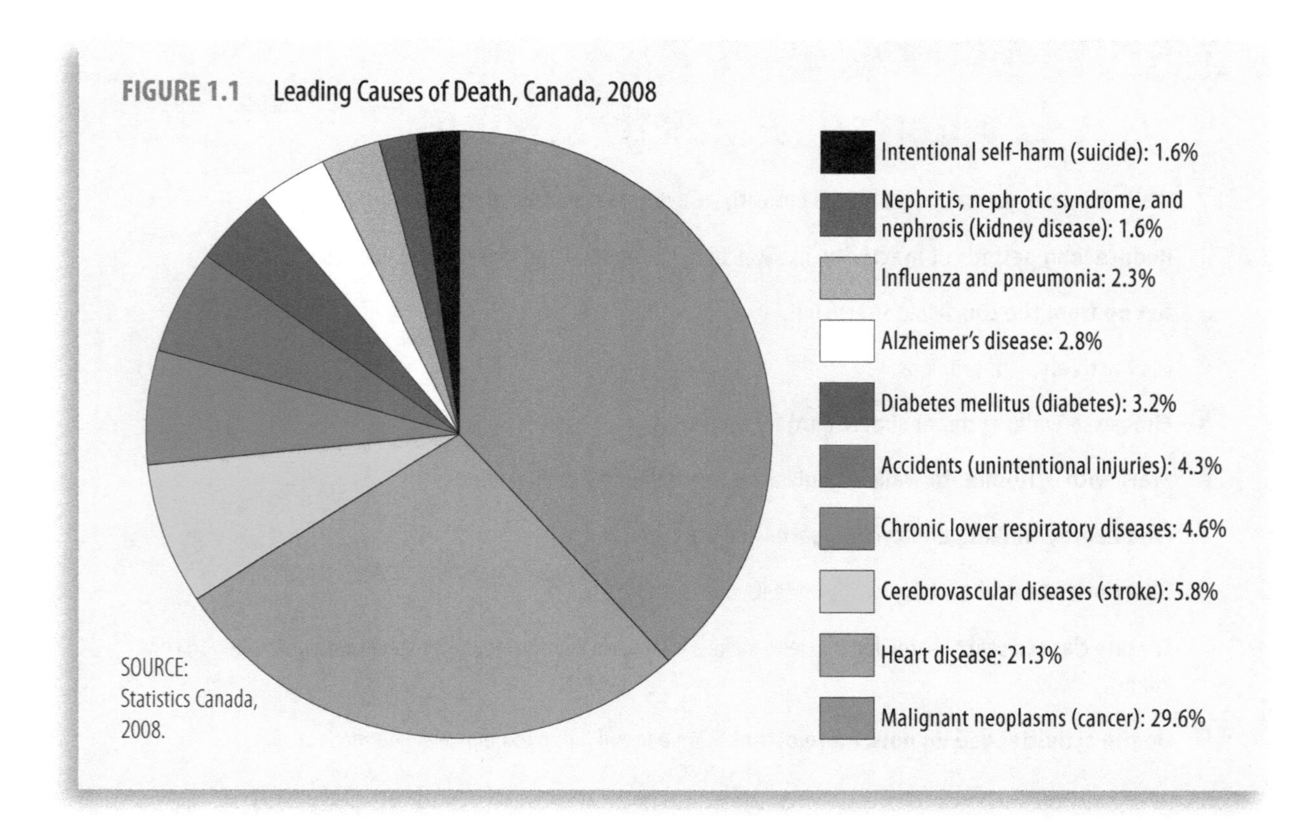

SOURCE: Statistics Canada, 2008.

levels, physical fitness, and muscular strength; improves endurance, flexibility, motor coordination, and general health; prevents disease; and reduces body fat.

Active living is also about finding opportunities to become physically active at home, school, work, and in the community. Getting involved in charity walkathons or joining the workplace baseball team, for example, can be an important part of active living. All activities of this kind provide physical, social, emotional, and spiritual benefits that lead to an improved quality of life. As a result, the Public Health Agency of Canada (PHAC, 2004) took a federal role in encouraging and assisting

PERSONAL PERSPECTIVE

Curriculum and Fitness Concerns

In the early 1980s, when I first started teaching in the Law and Security Administration (LASA) program at Georgian College in Barrie, Ontario, fitness was a mandatory course. The police and firefighting services were the only two employers in Ontario to enforce fitness standards at that time. All students in the LASA program had to meet police fitness standards, even if policing was not their career choice.

During the mid- and late 1990s, we re-addressed the program's fitness requirements. In the first-year curriculum, fitness instruction took on a wellness and active living approach. It became the students' responsibility to meet set fitness criteria that would enable them to continue into a second-year fitness class. Some students self-selected into different careers based on their ability to meet the standards in the policing, corrections, and security fields. For many individuals, this was their first exposure to a demanding regime meant to test their fitness to do their job.

With the change in the college curriculum, in order to address many students coming out of high school with only Grade 9-level fitness, we created a healthy living lecture component to teach basic concepts in health and fitness that many of our students were missing, as well as a basic fitness component in first year to address the cardiovascular and endurance standards necessary to achieve the Bona Fide Occupational Requirements (BFOR, discussed as part of the Physical Readiness Evaluation for Policing [PREP] and the Physical Abilities Requirement Evaluation [PARE] later in this chapter and in Chapter 15).

One of the positive outcomes of this new approach was some students' stronger lifelong commitment to fitness. The negative side of an optional second-year fitness course was the number of students who quickly lost interest in maintaining a healthy weight and lifestyle. Again, it became an issue of extrinsic motivation (surviving first-year fitness) rather than an intrinsic commitment to themselves (keeping active throughout their lives).

Students face a great responsibility to meet the fitness requirements of the career they have chosen. Standards now exist for police, corrections workers, and private and court security officers. With a responsibility to achieve the BFOR, there is a greater onus on students to maintain their fitness at the required levels. Note that being fit is not necessarily the same as meeting the minimum requirements of the various police and correctional services standards. Students who are fit, however, easily meet the required standards when they apply for a career in law enforcement.

In the fall of 2001, the Ontario Police Service's Physical Readiness Evaluation for Policing (PREP) reduced the graduation requirement in the shuttle run from level 7.5 to the applicant standard of level 6.5. As a result of this change, we are seeing new concerns from a fitness perspective. Are applicants as fit as they should be for the physical demands and lifestyle of law enforcement? There has been a significant reduction in physical fitness training at the Ontario Police College owing to the changing demands of law enforcement. Under the current curriculum, students participate in fewer than 15 workouts over a 12-week program. Some can barely pass level 6.5 when they graduate from the Ontario Police College. What happens in six months, two years, five years, and ten years from now? Will this reduction of the exit requirement result in health issues and real costs down the road, in terms of sick days and higher rates of injury, to police agencies that may not have as fit a workforce? These questions remain a major concern to the Police Fitness Personnel of Ontario, who are the fitness promotion body for Ontario police officers.

Canadians to be physically active through awareness and programs meant to facilitate the integration of physical activity within communities throughout Canada. In 2010, the Public Health Agency of Canada supported the Canadian Society for Exercise Physiology in developing physical activity guidelines for every age group (CSEP, 2011a, 2011b, 2012). Other programs that CSEP has implemented include the Pedometer Challenge and Active Living in Your Neighbourhood, which are held in parks, schools, and community centres in various communities. Global Advocacy for Physical Activity (2011) states that "active transportation" is the most practical and sustainable way to increase physical activity on a daily basis while simultaneously improving air quality, reducing traffic congestion, and reducing carbon dioxide emissions. The benefits include more land use for footpaths and bikeways to promote more physical activity.

So how does this information affect potential employees in the field of law enforcement? How should law enforcement promote the importance of physical fitness as it relates to the demands of the job? Is the onus solely on potential employees to ensure that they can meet the demands of the job? How do law enforcers maintain a proper level of fitness? Should employers ensure that their employees maintain a healthy level of fitness by providing facilities or opportunities to participate in various forms of physical activity? Should services test employees yearly to ensure that they are fit enough to do their job? Ultimately, who is responsible for fitness? The box on the previous page provides a perspective on these issues.

The Health Benefits of Physical Activity: A Summary

Health experts who want to convince people to follow a more active lifestyle and make healthier choices must convince those people that physical activity is an integral part of a healthier life. The following are some of the health benefits of a lifestyle that includes regular physical activity (Pitts, 1996; Bouchard & Shephard, 1991; Klonoff, 1994):

- reduced risk of coronary heart disease, non-insulin-dependent diabetes, obesity, osteoporosis, reproductive and colon cancer, hypertension (high blood pressure), and stroke
- help with maintaining a healthy body weight and more desirable body image
- increased strength, energy, and stamina
- improved cardiorespiratory function
- improved functioning of the digestive and excretory organs
- improved agility, speed, and coordination
- increased range of motion in joints
- improved general posture
- increased resistance to mental fatigue
- greater ability to cope with the intellectual demands of college and full-time or part-time jobs
- better stress management
- reduced anxiety and depression
- improved sleep
- higher self-esteem and perceived quality of life

DID YOU KNOW?

Each 500 kcal of additional leisure-time physical activity per week has been associated with a 6 percent decrease in the risk of developing non-insulin-dependent diabetes.

SOURCE: Bassuk & Manson, 2005.

Turn to **assignment 1.1** (in the appendix). Complete the questionnaires to determine how ready you are to make healthier choices concerning habits, nutrition, stress management, and physical activity.

The Seven Dimensions of Health

Originally, health was defined as the absence of disease. Many exercise physiologists, kinesiologists, and health educators have concluded that this definition is too restrictive. They have decided that good health should be defined as wellness and equated with healthy living. According to the Physical Activity, Fitness, and Health Consensus Statement (Quinney, Gauvine, & Wall, 1994), health has physical, social, and psychological dimensions, each of which lies along a continuum. Positive health is associated with a capacity to enjoy life and to withstand challenges; it is not merely the absence of disease.

There are seven dimensions to health, and all must work together to create good health. One weak dimension can affect all the others. This integrated approach empowers individuals to make positive choices. It avoids "ideals" and specific body types, focusing instead on healthy eating and regular, varied physical activity to promote overall personal well-being, enhanced quality of life, and better nutritional choices to maintain a healthy weight.

The seven dimensions of health are as follows:

1. *Physical* health involves looking after your body as best you can. This means eating properly, exercising, avoiding unhealthy behaviours and substances, making responsible decisions about sex, being aware of the symptoms of disease, having regular checkups, and taking steps to prevent injuries.
2. *Emotional and psychological* health involves maintaining a positive self-concept; dealing constructively with feelings; developing such qualities as optimism, trust, and self-confidence; and being able to cope with the challenges of daily stressors. It also entails self-acceptance, controlling your emotions, and knowing when to seek support.
3. *Intellectual* health involves valuing lifelong learning and challenging yourself while searching for answers and solutions. It also involves being able to analyze and evaluate a situation so that you can propose alternatives or solutions. As well, intellectual health includes self-awareness and learning from life experiences.
4. *Spiritual* health entails searching for meaning and purpose in your life. It also involves coming to terms with what is right and wrong, whether through religion, meditation, art, or some other practice. Spiritual health may involve developing faith in a being or power beyond yourself, as well as the capacity for compassion, altruism, joy, and forgiveness. Research has found that "intrinsic religiosity" plays a role in speedier recovery from depression, anxiety, and illness, and can contribute to a longer life expectancy (Hummer, Rogers, Nam, & Ellison, 1999).
5. *Social and interpersonal* health involves being able to develop meaningful relationships, cultivating a network of supportive friends and family members, and contributing to the community. It also includes valuing

diversity—accepting people for who they are. Statistics show that people who are socially isolated are at higher risk of illness and death (Cacioppo et al., 2002).

6. *Environmental* health involves respecting and protecting the environment at the local level and beyond, protecting yourself from environmental hazards, and minimizing the negative impact of your behaviour on the environment.
7. *Occupational* health involves deriving satisfaction from the accomplishments and challenges of your job while maintaining a balance between work and the rest of your life.

Law enforcement officers deal with the physical demands of altercations, the emotional demands of domestic calls, the intellectual demands of having to make sound decisions (sometimes almost instantly), the spiritual demands of coming to terms with deaths and other tragic events they witness, the interpersonal demands of dealing with the public, the environmental demands of working in all weather and under other difficult conditions, and the occupational demands of encountering society at its best and worst. It is important to be healthy in all these areas in order to do your job effectively and safely. Ultimately, you have a healthy lifestyle if you engage in regular physical activity, eat well, manage your time, avoid destructive habits, manage stress, and adopt good health and safety habits, including learning first aid and being an informed consumer.

mortality
number of deaths in a population, usually expressed as an annual rate

morbidity
number of ill people in a population, usually expressed as an annual rate

Today, with advances in health care that help to cure or reduce the spread of infectious diseases, we have seen the **mortality** (death) rate decline. People live well into their 70s and 80s, and more people will reach 100 years old in the 21st century than ever before. **Morbidity** (illness) rates show us that people are becoming ill less from common infectious diseases than in past generations.

However, just because we are living longer does not mean that we are healthier. It has been estimated that more than 67 percent of our youth are inactive, and 50 percent are not active enough to receive the health benefits associated with exercise (de St. Auboin, 1997). This inactivity, combined with more sedentary behaviours (CSEP, 2011b), has led to a generation that is less active than 30 years ago (Anderson, 2000). With the academic changes in high school curricula in Ontario, there are fewer physical fitness classes and an apparent devaluing of the importance of physical activity in young people's lives.

The 2011 *Active Healthy Kids Canada Report Card* found that from 3 p.m. to 6 p.m.—the time between the end of the school day and before the dinner hour—6- to 19-year-olds in Canada get only 14 minutes of moderate to vigorous physical activity (for example, aerobics, jogging, running), while they spend an average of 107 minutes in light activity (light play, walking less than 3.2 km/h) or sedentary pursuits (such as motorized transportation, sitting, or standing idle). Only 7 percent of children and youth (6 to 19 years of age; 9 percent of boys and 4 percent of girls) get at least 60 minutes of moderate to vigorous physical activity 6 days of the week, as recommended by the *Canadian Physical Activity Guidelines* (CSEP, 2011a).

It is important to make cognitive choices based on family history, disabilities, aging, and knowledge of our health-care system. Self-management is key to problem-solving and making informed decisions. It is important for schools and parents to play an integral role in providing programs outside regular physical education classes. Similarly, it is important that you get involved with intramurals, sport teams, and fitness classes that are offered at your school.

This is why the federal government has pushed for education programs like Active Living, the *Canadian Physical Activity Guidelines*, and Healthy Living, which are all aimed at addressing health and wellness. By informing people about the seven dimensions that work together for good health, we may improve the quality of Canadians' lives.

The Wellness Continuum

Wellness applies to all ages, socio-economic groups, and levels of ability or disability. Wellness relies on personal empowerment—people taking charge of their lives. Many disabled people, for example, find ways to live healthy, physically active lives. As Ardell (1987, p. 131) has pointed out, "Wellness is not a goal to be attained but a process to be maintained." It runs along a continuum (see Figure 1.2).

At each phase of your life, physical fitness, active living, and wellness take on different degrees of importance. For those entering the field of law enforcement, physical skills and abilities are becoming a prerequisite for employment. During the middle and later phases of a law enforcement career, active living and health-related issues come to the fore. Physical activity also becomes an employer's issue when it is associated with sick days and Workplace Safety and Insurance Board claims.

FIGURE 1.2 Wellness/Illness Continuum

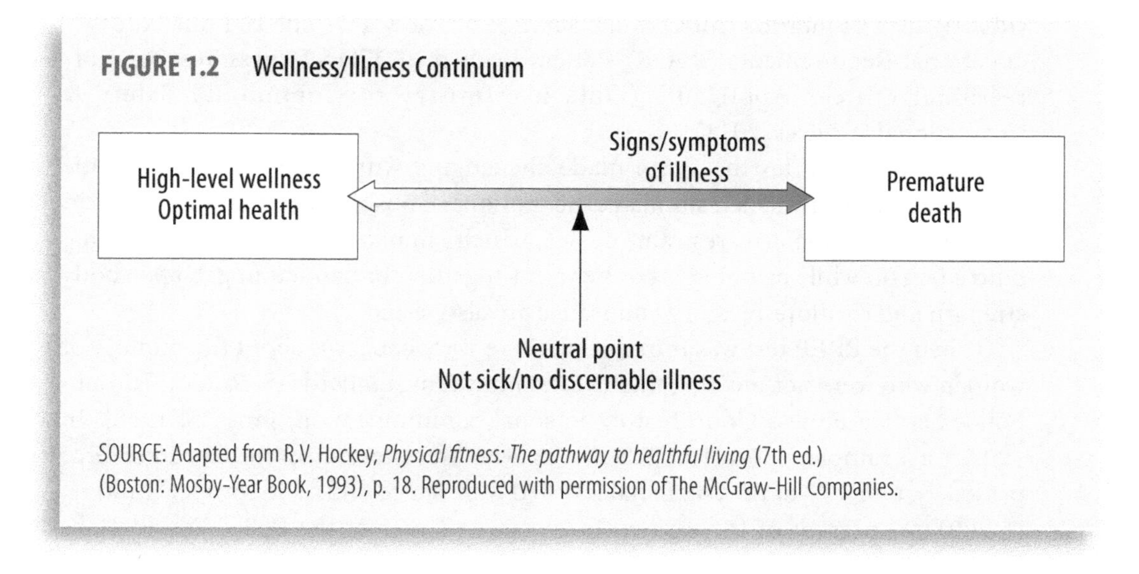

SOURCE: Adapted from R.V. Hockey, *Physical fitness: The pathway to healthful living* (7th ed.) (Boston: Mosby-Year Book, 1993), p. 18. Reproduced with permission of The McGraw-Hill Companies.

Fitness for Law Enforcement Officers

A healthy lifestyle improves feelings of wellness that are key to optimal health. It is important that you make choices throughout your career that keep you balanced and focused so that not only can you do your job effectively, but you have good quality of life during and after retirement.

Decades ago, fitness in the law enforcement context was treated exclusively as a hiring issue, but today it is viewed more broadly. We now see campaigns to address fitness throughout a person's law enforcement career. For example, Ontario Police College fitness staff and the Police Fitness Personnel of Ontario (PFPO; see the box

FYI

Police Fitness Personnel of Ontario

The PFPO, an organization sanctioned by the Ontario Association of Chiefs of Police, has a mandate to promote fitness and health awareness within the policing community. In addition to its yearly fitness lapel-pin awards, the PFPO offers awareness programs on topics such as maintaining a healthy back, nutrition, fitness and shiftwork, and cardiovascular disease (for more information, see PFPO, 2009).

on this page) have implemented a yearly fitness lapel-pin initiative to encourage ongoing fitness for all officers. Since 1988, the PFPO has rewarded officers who meet the criteria with the pin to recognize their commitment to fitness. Close to 40,000 fitness tests have been performed over the years since the program's inception, an average of 3,000 to 5,000 pins annually; 2012 marked the 25th year that the pin has been worn by police officers in Ontario.

During the mid- and late 1980s, we at Georgian College had to rethink our standards for two reasons. First, fewer students were entering policing and other fields with less stringent standards. Second, students were arriving at college less fit than their predecessors, because fitness programs were no longer mandatory throughout the high school years. As a result, the program lowered its fitness standards, although we continued to encourage students to meet police standards through the academic advisory process.

Since the 1980s, the physical and occupational skills of various public employees have been tested by the Ontario Police Service's Physical Readiness Evaluation for Policing (PREP) (Ontario Ministry of Community Safety & Correctional Services, 2007) and the RCMP's Physical Abilities Requirement Evaluation (PARE) (RCMP, 2011). Ontario's Correctional Services has now developed a Bona Fide Occupational Requirements (BFOR) standard called FITCO—Fitness Test for Correctional Officer Applicants (Ontario Ministry of Community Safety & Correctional Services, 2011).

Ontario's PREP test has been made challenging with the introduction of the push–pull machine, which simulates the motions of pushing and pulling during an altercation, and the arm-restraint device, which simulates the motion of holding onto a person while bringing his or her arms together for handcuffing. Upper-body strength and cardiorespiratory endurance are also tested.

When the PREP test was introduced, there were concerns about the number of women who were not meeting the PREP's minimum standards (S. Ruttan, Toronto Police Service Fitness Coordinator, personal communication, June 25, 1998). In 1998, for example, 656 of the 739 males who were tested by the Toronto force passed, but only 73 of the 148 females tested were successful. With proper training, in 2001, 94 percent of the women in the second year of the Police Foundations Program at Georgian College met the graduation standards for both the PREP and the PARE. There is a definite learning curve for these machines, but upper-body strength and **aerobic conditioning** are also important. However, if people are physically motivated as well as educated about the requirements, they should have no difficulty passing by the time they graduate from their law enforcement program. The keys to success lie in familiarity with the equipment and a commitment to a personal fitness program designed to meet the standards, including a strong aerobic and strength-training program. Today, most students are able to get through the pursuit and restraint component; however, a greater percentage of individuals find it aerobically challenging to get to level 6.5 on the shuttle run and to continue to maintain or improve above that level. It is important that individuals train above the accepted standard in order to achieve the standard on the day of testing.

aerobic conditioning an exercise program that incorporates activities that are rhythmic in nature, using large muscle groups at moderate intensities for 4 to 7 days per week

How can law enforcement officers be convinced to integrate physical fitness into their lives? Simply telling people that physical activity is good for them is not sufficient motivation. There must be some intrinsic or extrinsic motivation for becoming and remaining fit (see the box below). A commitment to lifelong wellness and fitness is an integral part of achieving your career goals. This textbook provides information that will allow you to make positive health and lifestyle changes, but ultimately, it is up to you to make the choice regarding your health and fitness level.

Requirements for Ontario Police Officers

The following pages provide an overview of some of the standards for a police officer in the province of Ontario (OPP, 2002). See if you have these skills and abilities, and look very carefully at the medical requirements to see whether you can pass the tests.

In 1996, the Ontario Association of Chiefs of Police (OACP) developed a standardized police applicant process. From this process, they developed one set of standards that police services could use to look for applicants through a centralized system. They stated:

PERSONAL PERSPECTIVE

It's Never Too Late

At 37, my father had his first angina attack while visiting Expo 67. Then, in 1970, when he was 40, he suffered a massive heart attack caused by a blockage of the left coronary artery.

I now know that my father was a time bomb waiting to go off. He led a sedentary life and was a meat-and-potatoes man who worked six days a week, walked only a few short steps to work, and smoked two-and-a-half packs of cigarettes a day.

After his heart attack, my father spent six weeks in hospital. Today, heart attack patients are out of the hospital in days, but in 1970, heart research was in its infancy. By the time my father was discharged, he had given up smoking and had begun daily one-hour walks covering up to 6 kilometres; he has stuck to this walking program ever since.

In 1983, two days before my mid-term exam on the physiology of heart disease, my father suffered another heart attack. Although he had taken a stress test a week earlier, there was no sign of an impending heart attack (a stress test uses exercise to evaluate whether the heart and blood vessels are working properly). I remember how he denied that he was having another heart attack. Mental stress—not problems with eating or exercise—caused this attack. Afterward, my father made further changes to his lifestyle and outlook on health.

In December 2003, my father suffered his third heart attack at 73 years of age and had quadruple bypass surgery. He was sent home three days later. It truly is amazing that after three heart attacks, an aortic aneurysm, and kidney problems, technology has advanced far enough to enable my family to continue to have him with us. He now suffers from congestive heart failure, but walks every morning. He appreciates that if he had made healthier choices and been physically active, his quality of life would have been better.

Law enforcement officers sometimes get caught up in their careers and forget about their health; for example, they eat on the run and fail to maintain a balanced diet. Shiftwork, court appearances, and overtime all take their toll, and many officers become run down from lack of sleep. Fitness seems to be the first thing that is left out of people's daily routine when they become overwhelmed. The most common excuse that I hear from officers is that they do not have time for fitness. As a result, I see many who are overweight, have back problems, and suffer from stress-related issues that should not be a factor at their young age. Fitness is not just about the number of years you are able to be employed, but the quality of life you have during and after your career.

I hope that reading this book will lead you to a greater appreciation of the importance of fitness. Taking care of your health is an important part of leading a long, productive, and rewarding life. We work to enjoy the rewards of retirement. Make sure that you are healthy enough to enjoy those rewards.

> [a] career in policing is primarily about one thing: working with people to ensure public safety through crime prevention and law enforcement. … Police work is demanding. A police constable must work shifts, including evenings, nights, and weekends, at all times of the year. It affects an individual's health, perspective on life, and family life. This is not a job that everyone will like or can do well. Many cannot work shifts.

In Ontario, you must meet certain minimum requirements as outlined in Ontario's *Police Services Act*. One of these is for you to "be physically and mentally able to perform the duties of the position, having regard to your own safety and the safety of members of the public."

Competencies

In addition to the minimum requirements set out in the *Police Services Act*, you must possess specific competencies, which are skills, abilities, behaviours, and attitudes that are essential to law enforcement work. The two categories specified for the job of policing are essential competencies and developmental competencies (OPP, 2002).

Eight *essential competencies* must be demonstrated before you can become a police officer (OPP, 2002):

1. *Analytical thinking* The ability to analyze situations and events in a logical way, and to organize the parts of a problem in a systematic way.
2. *Self-confidence* A belief in your own abilities and judgment, and recognition of personal limitations and development needs.
3. *Communication* The ability to demonstrate effective listening, verbal, and written communication skills.
4. *Flexibility/Valuing diversity* The ability to adapt your approach in a variety of situations, and to work effectively with a wide cross-section of a community representing diverse backgrounds, cultures, and socio-economic circumstances.
5. *Self-control* The ability to keep your emotions under control and to restrain negative actions when provoked or when working under stressful conditions.
6. *Relationship building* The ability to develop and maintain a network of contacts, both inside and outside the police service.
7. *Achievement orientation* The desire for continuous improvement in service or accomplishments.
8. *Medical/Physical skills and abilities* Job-related medical/physical skills and abilities, including vision, hearing, motor skills, **cardiovascular fitness**, and upper-body strength (see Physical Skills and Abilities, below).

cardiovascular fitness the ability to transport and use oxygen during prolonged, strenuous exercise or work; it reflects the combined efficiency of the lungs, heart, vascular system, and exercising muscles in the transport and use of oxygen

Developmental competencies can be acquired through training after you have been hired as a police officer. However, some police services may require these competencies in new applicants, thus making them conditions for hiring. The following 11 competencies have been identified as developmental:

1. *Information seeking* The ability to seek out information from various sources before making decisions.

2. *Concern for safety* The ability to exercise caution in hazardous situations in order to ensure the safety of self and others.
3. *Assertiveness* The ability to use authority confidently and to set and enforce rules appropriately.
4. *Initiative* Demonstrated ability to be self-motivated and self-directed in identifying and addressing important issues.
5. *Cooperation* The ability to collaborate with others by seeking their input, encouraging their participation, and sharing information.
6. *Negotiation/Facilitation* The ability to influence or persuade others by anticipating and addressing their interests and perspectives.
7. *Work organization* The ability to develop and maintain systems for organizing information and activities.
8. *Community service orientation* Proven commitment to helping or serving others.
9. *Commitment to learning* Demonstrated pattern of activities that contribute to personal and professional growth.
10. *Organizational awareness* Understanding of the dynamics of organizations, including the formal and informal cultures and decision-making processes.
11. *Developing others* Commitment to helping others improve their skills.

Physical Skills and Abilities

When you apply to become a police officer in Ontario, you will also have to go through a medical/physical skills and abilities test (OPP, 2002). These abilities are equally important to determine prior to applying to the service. It is prudent to do these tests while you are still in school to ensure that you have the ability to apply and meet these standards:

- *Vision* Uncorrected (no eyeglasses or contact lenses) visual acuity must be at least 20/40 (6/12) with both eyes open. Corrected visual acuity must be at least 20/20 (6/6) with both eyes open. There are also minimum requirements for farsightedness, colour vision, depth perception, peripheral vision, and other vision-related areas.

  Don't wait until you apply to find out whether you meet these standards. Too many students who have not done their own research have found out after two years of college that they will never be able to meet the standards, especially for colour vision. Statistically, more males are colour-blind than females.
- *Hearing* You must have normal hearing at frequencies of 500 to 4,000 Hz, as measured by an audiometer.
- *Physical fitness* This part of the test assesses whether you have the physical skills and abilities to pass the PREP in 162 seconds or less, with a shuttle run to a level of stage 6.5 (this is explained in more detail in Chapter 15). This test does *not* assess your fitness level.

  This is the one test over which you have total control. Some people require only one or two attempts to acquaint themselves with the equipment and successfully meet the standard. Others may need the entire two years of training at college to gain the required physical strength, coordination, and aerobic endurance. Ultimately, you are the only one who can ensure your success. (For more information on the constable selection process, see Ontario Ministry of Community Safety & Correctional Services, 2007. Links at that website provide specific information about individual services.)

Informed Consent for Fitness Testing

Part of the requirement prior to testing for police services is to ensure that you are medically safe to do the testing. By completing the Physical Activity Readiness Questionnaire (PAR-Q), you will assure the assessor that you are physically able to do the test without limitations. Informed consent takes that process one step further in addressing due diligence to ensure that you know about the test protocols and are aware of the stress that they may put you under. Informed consent also ensures that you have followed appropriate guidelines to affirm that you are able to perform the tasks safely.

Turn to **assignment 1.2** (in the appendix). Carefully read the informed consent form, sign it, and return a copy to your instructor. If you require further clarification, be sure to ask your instructor.

Local Needs of Police Services

Apart from the competencies listed above, police services may require certain special skills and abilities in order to address urgent issues pertaining to the specific service or community. A local need may be a second language, a special type or level of computer skill, prior experience in working with abused women or troubled youth, volunteering in your community, the ability to relocate, and so on.

As you go through the chapters of this book, think about some of these competencies. When you set your goals in Chapter 2, you may have to include some competencies to work on so that you can demonstrate those skills to the agency to which you apply. Ultimately, you will have to determine whether you have chosen the right career.

KEY TERMS

active living, 8
aerobic conditioning, 16
cardiovascular fitness, 18
exercise, 7
health, 4
health-related fitness, 7
healthy living, 5
metabolic syndrome , 6
moderate-intensity physical activity, 6
morbidity, 14
mortality, 14
musculoskeletal fitness , 7
performance/skill-related fitness, 7
physical activity, 5
physical fitness, 7
resistance training, 8
vigorous-intensity physical activity, 6
wellness, 4

EXERCISES

Multiple Choice

1. Physical inactivity is associated with
   - **a.** occupational sitting, TV watching, eating, and moderate physical activities
   - **b.** occupational sitting, TV watching, eating, and vigorous physical activity
   - **c.** TV watching, eating, occupational sitting, and computer game activity
   - **d.** TV watching, eating, occupational sitting, and low physical activity
   - **e.** eating, TV watching, occupational sitting, and dancing
2. It is important that we encourage children and youth to become moderately physically active to prevent
   - **a.** high blood pressure
   - **b.** obesity
   - **c.** metabolic syndrome
   - **d.** depression
   - **e.** all of the above
3. The 2010 *Canadian Guidelines for Physical Activity* for adults recommend
   - **a.** 150 minutes per week of moderate to vigorous physical activity accumulating in bouts of at least 10 minutes each
   - **b.** 150 minutes per week of moderate to vigorous physical activity accumulating in bouts of at least 20 minutes each
   - **c.** 150 minutes per day of moderate to vigorous physical activity accumulating in bouts of at least 10 minutes each
   - **d.** 120 minutes per week of moderate to vigorous physical activity accumulating in bouts of at least 10 minutes each
   - **e.** 120 minutes per day of moderate to vigorous physical activity accumulating in bouts of at least 20 minutes each
4. The wellness concept emphasizes which of the following?
   - **a.** reliance on the health-care system
   - **b.** personal responsibility for well-being
   - **c.** a complete absence of disease
   - **d.** adequate medical insurance coverage
   - **e.** exercising to maximum heart rate every day
5. Which of the following is one of the dimensions of health?
   - **a.** wellness
   - **b.** sexual health
   - **c.** environmental health
   - **d.** cardiovascular health
   - **e.** nuclear health
6. Which of these statements about a wellness lifestyle is true?
   - **a.** the rewards of wellness are delayed
   - **b.** living to an old age is a benefit to living a wellness lifestyle
   - **c.** college is a time to think about wellness
   - **d.** wellness involves gaining control of your life
   - **e.** all of these choices are true

7. The wellness/illness continuum identifies a neutral point. This neutral point is where
   a. premature death occurs
   b. no discernible illness exists
   c. medical intervention is important
   d. a person is physically fit
   e. a high level of wellness is enjoyed
8. Wellness includes concepts such as
   a. embracing big, positive changes in order to get fit
   b. taking steps to ensure your wealth when you can finally retire
   c. compromising lifestyle habits to enjoy yearly vacations
   d. allowing someone to dictate how your leisure time is spent
   e. embracing small, positive changes in order to have a healthy attitude and lifestyle
9. Behaviours and habits to ensure wellness in your life do NOT include
   a. taking responsibility for your own health
   b. choosing to drink and smoke only on special occasions every week
   c. learning to manage stress effectively
   d. maintaining self-esteem
   e. eating well and exercising daily
10. The practice of "leaving work at work" is an example of which dimension of health?
   a. social
   b. spiritual
   c. occupational
   d. emotional
   e. intellectual
11. Dealing effectively with a stressful situation is an example of which dimension of health?
   a. social
   b. spiritual
   c. occupational
   d. emotional
   e. intellectual
12. Taking time to read up on a subject that interests you is an example of which dimension of health?
   a. social
   b. spiritual
   c. occupational
   d. emotional
   e. intellectual
13. Developing a good network of friends both within and outside your career is an example of which dimension of health?
   a. social
   b. spiritual
   c. occupational
   d. emotional
   e. intellectual
14. Finding a rewarding career in law enforcement is an example of which dimension of health?
   a. social
   b. spiritual
   c. occupational
   d. emotional
   e. intellectual
15. Which of the following is a benefit of regular physical activity?
   a. greater resistance to mental fatigue
   b. reduced risk of heart disease
   c. better stress management
   d. improved agility
   e. all of these

Short Answer

1. Define "healthy living."

2. What are the seven dimensions of good health?

3. Why is it important to put equal emphasis on each dimension of good health?

4. How does wellness apply to law enforcement?

5. What does physical fitness mean to you?

6. What is the difference between health-related

7. Describe the difference between active living and physical inactivity/sedentary behaviour.

8. List some of the ways you can improve your health based on the information in this chapter.

9. Which of the 8 essential and 11 developmental competencies required of Ontario police officers do you possess? Which ones do you need to work on?

10. What are some of the concerns that police have when dealing with issues around being overweight or obese?

11. What are some of the benefits of reducing weight?

REFERENCES

Active Healthy Kids Canada. (2011). Don't let this be the most physical activity our kids get after school. *The Active Healthy Kids Canada 2011 report card on physical activity for children and youth*. Toronto: Author. http://dvqdas9jty7g6.cloudfront.net/reportcard2011/ahkc2011_shortform_eng_final.pdf.

Anderson, R.E. (2000). The spread of the childhood obesity epidemic. Commentary. *Canadian Medical Association Journal*, *163*(11), 1461–1462. http://www.cmaj.ca/content/163/11/1461.full.

Anis, A.H., Zhang, W., Bansback, N., Guh, D.P., Amarsi, Z. & Birmingham, C.L. (2009). Obesity and overweight in Canada: An updated cost-of-illness study. *Obesity Reviews, 11*(1), 31–40.

Ardell, D. (1987). The health benefits of exercise (part 1): A round table. *The Physician and Sportsmedicine, 15*, 131ff.

Bassuk, S., & Manson, J. (2005). Epidemiological evidence for the role of physical activity in reducing risk of type 2 diabetes and cardiovascular disease. *Journal of Applied Physiology, 99*, 1193–1204.

Bouchard, C., & Shephard, R.J. (1991, August 22). *Physical activity, fitness, and health: A model and key concepts.* Consensus document #017 prepared for the International Consensus Symposium on Physical Activity, Fitness and Health.

Cacioppo, J.T., Hawkley, L.C., Crawford, L.E., Ernst, J.M., Burleson, M.H., Kowalewski, R.B., et al. (2002). Loneliness and health: Potential mechanisms. *Psychosomatic Medicine, 64*, 407–417.

Cady, L.D. (1985, February). Program for increasing health and physical fitness of fire fighters. *Journal of Occupational Medicine, 27*(2), 110–114.

Canadian Society for Exercise Physiology (CSEP). (2011a). *Canadian Physical Activity Guidelines.* http://www.csep.ca/english/view.asp?x=1.

Canadian Society for Exercise Physiology (CSEP). (2011b). *Canadian Sedentary Behaviour Guidelines.* http://www.csep.ca/english/view.asp?x=1.

Canadian Society for Exercise Physiology (CSEP). (2012). *Canadian physical activity and sedentary behaviour guideline handbook.* http://www.csep.ca/guidelines.

Colley, R.C., Garriguet, D., Janssen, I., Craig, C., Clarke, J., & Tremblay, M.S. (2011a). Physical activity of Canadian adults: Accelerometer results from the 2007–2009 Canadian Health Measures Survey. *Health Reports, 22*(1). Catalogue no. 82-003-XPE. Ottawa: Statistics Canada.

Colley, R.C., Garriguet, D., Janssen, I., Craig, C., Clarke, J., & Tremblay, M.S. (2011b). Physical activity of Canadian children and youth: Accelerometer results from the 2007–2009 Canadian Health Measures Survey. *Health Reports, 22*(1). Catalogue no. 82-003-XPE. Ottawa: Statistics Canada.

Constance, S., Sullivan, B., & Shimizu, K.T. (1988). Epidemiological studies of work-related injuries among law enforcement personnel. *Occupational Medicine, 38*, 33–40.

de St. Auboin, B. (1997, Winter). Get serious! Promote physical activity. *Ontario Physical and Health Education Association Newsletter,* 24–25.

First Nations Regional Longitudinal Health Survey 2002/03. (2007, March). *Results for adults, youth, and children living in First Nations communities.* Ottawa: Assembly of First Nations/First National Information Governance Committee.

Fitness Canada. (1991). *Active living: A conceptual overview.* Ottawa: Government of Canada.

Garriguet, D. (2004). *Nutrition: Findings from the Canadian Community Health Survey.* Catalogue no. 82-620-MIE. Ottawa: Statistics Canada.

Garriguet, D. (2007). Canadians' eating habits. *Health Reports, 18*(2), 17–32. Catalogue no. 82-003. Ottawa: Statistics Canada. http://www.statcan.gc.ca/pub/82-003-x/2006004/article/habit/9609-eng.pdf.

Global Advocacy for Physical Activity (GAPA), Advocacy Council of the International Society for Physical Activity and Health (ISPAH). (2010, May 20). *The Toronto Charter for Physical Activity: A global call to action.* http://www.globalpa.org.uk.

Global Advocacy for Physical Activity (GAPA), Advocacy Council of the International Society for Physical Activity and Health (ISPAH). (2011, February). *NCD prevention: Investments that work for physical activity.* http://www.globalpa.org.uk/pdf/investments-work.pdf.

Heart and Stroke. (2010). *A perfect storm of heart disease looming on our horizon.* http://www.heartandstroke.ca.

Hockey, R.V. (1993). *Physical fitness: The pathway to healthful living* (7th ed.). Boston: Mosby-Year Book.

Hummer, R.A., Rogers, R.G., Nam, C.B., & Ellison, C.G. (1999). Religious participation and U.S. adult mortality. *Demography, 30*(2), 273–285.

Klonoff, E.A. (1994). Predicting exercise adherence in women: The role of psychological and physiological factors. *Preventive Medicine, 23*, 257–262.

Ontario Ministry of Community Safety & Correctional Services. (2007). *Physical Readiness Evaluation for Police (PREP).* http://www.mcscs.jus.gov.on.ca/english/police_serv/const_select_sys/const_select_info/prep/prep_contents.html.

Ontario Ministry of Community Safety & Correctional Services. (2011). *Frequently asked questions about Ontario correctional officer recruitment.* http://www.mcscs.jus.gov.on.ca/english/corr_serv/careers_in_corr/FrequentlyAskedQuestions/Corr_career_FAQs.html.

Ontario Provincial Police (OPP). (2002). *To be a constable.* http://www.opp.ca.

Pitts, E.H. (1996). The surgeon general's call to action. *Fitness Management, 12*(9), 36–38.

Police Fitness Personnel of Ontario (PFPO). 2009. http://www.pfpo.org/home.

Police Services Act, RSO 1990, c. P.15, as amended.

Public Health Agency of Canada (PHAC). (2004). *Healthy Living Unit.* Ottawa: Supply and Services Canada.

Public Health Agency of Canada (PHAC). (2005a). *Healthy Living Strategy*. Ottawa: Supply and Services Canada. http://www.phac-aspc.gc.ca/hl-vs-strat/index.html.

Public Health Agency of Canada (PHAC). (2005b). *Integrated Pan-Canadian Healthy Living Strategy.* http://www.phac-aspc.gc.ca/hp-ps/hl-mvs/ipchls-spimmvs/index-eng.php.

Public Health Agency of Canada (PHAC). (2012). *Healthy Living.* http://www.phac-aspc.gc.ca/hp-ps/hl-mvs/index-eng.php.

Quinney, H.A., Gauvine, L., & Wall, A.E.T. (Eds.). (1994). *Toward active living: Proceedings of the International Conference on Physical Activity, Fitness and Health.* Champaign, IL: Human Kinetics.

Royal Canadian Mounted Police (RCMP). (2011). *PARE—Physical Abilities Requirement Evaluation.* http://www.rcmp-grc.gc.ca/recruiting-recrutement/htm-form/pare-tape-requirement-exigences-eng.htm.

Shields, M., Carroll, M.D., & Ogden, C.L. (2011, March). *Adult obesity prevalence in Canada and the United States.* NCHS Data Brief no. 56. Hyattsville, MD: U.S. Department of Health & Human Services.

Shields, M., Tremblay, M.S., Lavoilette, M., Craig, C.L., Janssen, I., & Connor Gorber, S. (2010). Fitness of Canadian adults: Results from the 2007–2009 Canadian Health Measures Survey. *Health Reports, 21*(1), 1–15. Catalogue no. 82-003_XPE. Ottawa: Statistics Canada.

Statistics Canada. (2008). Mortality by selected cause of death (ICD-10) and sex, Canada, provinces and territories, annual (age-standardized rate per 100,000 population). Catalogue no. 84F0209X. Ottawa: Author.

Statistics Canada. (2009). Musculoskeletal fitness in Canada 2007 to 2009. http://www.statcan.gc.ca/pub/82-625-x/2010001/article/11089-eng.htm.

Statistics Canada. (2011, March). Physical activity of Canadian adults: Accelerometer results from the 2007 to 2009 CHMS. Research article. *Health Reports, 22*(1). Catalogue no. 82-003-XPE. Ottawa: Author.

Tremblay, M.S., Colley, R., Saunders, T.J., Healy, G.N., & Owen, N. (2010). Physiological and health implications of a sedentary lifestyle. *Applied Physiology, Nutrition and Metabolism, 35*(6), 725–740.

Tremblay, M.S., Esliger, D.W., Tremblay, A., & Colley, R.C. (2007). Incidental movement, lifestyle-embedded activity and sleep: New frontiers in physical activity assessment. *Applied Physiology, Nutrition and Metabolism, 32*, 1–10.

Tremblay, M.S., Warburton, D.E.R., Janssen, I., Paterson, D.H., Latimer, A.E., Rhodes, R.E., et al. (2011). New Canadian Physical Activity Guidelines review. *Applied Physiology, Nutrition and Metabolism, 36*, 36–46.

Tremblay, M., Wolfson, M., & Connor Gorber, S. (2007). Canadian Health Measures Survey: Rationale, background, and overview. *Health Reports, 18*(Suppl.), 7–20. Catalogue no. 82-003. Ottawa: Statistics Canada.

Warburton, D.E.R., Charlesworth, S., Ivey, A., Nettlefold, L., & Bredin, S.S.D. (2010). A systematic review of the evidence for Canada's Physical Activity Guidelines for adults. *International Journal of Behavioral Nutrition and Physical Activity, 7*, 39.

Warburton, D.E., Gledhill, N., & Quinney, A. (2001a). Musculoskeletal fitness and health. *Canadian Journal of Applied Physiology, 26*, 217–237.

Warburton, D.E., Gledhill, N., & Quinney, A. (2001b). The effects of changes in musculoskeletal fitness on health. *Canadian Journal of Applied Physiology, 26*, 161–216.

World Health Organization (WHO). (2008). *The global burden of disease: 2004 update.* Geneva: Author.

World Health Organization (WHO). (2009.) *Global health risks: Mortality and burden of disease attributable to selected major risks.* Geneva: Author. http://www.who.int/healthinfo/global_burden_disease/en/.

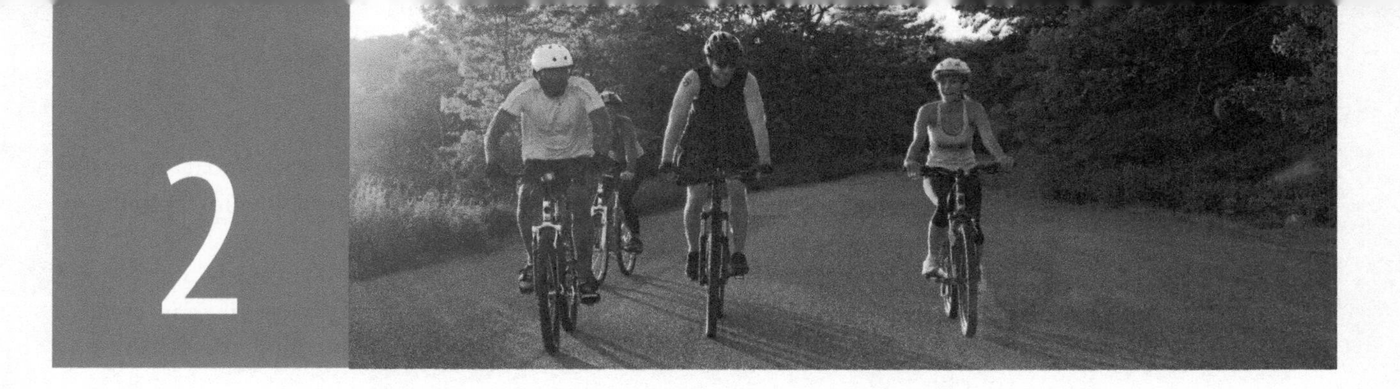

Goal Setting

LEARNING OBJECTIVES

After completing this chapter, you should be able to:

- Understand how self-esteem, self-efficacy, attitude, and intentions play a role in participation in physical activity.
- Understand the process of setting short- and long-term goals that are specific, measurable, attainable, relevant and realistic, and timed (SMART).
- Assess your values and formulate goals that reflect those values.
- Identify and develop strategies to change and maintain lifestyle behaviours that promote health.
- Create a mission statement that will give direction to the decisions you make throughout the course of your life.

OVERVIEW

As a law enforcement student, you are working toward various goals. Your first goal was achieved when you were admitted into your law enforcement program. To achieve your other goals, you must set up pathways to success. In this chapter, you will assess your values, set short- and long-term goals for yourself, devise strategies for adopting and maintaining healthy behaviours, and create a mission statement. These steps will help you find more meaning and direction in your life.

Remember that you are in charge of your law enforcement career. Managing it will be a lifelong process. You will have to strike a balance that is right for you and the people around you.

The Stages and Processes of Change

As the demands of law enforcement change, employers are looking for people with both academic training and practical life experience gained through paid or volunteer work. Law enforcement agencies want independent decision-makers and self-directed learners who have a positive attitude toward work. Candidates need a well-rounded education (including math and computer literacy), communication skills (including a good command of vocabulary and grammar), interpersonal and time-management skills, flexibility, dependability, and a lifelong commitment to physical activity. To be successful, people in law enforcement must be able to adapt to the changing demands of their field and set their goals accordingly.

Behavioural psychologists have undertaken a great deal of research to understand why people find it difficult to follow through on major lifestyle changes or goals. Lifestyle behaviours can have a negative effect on people's ability to stay healthy and free from disease or disability. Unfortunately, many people succumb to behaviours that lead to illness, including alcohol and drug abuse, smoking, inappropriate dieting, and insufficient physical fitness.

After studying people who committed themselves to health-related behavioural changes, Prochaska, Norcross, and DiClemente (1994) discovered that people pass through five distinct stages of change: pre-contemplation, contemplation, preparation, action, and maintenance and termination (with relapse possible at any point; see below). Some people pass through all five stages in sequence, whereas others bounce back and forth between stages or get stuck at one stage. Some people never achieve their goals. Behavioural change is largely a matter of self-management. It is important, therefore, to recognize barriers and move toward ideas, feelings, and actions that support change. Table 2.1 describes the five stages of change.

Another stage sometimes included in this model is relapse. Prochaska and Velicer (1997) conceptualized this not so much as a stage as a "return from Action or Maintenance to an earlier stage." That is, the individual falls back into old behaviours after going through some or all stages. At this point, he or she must re-evaluate the triggers for relapse, reassess motivation and barriers, and plan stronger coping strategies for success.

One of most common relapses occurs when students go home for Christmas holidays or the summer and diverge from their normal workout routines. It is important to find ways to continue to work out when you are away from your usual surroundings and familiar workout facilities, and to resist the tendency to fall back into old habits.

TABLE 2.1 The Five Stages of Change

PROCESSES	DESCRIPTION	EXAMPLES
1. Pre-contemplation	The individual does not believe that a problem exists and resists changing his or her behaviour.	• "Why should I quit smoking? Winston Churchill drank and smoked into his nineties." • "Why should I exercise? My weight is the same as it was ten years ago."
2. Contemplation	The individual understands and appreciates the importance of changing his or her behaviour, but is unable to take that step.	• "I know that I should stop smoking, but right now I'm too stressed out to try." • "I know that if I exercised I would have more energy, but I don't have the time for an exercise program."
3. Preparation	The individual intends to act on his or her goals.	• "I've marked a weight-control session on my calendar." • "I've set aside three hours next week to work out."
4. Action	The individual commits time and energy to realizing his or her goals.	• "I worked out four times this week." • "I'm doing upper-body exercises, including chin-ups and push-ups, so that I will be able to complete the push–pull component of the PREP test without any difficulty."
5. Maintenance/ Termination	The individual has realized his or her goals and is now working to safeguard these accomplishments.	• "I've been able to stay at my target weight for the last six months and I'm going to continue my weight-control program because I feel better than I've ever felt." • "I look at that two-year-old pack of cigarettes in the cupboard and realize that cigarettes don't control my life anymore."

SOURCE: Prochaska et al., 1994. Reprinted by permission of HarperCollins Publishers.

One factor that affects the likelihood of relapse is whether the individual is intrinsically or extrinsically motivated. **Extrinsic motivation** depends on an external reward or outcome, such as losing weight, quitting smoking, being physically fit, and being less prone to disease. Unfortunately, this kind of motivation does not keep people participating in exercise programs for long. They can become so focused on the outcome that they ignore the process (why they are exercising). In contrast, those who are **intrinsically motivated** to exercise regularly or lose weight are motivated by the activity itself—that is, exercise for exercise's sake. This is why most people lose interest in participating in regular physical activity or sticking to a smoking cessation program within the first six months of trying: they quickly lose their motivation when they are not realizing their goals. Those individuals who successfully adopt attitudes and behaviours for a healthy lifestyle usually have a positive attitude toward themselves and others, as well as a zest for life. They enjoy physical activity as part of their daily routine.

extrinsic motivation motivation to perform a task or goal based on external rewards

intrinsic motivation motivation to perform a task or goal based on enjoyment of doing the task itself

Prochaska, DiClemente, and Norcross (1992) have identified ten processes of change that affect a person's ability to progress through the five stages of change (see Table 2.2). These processes of change include both obvious and non-obvious activities, events, and experiences that affect individuals who are attempting to change their behaviour. This means that you have to be doing the right things at the right time and at the right stage in order to see positive change. Unless you are ready to embrace the steps necessary for success, the change will not happen. Are you ready to see your efforts through to completion?

self-esteem how one feels about oneself and one's characteristics

We know that lifestyle behaviours are affected by an individual's thoughts and feelings and the impact of family, friends, and colleagues. **Self-esteem** (how one feels about oneself and one's characteristics) is at the centre of personal success. If an individual has negative feelings including depression, helplessness, and loneliness, he or she may be unable to develop positive lifestyle behaviours. We know that those who succeed in developing and maintaining healthy behaviours have high self-esteem. They regularly engage in physical activities and maintain good dietary practices.

Several dimensions help to determine a person's self-esteem. Intellectual, social, emotional, and physical dimensions combine to affect behaviour, and our percep-

PERSONAL PERSPECTIVE

Intrinsic Motivation

A few years ago, I had an opportunity to talk to a grad who was doing background checks for her police service. After our interview, she shared with me something that I have been keenly aware of in my students for years. She told me that although she had hated fitness classes when I made her run, she really enjoyed running now and could see why I had advised her to make fitness part of her everyday life. In fact, she had just completed her first half-marathon, and she wanted me to know what a difference doing fitness for personal reasons had made in her life.

I realized two things: first, that students often believe it is someone else's responsibility to make them successful (or not). Second, rewarding students extrinsically through marks is less effective than helping them to see the intrinsic rewards of fitness. This principle can apply to just about anything, from success in fitness, to academics, to goals in everyday life. We need to identify the values that are important to us and shift from extrinsic motivation (outcomes) to intrinsic motivation (process for its own sake) if achieving our goals is to become part of our daily life. So, where does *your* motivation come from?

TABLE 2.2 The Ten Processes of Change

PROCESSES	DESCRIPTION	EXAMPLES
1. Consciousness raising (increasing awareness; belongs to stages 1 and 2)	The individual seeks out information that will assist him or her in reaching a goal. The individual is able to create self-motivation—find the reason for change.	• Learning to use the push–pull machine • Understanding that you will not be physically fit unless you work out three or more times a week • Analyzing the information provided for your school's alcohol awareness week
2. Dramatic relief (emotional arousal; belongs to stages 1 and 2)	The individual draws on emotional experiences to instigate changes in behaviour. It is important that the person be able to express his or her feelings about the problem and solution.	• Watching a family member go through a similar situation that does not result in a positive outcome • Taking part in a media or awareness campaign that includes personal testimonies or role playing
3. Environmental re-evaluation (reassessment; belongs to stages 1 and 2)	The individual combines cognitive information with emotional assessment of how his or her target behaviour affects others. This may include awareness of serving as a positive or negative role model.	• Taking note of when, where, and how the target behaviour occurs, and what prompts it • Thinking, "When I'm around a certain group of people, I'm more likely to overeat and smoke. I need to develop strategies for avoiding these activities when I'm around them."

PROCESSES	DESCRIPTION	EXAMPLES
4. Social liberation (environmental opportunities; belongs to stages 1, 2, 3, and 4)	The individual implements alternatives for ensuring success.	• Encouraging group participation in running • Identifying alternative fitness activities on campus that will help you become fit
5. Self-re-evaluation (belongs to stages 2 and 3)	The individual weighs the benefits against the drawbacks. He or she needs to ensure that the behavioural change is in line with the goals. The task is to get out of stage 2 ("yes, I need to do this") and actually act on the behavioural change.	• Telling yourself, "If I give up smoking I will be able to run without relying on my puffer." • Asking yourself, "What will happen if I accept a ride from this person, whom I know has been drinking?"
6. Self-liberation (commitment; belongs to stages 3, 4, and 5)	The individual now believes in him- or herself and assumes responsibility for changing the target behaviour. He or she recognizes what impact the behaviour will have. This stage is self-liberating, where the person believes in his or her ability to change, make a commitment, and plan the change.	• Creating an action plan and following through on it • Setting specific time limits for achieving your goals • Resolving, "I want to set a healthy example for my family."
7. Counter-conditioning (substituting; belongs to stages 3, 4, and 5)	The individual is prepared to initiate further behavioural changes if the original changes do not work. He or she also must work on counter-thoughts that undermine the ability to change.	• Using a treadmill as an alternative to exercising outdoors when it is raining • Asking another person to help you complete a task that you cannot complete on your own • Understanding what barriers have prevented your success in the past and using tools and support in order to become successful
8. Stimulus control (environmental control; belongs to stages 4 and 5)	The individual alters his or her environment to avoid being tempted by problem behaviours. It is important to avoid negative triggers and stimuli and cue positive behaviours to increase the odds of change.	• Waking up half an hour early to have time for a workout • Writing a note to yourself about not forgetting your workout • Avoiding those individuals who sabotage your success and replacing them with others who will assist you • Recognizing cues that lead you to eat and replacing eating with an activity
9. Contingency management (reinforcement; belongs to stages 4 and 5)	The individual rewards him- or herself for changing the target behaviour.	• Feeling good about yourself and encouraging yourself to succeed • Putting incentives in place to encourage yourself to move forward along the road to success
10. Helping relationships (belongs to stages 3, 4, and 5)	The individual solicits support from family and friends to change problem behaviours. It is important to seek others who are supportive in order to change a behaviour.	• Enlisting a friend as a workout partner • Entering into a written workout "contract" with a friend

SOURCE: Prochaska & Velicer, 1997: 39–40.

tion of this behaviour will influence a healthy lifestyle. People who have a positive perception of themselves (that is, a higher level of self-esteem), even if they are not in great shape, will still have positive outcomes from their physical activity. However, people who possess a negative perception (that is, a poor self-image due to unrealistic cultural, media, and peer pressure) may have unrealistic expectations and, as a result, may make poor lifestyle choices.

self-efficacy
one's ability to take action and perform a specific behaviour

Confidence in your ability to take action and perform a specific behaviour is known as **self-efficacy**. Those who are successful have the confidence to believe that they have internal control over their behaviour. They believe in themselves and do not allow external influences to sabotage their efforts toward change. They have the ability to visualize the success they will achieve, and reinforce that success with positive self-talk (such as, "I am a strong person who is committed to seeing these changes in myself"). Those who have strong self-efficacy also surround themselves with people who support these changes, encourage their attempts, and revel in their successes.

Factors That Affect Participation in Physical Activity

Ultimately, there are three main reasons why people participate in physical activity. These include health benefits (for example, preventing a heart attack), enjoyment, and self-image (for example, losing weight).

health benefits
improvements to physical, mental, and psychological health

Health benefits are easy to recognize—"I want to get in shape," "I want to be able to see my child graduate," "I want to feel better." Many people are looking for improved strength and stamina, stress reduction, or reduced risk of certain diseases. Often this motivation comes when someone experiences a serious illness or health problem.

belief
acceptance of an idea on the basis of knowledge and conviction

Belief that physical activity will lead to this success is key. Through personal experience, observation, and education, those who commit to physical activity have determined expected outcomes and believe they will succeed (self-efficacy).

attitude
value added to one's beliefs

Having the right **attitude** (value added to one's beliefs) when starting a fitness program is also a key to success. Going into any activity with a positive attitude will help the success of the outcome.

intention
a determination to achieve an aim

The right **intention** is important, too. Those who have made informed decisions, designed a plan of action, and made a commitment are more likely to stick with a fitness program. For such intentions to work, the plan must be realistic. Individuals need to be aware of the obstacles they may face (for example, shiftwork, which does not allow them to work out at the same time each day), and should determine success markers, sources of support, and rewards for their successes. People must also enjoy the physical activity they are doing—very few people who hate running, for example, will ever complete a marathon.

Self-Management Behavioural Strategies

self-management behavioural strategies
having the ability to shift your attention from barriers and toward ideas, feelings, and actions that support change

In order to be successful, individuals need to shift their attention from barriers and toward ideas, feelings, and actions that support change. The following **self-management behavioural strategies** will help increase participation in regular physical activity and lead to change:

- *Self-monitoring* It is important to keep track of what you are doing and how you feel (both when making a change and when avoiding it).
- *Goal setting* Set realistic daily, specific, and achievable goals (small baby steps rather than leaps).
- *Cognitive change technique* This involves changing your mind, attitudes, and feelings (that is, taking negative behaviours such as stress, loss of confidence, and disappointment from not seeing instant gains and turning them into positive attitudes—for example, by developing strategies to deal with stress, surrounding yourself with people who make you feel more confident, and ensuring that your goals are realistic).
- *Corrective feedback* Consciously exchange unhealthy behaviours for healthier ones. For example, instead of stopping off for fast food after work, pack some fruit for the ride home to tide you over till you can make supper.

Understanding Your Goals

Once you are able to make positive changes in your behaviour, you will have a greater chance of achieving your goals. To achieve your goals, you must understand what they are and why they are important to you. Take, for example, your long-term goal of a career in law enforcement. One possible reason you are attracted to this field is that you like the physical challenges it presents. You know you can meet these challenges because you value physical fitness and have made it a part of your life. Therefore, what you value is reflected in your goal. **Values** are the things that matter most to us and guide our daily behaviour, activities, and decisions. **Assignments 2.1**, **2.2**, and **2.3** are designed to help you set your goals (see the appendix).

values
the things that matter most to us and guide our daily behaviour, activities, and decisions

Assignment 2.1 begins the process by asking you to assess your values. Turn to it now.

Short- and Long-Term Goals

Clear and compelling goals are important to the success of your personal development. Values define what you are about. Simply put, we need to know who we are and where we want to go in order for our goals to become reality.

In setting your goals, you need to look at short-term goals (for example, goals for next semester, next year, or the next two years) and long-term goals (goals for five and ten years down the road). Short-term goals are as simple as passing the test on Thursday, meeting fitness requirements for the semester, or earning a 3.4 grade-point average for the year. Short-term goals are smaller and more manageable than long-term goals and exist within limited time frames. Long-term goals can last a lifetime and are a better reflection of who you are as a person and where your interests lie. Long-term goals may have to be adjusted owing to changing circumstances in one's life (for example, adjusting when you will take time off to travel for a job opportunity).

Five kinds of goals (both short- and long-term) drive your life:

1. ***Personal goals*** These reflect your personality—who you are, how you think, and how you look. Are you prepared to make fitness a lifelong commitment? Do you value your health? Do you have short- or long-term goals that include overcoming personal obstacles?

personal goals
goals that reflect personality—who we are, how we think, and how we look

2. *Family and relationship goals* Have you thought about relationships? What kind of lifestyle are you interested in? Will it involve a significant other or children? Do you get on well with your family? What does "family" mean to you? Are your goals the same as those of your significant other (if you have one)?

professional goals goals that reflect career aspirations

3. ***Professional goals*** These reflect your career aspirations. What career would you like to pursue? Do you have the academic background and basic skills that law enforcement requires? Are you prepared to do whatever your course of study demands to achieve your career goals? Do you have the basic skills to successfully pass the police selection process in Ontario, Corrections Canada aptitude testing, or private security screening? Do you have the medical clearance that agencies require (that is, have you had a full medical examination, had your eyes tested for vision and colour-blindness, and so on)?
4. *Financial goals* Are you choosing a career that will financially support the lifestyle you want? Can you handle loans, credit cards, and other financial obligations? Have you demonstrated a good credit rating?
5. *Lifestyle goals* Do you want to travel before getting a full-time job? Where do you want to live? Are you prepared to move anywhere in the province or country to have the career of your choice? Will you commit some of your leisure time to volunteer work with the Girl Guides, the Scouts, sports teams, Neighbourhood Watch, a crisis-intervention team, or similar groups?

Go to **assignment 2.2** (in the appendix) and begin to determine which goals are important to you and what being successful means to you.

Choosing Effective Goals

Understanding values makes us aware of why we choose certain goals and prepares us to make more effective decisions about our lives. According to the Canadian Society for Exercise Physiology (2003) and Meyer (2003), effective goals are specific, measurable, attainable, relevant and realistic, and timed (SMART).

- *Specific goals* are goals that are clearly formulated. If your goals are not specific, you will not have a sense of direction or purpose. For example, you might set your goal at running a 5-kilometre run this semester with the goal of running a half-marathon by the end of the year.
- *Measurable goals* are necessary for gauging your progress. If you cannot measure your progress, how will you know when you have attained your goal? For example, you might set a goal of starting to run 5 kilometres in 40 minutes. Measuring progress this way will help you stay on track, reach your target date, and experience the exhilaration of achievement.
- *Attainable goals* are realistic in terms of your current abilities. You may need to stretch yourself to achieve them, but they are not totally out of reach. For example, if you are sedentary, beginning an exercise program in which you engage in physical activity just three times a week, while working up to six

to seven times a week over the school year, may be a realistic choice for you and allow you to see results. Choosing unrealistic goals may discourage you from continuing and is therefore self-defeating. It is often better to set a number of small goals that work incrementally toward achieving your ultimate goal.

- *Relevant and realistic goals* are meaningful goals—they matter to you. The desire to achieve them gives you the drive to persist until you succeed. For example, you might choose a fitness regime that you like to do and that realistically fits into your lifestyle (say, making time to jog, play hockey, or swim at least twice a week to begin getting into shape).
- *Timed goals* relate to setting realistic timelines that will ensure your success. Having a set time frame for achieving your goal will help keep you on track despite the day-to-day demands of your work and personal life. For example, if you are running three times a week, you might plan to build up your distance from 2 kilometres to 5 kilometres over the next semester. Schedule your running dates on a calendar to help ensure that you stay on track.

SMART GOALS are ...

Specific:	You can answer what, when, where, and how you wish to accomplish a goal
Measureable:	You know when a goal has been accomplished
Attainable:	The goal is possible for you to achieve
Relevant and Realistic:	The goal is important to you and realistic in terms of your circumstances, lifestyle, budget, and tools available to you
Timed:	You have set a time frame for achieving your goal

Now that you know something about choosing effective goals, go to **assignment 2.3** (in the appendix) to see whether your prioritized goals meet the criteria of effectiveness. Use the chart "Smart Goal Setting and Action Planner" to develop your action plan. You will determine what steps to take to work toward your goals and what indicators will show you that you have succeeded. Also determine some rewards to keep yourself motivated. Two to three weeks before the end of the semester, look at **assignment 2.4** and determine how things went.

DID YOU KNOW?

Fifty percent of people who start a fitness program are no longer participating in it 6 months later (Gledhill, 2001). How can you ensure that you do not become one of those statistics?

The first time most people set goals, they usually do not succeed in listing all of them. Some people have difficulty thinking beyond the next semester. If you are having trouble setting goals, simply take a break and return to this task when you feel fresher. Setting goals is an important step in the process.

As you work on your goals, focus on the effects that are most meaningful to you. Remember that in order for these goals to be successful, they must be tied to your values of success. Expect and anticipate obstacles. Make sure that you acknowledge the challenges that you face and assess your readiness for change. Build and maintain rapport with individuals who will help support your goals. Finally, re-evaluate your goals on a regular basis to ensure that you have the appropriate behavioural strategies in place to succeed.

Table 2.3 may help you develop strategies to ensure effectiveness in changing your behaviours.

TABLE 2.3 Strategies to Change Behaviour

TIMELINE	STRATEGY
Initial stage 4–6 weeks	• Set goals that focus on being active (e.g., "I will go the gym 3–4 times per week for the next 6 weeks"). • Enhance self-efficacy via education, mastery experiences, and encouragement. • Develop a positive attitude toward physical activity. • Develop a plan to overcome initial barriers (e.g., "I will work on the push–pull machine 3 times a week until I can do 6 rotations at 50 lb"). • Find a buddy to work out with. • Try the fitness courses that are offered before and after school. • List your gains/losses associated with exercise. • Sign an exercise contract and record your exercise sessions. • Decide on a reward if your meet your initial goals.
Conditioning stage 12–20 weeks	• Enhance self-efficacy via modelling and continuing to mastery-level experiences. • Continue to foster a positive attitude. • Set goals focused on the activity (e.g., go to the gym 4–5 times per week and add 1–2 days of specific weight training). • Re-evaluate your goals to see if they are realistic and attainable. • Develop a plan to deal with any barriers encountered (e.g., "I will come in an hour before classes to do fitness training or work on the push–pull machine 3 times a week until I can do 6 rotations at 50 lb"). • Continue to record your sessions and re-evaluate your progress. • Reward yourself when you meet your goals. • Redefine your goals if they are unachievable. • Encourage someone to be active with you.
Maintenance stage 6 months and beyond	• Continue to challenge yourself with different workouts. • Assess your goals using positive feedback. • Set goals focused on performance (e.g., "I will reduce my time for the 1.5-mile [2.4-km] run by 30 seconds for the next 4 weeks"). • Develop creative ways to overcome barriers and prevent relapse. • Maintain progress monitoring. • Identify/discuss "high-risk" situations and preventive solutions. • Continue to seek support or provide support for others.

SOURCE: White, Mailey, & McAuley, 2010.

Staying on Track

We inevitably put up obstacles and resistance when we are trying to change. Here are some suggestions to help you deal with this problem.

- When your desire to continue a negative behaviour is stronger than the motivation and commitment to change, remember that change does not typically happen overnight. In fact, the behaviour may have to become more annoying or a greater health risk before you are able to change. Smokers, for example, usually make three or four attempts to break their habit. Don't be too hard on yourself.

- Be aware that making lifestyle changes carries costs as well as benefits. For example, the time commitment to physical activity may require you to reschedule or even abandon other activities. You will need to weigh the short-term costs against the long-term gains, such as decreased risk of cardiovascular diseases, cancers, diabetes, and premature death.
- **Social involvement** is a key issue in achieving goals. Many people, especially young people, pursue activities based more on whom they do them with rather than the activity itself. In this case, the buddy system keeps people involved in the activity. If you have the support of family and friends in the early stages of a fitness program, you will be more likely to succeed in making behavioural changes and to have continued commitment to maintaining them. Find the support you need. If your family or close friends cannot offer you support, find a support group that will. Monetary commitment to an aerobics class, for example, keeps many people going until they learn to exercise for other reasons.

social involvement the support of other people to assist you in achieving your goals

- If an activity just is not for you, try something else. People who have been turned off aerobics classes, for example, can get the same benefits from a program that incorporates martial arts into the exercises.
- Although physical activities can reduce stress, you may have to take time out from one if you feel it is adding stress to your life. Try something new, or take a small break and then approach the activity again from a different angle.
- Focus on the real problem. Some people blame others for their inability to change, making excuses and putting things off. Accepting responsibility for your actions and refocusing on the goal may help you succeed.
- Track your efforts in your chosen activity so that you can review your action plan for the goals you have set to ensure that you are monitoring the small gains.

Rewarding Yourself

Behaviours that are rewarded tend to be repeated. Building in different types of rewards to reinforce your efforts will increase your chances of success. Rewards can include treats, breaks from other tasks, monetary rewards (such as a new outfit), and special activities (such as a movie). Remember that everyone has setbacks. Learn from each experience, and try to avoid negative thoughts and comments. Focus on the positive, and move on from there.

THE "FIVE Cs"

What makes physical activities enjoyable and achievable? Consider the "Five Cs":

1. Competence: People are more likely to engage and maintain participation in a program that makes them feel competent while they learn new skills.
2. Challenge: The skill being learned needs to match the ability of the individual. If the challenges are too hard, most people will give up quickly. Conversely, to keep motivation up, the skill must constantly become more challenging.
3. Control: A sense of personal control leads to higher motivation. This goes back to intrinsic motivation (for example, improving one's time in the 1.5-mile [2.4-km] run) rather than extrinsic motivation (for example, passing the requirements of a course).
4. Choice: By choosing a variety of activities to achieve a goal, people have a greater chance of accomplishing it.
5. Commitment: People who have sufficient competence and are involved in a challenging situation that they choose are more likely to stay motivated and committed to the activity.

SOURCE: Canadian Society for Exercise Physiology, 2003.

Your Mission Statement

mission statement
a concise statement of major values and goals that is meant to give direction to the decisions a person will make throughout his or her life

Having assessed your values, priorities, and long-term goals, you are ready to begin creating your **mission statement**. Your mission statement will reflect your values and goals and be a road map that guides you through life for the next five years.

It may take a few attempts to create a mission statement that accurately reflects your values and goals. A mission statement is a very personal document about what you want out of life and what you are striving to achieve. Make sure that your mission statement is dynamic—that is, flexible enough to respond to changes in your life. As your life progresses, so will your goals and mission statement. Remember to think in terms of both professional and personal priorities.

The following is an example of a mission statement:

> My mission is to help educate, motivate, and support students and individuals who work in the law enforcement field with a positive attitude to help them plan and attain measurable and realistic goals. I aim to help them optimize a successful experience in planning and implementing a valuable fitness and nutrition program as part of their overall lifestyle that will assist them in realizing their dreams. I will work toward inspiring people to be more physically active and committed to being lifelong learners in the areas of fitness and nutrition. I will strive to balance work with family time, physical activity, and independent growth, while remembering that my family and friends are my first priority.

Remember that your mission statement is exclusively yours. It empowers you to have control over the decisions you must make. The mission statement must truly reflect your goals and guide your everyday decisions.

Turn to **assignment 2.5** (in the appendix) to create your mission statement.

Being Fit and Well for Life

Your first attempts at behavioural change may take a bumpy road. For some people, staying at the maintenance stage will be difficult the first time. To stay fit and be ready for a career in law enforcement takes a great deal of determination and work. When you are able to maintain your healthy behavioural changes, you will realize that this empowerment will lead you forward to achieve new goals. Maintenance takes effort, and your goals will constantly change as new information and circumstances affect your choices.

Some of you may need two years to meet the standards of the various BFOR tests (for more information on these tests, see Chapter 15). Others will need to learn only the specific skills involved and then refine their ability to improve their results; if you are one of those people, you will need to focus on challenging yourself to continue to maintain and improve your fitness level.

Although you do not have total control over every aspect of your life, especially your health, you do have the ability to create a lifestyle that minimizes your health risks and improves your fitness level while maximizing your well-being and enjoyment of life.

Good luck!

> “Learn as if you will live forever. Live as if you will die tomorrow.”
>
> —Mohandas Gandhi

KEY TERMS

attitude, 32
belief, 32
extrinsic motivation, 29
health benefits, 32
intention, 32
intrinsic motivation, 29
mission statement, 38
personal goals, 33
professional goals, 34
self-efficacy, 32
self-esteem, 30
self-management behavioural strategies, 32
social involvement, 37
values, 33

EXERCISES

Multiple Choice

1. Prochaska and colleagues' five stages of change include pre-contemplation, contemplation, preparation, ________________, and ________________.

- **a.** goal setting, behavioural change
- **b.** consciousness raising, social liberation
- **c.** commitment, behavioural change
- **d.** motivation, support
- **e.** action, maintenance/termination

2. The stage of change where people acknowledge that they have a problem and are considering doing something about it is the ________________ stage.

- **a.** pre-contemplation
- **b.** contemplation
- **c.** preparation
- **d.** action
- **e.** there is no such stage

3. The stage of change in which a person is actively participating in a fitness program for two years is an example of the ________________ stage.

- **a.** pre-contemplation
- **b.** contemplation
- **c.** preparation
- **d.** action
- **e.** there is no such stage

4. People who deny that they need to practise for law enforcement evaluation tests or stop smoking to make the tests easier are in the ________________ stage.

- **a.** pre-contemplation
- **b.** contemplation
- **c.** preparation
- **d.** action
- **e.** there is no such stage

5. At the maintenance stage of making changes in your lifestyle, which behavioural change should you have already completed?

- **a.** continue to challenge yourself with different exercise programs
- **b.** set goals to focus on performance
- **c.** develop different ways to overcome barriers and prevent relapse
- **d.** continue to seek support to help you stay on track
- **e.** set goals toward becoming active

6. The key to effective behavioural change is

- **a.** writing a goal statement and posting it in a prominent place
- **b.** enlisting the help of those around you
- **c.** identifying the stage of change you are in and using the correct strategies for that stage
- **d.** setting up a reward system for each process
- **e.** having a lot of desire and willpower

7. Which of the following are *processes* in the change model of Prochaska and colleagues?
   a. emotional arousal, contemplation, social liberation
   b. counter-conditioning, self-liberation, consciousness raising
   c. maintenance, action, pre-contemplation
   d. motivation, reward, pre-contemplation
   e. preparation, action, self-liberation
8. Counter-conditioning is a process that involves
   a. rewarding yourself for making changes in your life
   b. weighing the benefits of a change against the consequences
   c. researching information regarding your goal
   d. being prepared to initiate further behavioural changes if the original changes do not work
   e. altering your environment to avoid being tempted by problem behaviours
9. Self-management behavioural strategies include all of the following except:
   a. self-monitoring
   b. cognitive change techniques
   c. accepting barriers
   d. corrective feedback
   e. goal setting
10. In the ten processes of change, social liberation involves
    a. researching information regarding your goal
    b. implementing alternatives to ensure success
    c. drawing on emotional experiences to change your behaviour
    d. weighing the benefits of the change against the consequences
    e. believing in yourself and assuming responsibility for changing your behaviours
11. Self-esteem
    a. is dependent on what people think about you
    b. is dependent on social behaviours and physical attributes
    c. is how you look at your emotional status
    d. is how you feel about yourself and your characteristics
    e. is not taken into consideration when someone tries to help motivate someone else into participating in fitness
12. The three major reasons why people participate in a fitness program are
    a. health benefits, self-image, and enjoyment
    b. health benefits, self-efficacy, and learning a new skill
    c. self-image, self-efficacy, and self-esteem
    d. self-image, learning a new skill, and determination
    e. to learn a new skill, to master that skill, and to meet people
13. Having the right intentions to participate in a fitness program includes
    a. having extrinsic motivation to keep you going
    b. making an informed decision, designing a program, and making a commitment
    c. designing a program, looking for extrinsic motivation, and setting goals for yourself
    d. having someone design a program that is based on extrinsic motivation with high-expectation goals
    e. designing a program that is based on extrinsic motivation with low-expectation goals
14. When it comes to values around physical activity, they are based on
    a. daily behaviours, attitude, and goal setting
    b. daily behaviours, fitness programs available, and physical prowess
    c. daily behaviours, individual decisions, and facilities available
    d. daily behaviours, activities available, and individual decisions
    e. daily behaviours, attitude, and physical prowess

Short Answer

1. What are values?

2. What five kinds of goals drive our lives?

3. Describe the five stages of change using an example from your life.

4. How can the ten processes of change help you achieve your goals?

5. Why is it important to understand values when choosing goals?

6. Describe the five characteristics that make goals attainable.

7. Define self-efficacy, and describe how you would boost your own.

8. List and give examples of the four self-management behavioural strategies required to be successful in fitness.

9. What is a mission statement? How can you apply a mission statement to a career in law enforcement?

REFERENCES

Canadian Society for Exercise Physiology (CSEP). (2003). *The Canadian physical activity, fitness and lifestyle approach: CSEP—health and fitness program's health-related appraisal and counselling strategy.* Ottawa: Author.

Gledhill, N. (2001, October 26). The latest research. Paper presented at the OASES 13th Annual Professional Development Day and Internet Conference, Toronto, Ontario.

Meyer, P.J. (2003). What would you do if you knew you couldn't fail? Creating S.M.A.R.T. goals. In *Attitude is everything: If you want to succeed above and beyond.* Scotts Valley, CA: The Meyer Group.

Prochaska, J.O., DiClemente, C.C., & Norcross, J.C. (1992, September). In search of how people change. *American Psychologist, 47*, 1102–1114.

Prochaska, J.O., Norcross, J.C., & DiClemente, C.C. (1994). The five stages of change. In *Changing for good* (pp. 36–50). New York: William Morrow.

Prochaska, J.O., & Velicer, W.F. (1997). The transtheoretical model of health behavior change. *American Journal of Health Promotion, 12*(1), 38–48.

White, S.M., Mailey, E.L., & McAuley, E. (2010). Leading a physically active lifestyle: Effective individual behavior change strategies. *ACSM's Health & Fitness Journal, 14*(1), 8–15.

3

Time Management

LEARNING OBJECTIVES

After completing this chapter, you should be able to:

- Understand the importance of time management.
- Evaluate your time-management skills.
- Demonstrate better time management by prioritizing tasks and creating and using action plans.
- Understand the effectiveness of scheduling with time-management tools.

OVERVIEW

Are you back at school after a number of years? Do you have one or more part-time jobs? Do you have time-consuming family or volunteer commitments? Are you on your own for the first time? If you answered yes to any of these questions, then as a student, you need to be aware of your time.

Many students discover the need to develop or hone their time-management skills when they come to college. Unlike high school, where teachers typically structured your class time and assignments, you will have less in-class time, more outside-class homework, and a great deal of freedom and flexibility. Students who fall behind in their work face the stress of trying to keep up. If you can keep up, not only will you be able to follow along with more confidence in class, but you will also experience less stress. If you can develop a balance between school, work, and family and social life, you will be successful in your endeavours.

In the previous chapter, you learned about setting short- and long-term goals. In this chapter, you will start to see how your goals can be achieved by managing your time well. Time management is essential for successful people in any line of work. In law enforcement, officers are expected to manage the time demands of shiftwork, court appearances, and personal life. Many people who do shiftwork struggle to maintain a normal routine in their personal life. Those who work 12-hour shifts soon realize that their four-day workweek seems to be consumed by work, travelling back and forth between home and work, and sleep. If court time is added to workdays or days off, organizing all these activities becomes a struggle. Paper workloads have increased exponentially. There is now a requirement to produce more detailed reports, answer emails, and be more accountable for your time. In high school, many of you had four courses per semester, but now have six to eight courses per semester. At times you can feel overwhelmed by twice the workload.

Setting goals, organizing your time, and adhering to a schedule are critical to a less stressful lifestyle. There is no excuse for officers who cannot carry out a job such as responding quickly to a call because they have mismanaged their time. As in any profession, failure to complete a task can have adverse career repercussions. To be effective, officers must be skilled at juggling different duties. Therefore, as someone pursuing a career in law enforcement, you must make a conscientious effort to manage your time effectively.

The Benefits of Time Management

Time management is a way of taking short-term goals and dividing them into manageable daily, weekly, and monthly increments, which in turn makes your long-term goals more achievable. Here are some other benefits of time management:

- Organizing your time gives meaning to daily activities by increasing your productivity, accountability, and commitment to the tasks at hand.
- It gives you a sense of order, progress, and success.
- It gives you a sense of control over your life.
- It distinguishes between priorities and non-priorities.
- It helps you deal with mundane tasks in a more effective manner.
- It helps you deal with the boredom of a task.

- It helps to improve your relationships both on and off the job.
- It allows you to do the things that have to be done while having time to do the things you want to do.
- It reduces stress and provides more enjoyment of everyday life.

At the heart of time management is an important shift in focus: you concentrate on results instead of on being busy. Many people spend their days in a frenzy of activity but achieve very little because they are not concentrating on the right things. Studies show that every interruption uses up to five minutes in addition to the actual time spent dealing with the interruption, because it takes this amount of time to get back to the task at hand (Georgian College Corporate Training and Consulting, 2001). Some people convert wasted time into a dollar amount (number of hours wasted times hourly salary) to see how much they "lost." Money lost can speak volumes, and usually helps motivate people to rethink how they use their day. Often a lack of time leaves us angry and hostile, unable to focus and maintain our productivity.

What remains unseen is the toll on people and organizations in terms of stress and even illness. Ultimately, those who have good time-management skills are those who enjoy their job.

The Stages of Time Management

According to Seaward (2004), time management should be broken down into three stages: prioritizing, scheduling, and implementing.

As was discussed in Chapter 2, you have to know what your goals are and why, and then prioritize them. The next step is to use a daily appointment book to schedule your activities. Scheduling adds clarity to your day. You must, of course, follow through on (implement) your scheduled activities, or your prioritizing and scheduling become pointless.

The remainder of this chapter will help you evaluate how well you manage your time and get you started on developing your time-management skills. Start by turning to **assignment 3.1** (in the appendix) and estimating where your time is spent over the course of a week. Then go on to **assignment 3.2** and actually monitor where you are spending your time. This assignment will help those who need to make better use of their time. Every last detail should be written down, including the time it takes to shower, dress, commute, attend meetings, wait in line, make phone calls, clean the house, cook dinner, pick up the children from school, take them to after-school activities, and eat meals. Also include time for entertainment or exercise, such as driving to the gym, going for a walk, watching TV, surfing the Internet, and answering emails and text messages.

Your self-assessment should make you aware of your time-management skills. If you over- or underestimate your hours, you may be overwhelmed in your attempts to prioritize. There are three common mistakes in setting priorities:

1. *technical errors*, such as tackling major assignments for school too early or late in the day for your energy levels, answering one more call or email before leaving for appointments or school, and misgauging the time necessary to complete a task

2. *external realities*, including disruptive environments (not studying in a quiet location), unrealistic schedules, or obligation to others (for example, promising you will help someone for an hour and three hours later the task is still not completed)
3. *psychological obstacles*, such as being chronically late because of poor judgment of dressing or driving time, or arriving too early and then sitting around waiting for others

An important first step in efficient time management is organizing your workspace or home. Even if your schedule is well ordered, if your office and filing system are a disaster, you will waste time trying to work efficiently in a disorderly place.

Prioritizing Your Activities

To get on track in your use of time, you need to devise an *action plan* or *to-do list* that arranges the tasks that need to be accomplished. Organize your list using the headings "Essential Activities," "Regular Activities," and "Optional Activities." Some people use calendars or meeting makers to schedule their time more effectively. If you write things down, you are less likely to forget an assignment, a meeting, or an activity.

- *Essential activities* are those that you must take care of no matter what, such as attending class, going to work, keeping a medical appointment, putting gas in your car, and paying bills.
- *Regular activities* are those that you normally carry out daily or a few days each week, such as preparing meals, working out, and doing homework. These activities are important but, in terms of scheduling, they offer more flexibility than essential activities.
- *Optional activities* include those you would like to do but can reschedule without much sacrifice, such as a trip to the mall, a social telephone call, or attending a sports event.

See if you can categorize the activities you have ahead of you this week.

Scheduling Your Activities

In addition to your action plan or to-do list, your daily appointment book should record the following:

- due dates for papers, projects, presentations, and tests
- birthdays, anniversaries, and other special occasions
- benchmarks for steps toward a goal, such as due dates for sections of a project, a deadline for losing 2 kilograms, or a date on which you need to contact someone
- important meetings, medical appointments, and due dates for bill payments
- your employment schedule (paid and volunteer work)
- your travel time to get to and from activities
- your workout schedule
- commitments of a personal nature

Turn to **assignment 3.3** (in the appendix) and determine your to-do list for this week. Figure out, based on importance, what needs to be done, or should or could be done this week, and then try mapping out the list on the activity chart. Here are some hints to ensure that your scheduling is effective:

- *Take time to think about time* Spending 10–15 minutes on time-management planning at the beginning of your day can save time later. Often when individuals write down every last activity, they find that there is very little time left for sleeping. The end result is that many activities must be pared down, eliminated, consolidated, or delegated. It is important to prioritize your activities.
- *Refer to your schedule* Make sure your daily appointment book and to-do list are easily accessible. Keeping a log may help you identify time-robbers. Word-processing programs contain calendars that can be easily accessed and put to effective use.
- *Develop a game plan* Allow for at least two evenings to study for a major test. Major research papers require more time. Set aside time to type papers, and make sure you have an extra cartridge for your printer before you start—you don't want to run out of ink a few hours before a paper is due.
- *Recognize the limits on your time* There are only 168 hours in a week. Don't set yourself up for failure by asking too much of yourself. Remember that self-discipline is important if you want to be successful.
- *Categorize a week's worth of hours* By estimating how many hours your regular activities will take this week, you will be able to determine how much time you have for other activities. Remember to leave some blocks of time open in case an activity takes longer than expected.
- *Get in the habit of setting time limits for tasks* Some tasks can consume your whole day (for example, reading or answering emails) if you let them, so set a limit of one hour a day for this task and stick to it.
- *Delete, delay, delegate, diminish* You may have to decide whether you need to delete some tasks because they are not worth doing, delay them if they are lower-priority tasks (this is not procrastination), delegate them to ease your workload, or diminish the time you spend on them (more is not always better).
- *Take a break when needed* It is important to make sure that you do not let stress derail your attempts to organize yourself. When you need a break, take one. This could mean taking quick stretches or going for a walk to clear your head.
- *Make the most of class* Read the assignment or chapter before class rather than reading just before a test. You will understand lectures better and be able to take better notes. Read your notes at the end of the day or at least at the end of each week.
- *Schedule downtime* Everyone needs time to relax and refresh. Make sure your downtime schedule includes activities you enjoy. Remember to enjoy life.
- *Keep your workspace in order* Piles of paper can be distracting, and you can spend a lot of time looking for misplaced notes or articles. Handle a paper

or bill only once—do not become a paper shuffler. Spending 10 minutes at the end of the day to get things in order can save valuable time and give you a fresh start on tomorrow.

- *Get plenty of sleep, eat a healthy diet, and exercise regularly* Leading a healthy lifestyle can improve your focus and concentration. This should help you improve your efficiency so that you complete tasks in less time.
- *Remember that practice makes perfect* Time management, like any new skill, takes time to perfect. Don't forget to review your overall approach to scheduling once in a while to see whether you need to make any changes.
- *Ask for professional help* If you feel that you are losing control of your time, your school counselling service has people who can assist you. Don't hesitate to use their services.
- *Reward yourself* Plan rewards for yourself for attempting to keep to a schedule and reducing wasted time.

Implementing Your Activities

After you have scheduled your activities, you must follow through on them. Otherwise, you will find yourself falling behind as new tasks arise.

It is important to develop a big-picture view of your day-to-day life in order to clarify what is driving particular activities and what motivates you to stay engaged with them. You will need to refer back to this overall view on a regular basis to ensure that you are on the right track.

People typically run into implementation problems by failing to prioritize activities or by setting an unreasonable schedule for themselves. You also need to avoid procrastination and other time traps (see Schafer, 1996; Steel, 2007; Wohl, Pychyl, & Bennett, 2010).

Procrastination and Other Time Traps

procrastination
the postponement of unpleasant or burdensome tasks

Many people fail to achieve their goals because they procrastinate over immediate tasks. **Procrastination** is postponing unpleasant or burdensome tasks. Procrastination is often deliberate, especially when you are facing a frightening prospect, such as having to get a major task done in very little time. Some of the most common tasks that people procrastinate over are paying bills, paying taxes, saving for retirement, and starting assignments. This tendency may reflect task aversion, where people dislike the task (such as cleaning the house), or boredom, where individuals are not interested in the task at hand (writing a paper on something that does not interest you). For others, the issue may stem from fear of failure, fear of success, perfectionism, self-consciousness, or evaluation anxiety. These factors all relate to harsh appraisal (Beck, Koons, & Milgrim, 2000). Still other reasons people procrastinate include fear of losing autonomy (wanting control over when and how you have to do something instead of following instructions) and fear of being alone (having to do a solitary activity without someone helping or being around). Whatever the reason, such fears can paralyze you and keep you from taking action, until discomfort and anxiety overwhelm you and force you to get the task done or give up (Burka & Yuen, 2004).

DID YOU KNOW?

It is estimated that about 15–20 percent of the general population and 80–95 percent of college students engage in procrastination.
SOURCE: Steel, 2007.

Many students report spending nearly a third of their days avoiding important tasks by texting, tweeting, watching TV, or sleeping (Pychyl, Lee, Thibodeau, & Blunt, 2000). This behaviour is tied to unhealthy sleep, diet, and exercise patterns. It does not indicate laziness or lack of discipline but instead usually results from unproductive, deep-seated habits.

Turn to **assignment 3.4** (in the appendix) to determine your level of procrastination. If you find yourself with no time left to revise and proofread a paper, feel a rush of adrenaline when you finish a paper ten minutes before it is due, and often pull all-nighters, you may have procrastination issues.

Here are some strategies for fighting procrastination. Remember, there are no quick fixes. You are not going to wake up tomorrow and never procrastinate again. However, you might figure out how to do one or two simple tasks that will help you finish a draft a little earlier or reduce your level of stress.

- Weigh the benefits of completing the task against the drawbacks of procrastinating. If you have two assignments that are due the next day, you may not be able to spend the time that you should on each, and will have to determine which one merits greater attention or is more beneficial (in terms of marks).
- Reward yourself for completing a task. Punishing yourself every time you put something off will not help you change. Try to be a little less critical of yourself.
- Ask for help with school, work, and domestic tasks. Learn to delegate (but don't dump all the work on someone else).
- Don't expect to be perfect—just do your best.
- Set goals that can realistically be accomplished in the time you have. Connect daily activities to your work and life goals.
- Adopt a positive attitude.
- Get started—the worst thing you can do is make excuses or distract yourself with other tasks simply to avoid the task you don't want to face.
- Analyze a task and break it down into manageable parts. Just as you have scheduled classes on specific days, you need to designate specific days or times to complete your tasks and assignments.
- Make time for exercise and relaxation so that you can rejuvenate and develop a fresh perspective.
- Screen telephone and text messages, email, TV and Internet use, and junk mail. If you are already overloaded, do not let these distract you from the task at hand. Ensure that you set aside time for these activities, but do not let them rule your time.

Here are some strategies to help prepare for tests:

- Refer to the course syllabus and pre-read the chapters that are going to be covered in a lecture so that you have some understanding of the material prior to class. This will help you take better notes and prepare questions relating to the material.
- Identify the best time to study, whether it is morning, afternoon, or early evening. If your classes do not start until afternoon, use your free time in the morning to get studying done.

- Find a homework-friendly location away from distractions (roommates, TV, cellphone, tweeting, and so on), where you can focus on your assignments.
- Review your notes after class. If they do not make sense, the information will still be fresh in your head to correct them, or to make a note to ask your instructor for clarification.
- Coordinate study time with friends and roommates. Students who coordinate their study times can support each other and work toward finishing assignments. Then, distractions such as TV watching can turn into rewards when the tasks are completed.
- Temporarily de-activate social media sites. If necessary, use free applications that block popular sites and online games for specific periods of time.
- Study the more challenging components first, when you are less fatigued. When you become tired, it is easier to cover the material you enjoy more.
- Study in the same place each time—you will be better able to focus on the task. Stay off the bed; ten-minute naps can easily turn into two-hour naps.
- If you are falling asleep, take a ten-minute nap. Put the alarm on loud enough to hear it immediately, and come back to the material more refreshed.
- Use waiting time (public transportation, the hour between classes) to learn small pieces of information, or write things out on cue cards that you can go over to help you memorize facts.
- Treat school as a full-time job. Remember that for every hour you are in class, you probably will be expected to do one to two hours of work outside the classroom. It takes time to read texts, read the chalkboard or whiteboard, review instructors' notes, and study for tests. If you have to work, know your limits and try to stick to set hours that you can handle.

Here are some time-management tips that may keep you from becoming overwhelmed in the first place:

- Don't say yes when you really don't have the time. Learn to say no graciously. Although this is one of the hardest skills to learn, you will experience less stress and be able to enjoy some time to yourself when you learn to say no to people.
- Avoid studying during those times of the day when you are the least productive. If you are a morning person, try to do your homework in the morning. Even if you have only a short time for homework in the morning, use that time effectively.
- Think ahead. By thinking ahead, you won't forget things or waste time. Don't be the student who tries to convince the teacher that it was the computer's fault for crashing ten minutes before your assignment was due.
- Limit your social time. Socializing is important, but going out five nights a week is not going to bring you success in school. Limit your phone conversations. Most importantly, do not give in to peer pressure.
- Ask for direction. If you are unable to self-manage or self-regulate, ask for structure. If you ask for the task to be broken down into components, you will find that smaller goals are easier to achieve.

- Focus on the future. If you start to lose concentration, focus on the benefits of working hard with regard to your short-term goals (grades) and your long-term goals (dream career and lifestyle).
- Delegate. Some things you must do for yourself, but there are times when you can ask for a favour (just be sure you do one in return). Be reasonable about how many tasks you can accomplish. Don't get to the point where you are overwhelmed; divide challenging tasks into smaller ones, or ask for help even if you are partway through a task.
- Don't try to do too much. Many people attempt too much and become stressed or suffer **chronic time urgency**. This occurs when people put pressure on themselves to perform an unreasonable number of tasks in too short a time. Such people often become agitated because they feel that they are always in a hurry and will let others down if they cannot complete everything they set out to do. Leave some time open for unplanned circumstances that are beyond your control.

chronic time urgency
a constant state of stress due to putting pressure on yourself to do too much in too little time

- Limit use of chat lines, text messaging, email, and your cellphone. Set aside a specific time frame for these activities, and stick to it even if you are not finished (for example, first thing in the morning, just before lunch, and an hour before shutting down your computer). Sometimes it's better to leave one detailed message explaining exactly what information you require rather than two or three additional messages.
- Do not multitask when on the phone or having face-to-face conversations. This strategy will reduce the conversation time as well as ensure that key information is conveyed.
- Ask for help. There are a multitude of people at your college who are there to assist you, including faculty, counsellors, learning strategists, and librarians. Learn what other resources your college has to offer. Many colleges have writing centres, math labs, and career centres. Some offer e-learning programs, such as SkillSoft E-Learning (Cisco Learning Network, 2012), that are designed to help with basic computer skills, word processing, and web design.

Try to realize that you must work at a pace that is conducive to health, and set only realistic goals. Step back now and then and ensure that your priorities are reasonable. Stop hurrying when there is no need to hurry.

Reward yourself when you finish tasks on time. The reward should reflect the difficulty of the task and the time spent on it. For example, reward yourself with time for social media, or take a break to enjoy a movie or workout.

Organizing Assignments

Here are some helpful tips for when you are working on an assignment with a deadline:

- There is no "right" way to break up your work tasks and get started—this depends on your personality.
- You can begin in the middle of the assignment and work outward, or start with the most difficult part, the most important part, or the most profitable part (the part that has the most marks attached to it).

- Nibble at the corners: ease into a tough assignment by doing the simple, routine, or more pleasant parts first.
- Consider the deadline. Some people work best "under the gun," while others suffer shell shock. Regardless, make sure you at least understand the task so that if you need information or equipment it will be there when the deadline looms. There is no excuse for running out of paper or printer ink.
- Some people work in bursts and intersperse other activities, such as a workout, before returning to a project. Others need to stay focused and work continuously to get it done. Schedule your time according to your strengths.

Ten Tips for Running an Effective Meeting

A well-run meeting proceeds efficiently from beginning to end. If it is well planned, has a defined purpose, follows an agenda, and proceeds crisply, it will be an effective meeting. Unfortunately, many meetings do not go well—they may be too long, deal too much with extraneous issues, include people who arrive late and disrupt the flow, and so on. Here are ten tips for having an effective meeting:

1. Give people ample notice so that they can prepare based on the agenda sent out, be able to notify you whether they can attend, and arrive on time.
2. Start at the appointed time, whether everyone is there or not. Ignore late arrivals—keep the agenda rolling and keep to the time limit you have set for the meeting.
3. Have a purpose that all participants know and understand (for example, to analyze or solve a problem, to achieve a training objective, to reconcile a conflict).
4. Have an agenda that is organized to achieve the purpose and that ensures everyone is "on the same page."
5. Include as participants only those who will contribute to or gain something from the meeting. Do not allow small groups to start up separate conversations.
6. Stick to the agenda, with no wasted time or motions. Restate the relevant points of the agenda when the discussion veers from the objectives.
7. Ask open-ended questions to obtain different points of view and to make sure that everyone's point of view is heard.
8. Encourage participants to understand their role, come prepared, and make contributions. Prevent individuals from dominating the discussion by asking them to allow others to speak.
9. Make sure that one person chairs the meeting. The chair should summarize what has been accomplished so that everyone has the same understanding.
10. Have a post-meeting follow-up where necessary. Include off-target subjects to be discussed at a later meeting.

Group Work and Delegation

One of the skills that a law enforcement employer is looking for is the ability to work effectively in groups. So much time can be wasted if you do not have the right group or have assigned the wrong person to a task. It can be very frustrating to be assigned by your instructor or boss to a group that you know has weaker individuals who have difficulty contributing. Here are some tips to help with group work:

- If you are allowed to choose your group, choose people who complement your work methods (not necessarily those who work the same way you do) and who work well in team settings.
- Decide what needs to be delegated. Determine what can and cannot be delegated, ensuring that both popular and unpopular components, and important and less important components, are delegated.
- Choose the right person for each job. Ensure that the workload is evenly distributed and that individuals are given authority over their work.
- Set goals for different tasks. Start with small projects to ensure that the group is on the right track. Define from the outset how the group wants each task accomplished—what are the criteria for a "good" job? Having this discussion will save frustration and time later. Agree on deadlines.
- As a group, agree who is in charge of overseeing the project. Plan periodic reviews and schedule them when you first start the assignment. Make sure everyone knows his or her role from the start. Then stand back and allow individuals to do their jobs.
- At the periodic reviews and when the final product is brought together, make sure to review the project as a team before handing it in. Hold people accountable for their contribution.
- Learn to conduct team meetings efficiently and effectively. Start and end on time, stick to an agenda, and keep any discussion on topic (see box on the previous page).

Final Thoughts on Time Management

Remember that the more you use your time-management skills, the closer you will be to achieving your long-term goals. It is very important to follow a schedule. If you fail to keep to your schedule, ask yourself why and attempt to change the behaviours that caused the problem. If you need help, ask. Every college campus has counselling services to help you make your academic career a success. A faculty member can point you in the right direction if you are unsure where to turn, such as choosing a topic for a project paper.

Remember that you have to find a balance between work and play. As stress-management expert Walter Schafer (1996, p. 493) has written, "Learn to live with unfinished tasks—only a corpse is completely finished."

KEY TERMS

chronic time urgency, 51
procrastination, 48

EXERCISES

Multiple Choice

1. Which of the following is a health-related consequence of an unrealistic schedule?
   - **a.** suffering from stress
   - **b.** being late for classes
   - **c.** missing your bus or car pool
   - **d.** failing to return calls
   - **e.** forgetting your textbooks in the cafeteria
2. Travel to and from school and work, household chores, and child care are examples of
   - **a.** free time
   - **b.** work time
   - **c.** committed time
   - **d.** lost time
   - **e.** valued time
3. What is the first step to managing time effectively?
   - **a.** analyzing your current time use
   - **b.** establishing priorities
   - **c.** making a schedule
   - **d.** monitoring your current time use
   - **e.** creating a calendar of your monthly events
4. Writing down your goals will help you to
   - **a.** organize them
   - **b.** evaluate them
   - **c.** remember them
   - **d.** publish them
   - **e.** share them with others
5. Managing your time by organizing and scheduling activities will
   - **a.** not make a difference
   - **b.** give you more control over daily stress
   - **c.** give you no more time for other activities
   - **d.** just be a paper exercise
   - **e.** let others see how busy you are
6. The three stages of good time management are
   - **a.** prioritizing, scheduling, and involving
   - **b.** scheduling, implementing, and assessing
   - **c.** scheduling, organizing, and implementing
   - **d.** prioritizing, organizing, and implementing
   - **e.** prioritizing, scheduling, and implementing
7. In recent years, the amount of time the average person spends at work has
   - **a.** decreased
   - **b.** increased
   - **c.** remained the same
   - **d.** fluctuated up and down
   - **e.** depended on each person's needs
8. Which is most likely to suffer due to a lack of time?
   - **a.** work
   - **b.** chores
   - **c.** sleep
   - **d.** relationships
   - **e.** travel time
9. Chronic time urgency refers to
   - **a.** teachers assigning you too much homework
   - **b.** putting too much pressure on yourself to perform a number of tasks
   - **c.** having your family expect you to help clean up around home before doing your homework
   - **d.** organizing a number of tasks in order to get them done on time
   - **e.** setting realistic goals for yourself

Short Answer

1. Why is it important to organize your time?

2. How does time management relate to goal setting?

3. Briefly describe the three headings under which activities can be prioritized.

4. What are some effective methods to assist you with your schedule?

5. What is procrastination? How can it be overcome?

6. What signs may indicate that you are procrastinating?

7. What are some other time traps? How can they be overcome?

8. What can you do to prevent multimedia and electronic devices from monopolizing your time?

9. What can you do to make studying time more effective?

10. How can you organize yourself to ensure that all your assignments are completed and handed in on time?

REFERENCES

Beck, B.L., Koons, S.R., & Milgrim, D.L. (2000). Correlates and consequences of behavioural procrastination: The effects of academic procrastination, self-consciousness, self-esteem and self-handicapping. *Journal of Social Behaviour and Personality, 15,* 3–13.

Burka, J.B., & Yuen, L.M. (2004). *Procrastination: Why you do it, what to do about it.* New York: Da Capo Press.

Cisco Learning Network. (2012). *SkillSoft E-Learning.* https://learningnetwork.cisco.com/docs/DOC-6622.

Georgian College Corporate Training and Consulting. (2001). *Time management training.* Barrie, ON: Author.

Pychyl, T.A., Lee, J.M., Thibodeau, R., & Blunt, A. (2000). Five days of emotion: An experience sampling study of undergraduate student procrastination. *Journal of Social Behavior and Personality, 15,* 239–254.

Schafer, W. (1996). *Stress management for wellness* (3rd ed.). Orlando, FL: Holt, Rinehart and Winston.

Seaward, B.L. (2004). *Managing stress: Principles and strategies for health and wellbeing* (4th ed.). Boston: Jones and Bartlett.

Steel, P. (2007). The nature of procrastination: A meta-analytic and theoretical review of quintessential self-regulatory failure. *Psychological Bulletin, 133*(1), 65–94.

Wohl, M.J.A., Pychyl, T.A., & Bennett, S.H. (2010). I forgive myself, now I can study: How self-forgiveness for procrastinating can reduce future procrastination. *Personality and Individual Differences, 48,* 803–808.

PART 2

Planning and Maintaining a Fitness Program

4

Principles of Exercise

OVERVIEW

LEARNING OBJECTIVES

After completing this chapter, you should be able to:

- Understand basic concepts of anatomy and physiology and how these apply to exercise.
- Explain how health-related and performance/skill-related fitness are important in law enforcement.
- Describe the physical and psychological benefits of exercise.
- Understand the principles of exercise and how to apply them in your fitness program.
- Explain the benefits of stretching and incorporate safe, effective stretching into your fitness program.
- Describe the proper way to start a fitness program.

The policing community promotes the importance of "fitness for duty, fitness for life," and the health benefits of being physically fit are widely acknowledged. Police services nationally strive to have officers in their best physical condition both when they are hired and throughout their careers, for a variety of reasons. These include maintaining a professional image, improving job performance, having the ability to handle shiftwork, reducing the likelihood of excessive force, and ensuring the quality of backup. The benefits of fitness for life include preventing health problems, reducing disability, increasing quality of life, and enjoying a longer life.

In this chapter, you will learn about the components of physical fitness, the many benefits of physical activity, and the principles of exercise. As you begin your studies toward a career in law enforcement, you must apply this information by starting a fitness program that will prepare you for the physical challenges of policing. The information in this chapter will serve as an important foundation for this training.

Introduction to Anatomy and Physiology

Before we look at the principles of exercise and its benefits, it is important to have a basic understanding of how the human body is structured and how it works. Many of the concepts that we will discuss later with respect to fitness standards and leading a healthy lifestyle—in particular, ways to improve our bodies' function and avoid harming them—will build on this knowledge. This section describes the basics of human **anatomy** and **physiology** so that you can develop skills to meet the physical demands of daily life, physical activities, sports, and job-related performance.

anatomy
the study of the structure and parts of the body in relationship to one another

physiology
the study of function of the human body, or how the parts work and carry out their life-sustaining activities

Cells, Tissues, and Organs

The human body is a complex system of parts that work together. The building blocks of all living organisms are cells. There are trillions of cells in the human body and they are grouped together into four basic kinds of tissue, each of which performs a specific function:

1. *Epithelial tissue* is made up of tightly packed cells. One of its most important functions is protection. It covers our whole body in the form of the outer layer of our skin, lines the digestive tract, and surrounds the organs, keeping them separate from one another and holding them in place.
2. *Connective tissue* adds support and structure to the body. There are several types of connective tissue, including tendons, ligaments, cartilage, blood, bone, and fat tissue.
3. *Muscle tissue* helps move parts of our bodies and helps transport substances through our bodies. For example, the biceps brachii muscle bends your arm, while your heart moves blood through your body.
4. *Nerve tissue* helps coordinate actions of other tissues by generating electrical signals and transmitting them down the spinal cord to the parts of the body.

Organs are structures that perform a function or functions in the body. They are made up of two or more types of tissue. All mammals possess these ten major organ systems:

1. The *circulatory system* transports oxygen, nutrients, and wastes through the body. It includes the heart, blood vessels, and blood.
2. The *lymphatic system* defends against disease by destroying viruses and microbes, and removes excess tissue fluid to the blood. It includes the lymph nodes, lymph, and white blood cells.
3. The *digestive system* breaks down food, absorbs nutrients, and eliminates non-useable materials. It includes the mouth, stomach, and intestines.
4. The *endocrine system* transmits chemical messages through the body, working with the nervous system. It includes the many glands in the body that secrete hormones, such as the thyroid and pituitary glands.
5. The *muscular system* allows us to move voluntarily, and controls involuntary movements in the body such as circulation. It includes the body's skeletal and smooth muscles.
6. The *nervous system* transmits electrical messages through the body to produce movement. It receives, processes, and reacts to stimuli, and with the endocrine system controls processes such as circulation and digestion. It includes the brain and spinal cord.
7. The *reproductive system* produces cells that allow humans to reproduce. It includes the ovaries in females and the testes in males.
8. The *respiratory system* exchanges gas between the blood and the outside environment, absorbing oxygen and expelling carbon dioxide. Among other organs, it involves the lungs and the nose.
9. The *skeletal system* provides structure and support for the body, and protects the organs. With the muscular system, it allows movement. It includes bone, cartilage, and ligaments.
10. The *excretory system* filters out wastes, toxins, and excess water. Among other organs, it involves the kidneys and bladder.

In the next section, we'll look more closely at the skeletal and muscular systems. We will explore the circulatory system in more detail in Chapter 5.

FYI

Metabolism

Chemical processes happen constantly within our bodies. Our metabolism converts the food we eat into the energy our bodies need to function, and also affects how efficiently we use that energy. It is controlled by our nervous system and by hormones secreted by the glands of the endocrine system.

Various factors determine our metabolic rate, or how quickly our metabolism works. These include our body size, age, gender, genes, amount of body fat and lean muscle tissue, level of physical activity, presence of illness, mental state, and drug use. Even though we cannot change some of these factors, we can increase our metabolic rate through exercise. Aerobic workouts can help burn more calories in the short term, and building up muscles through weight training helps increase a person's metabolic rate in the long term.

Bones and Muscles

There are 206 bones in the adult human body, including 29 in the skull, 26 in the spinal column, and 126 in the limbs. Our bones give our bodies form and serve a number of other functions, which help determine their individual sizes and shapes. Long bones in the arms and legs function as levers, while short ones (for example, in the wrist) provide additional flexibility. Other bones protect our organs, such as the sternum, which protects the lungs and heart, and the skull, which protects the brain.

The bones of the human body are shown in Figure 4.1.

Our bones meet at joints and are attached to each other by strong, fibrous connective tissue called **ligaments**. While some joints do not move (for example, the fixed joints in the skull), the most common kind, called synovial joints, function as pivot points, allowing for varying degrees of bending, twisting, or sliding and thereby permitting us to move. The full movement potential of a joint—that is, the degree to which it can move in each direction—is called its **range of motion**.

DID YOU KNOW?

The longest bone of your body is the femur, or thighbone, measuring approximately one-quarter of your height, while the smallest is the staples bone in your ear, measuring just one-tenth of an inch.

ligament
fibrous tissue that connects bones to other bones

range of motion
the distance and direction a joint can move to its full potential

FIGURE 4.1 Skeletal Front and Back Views

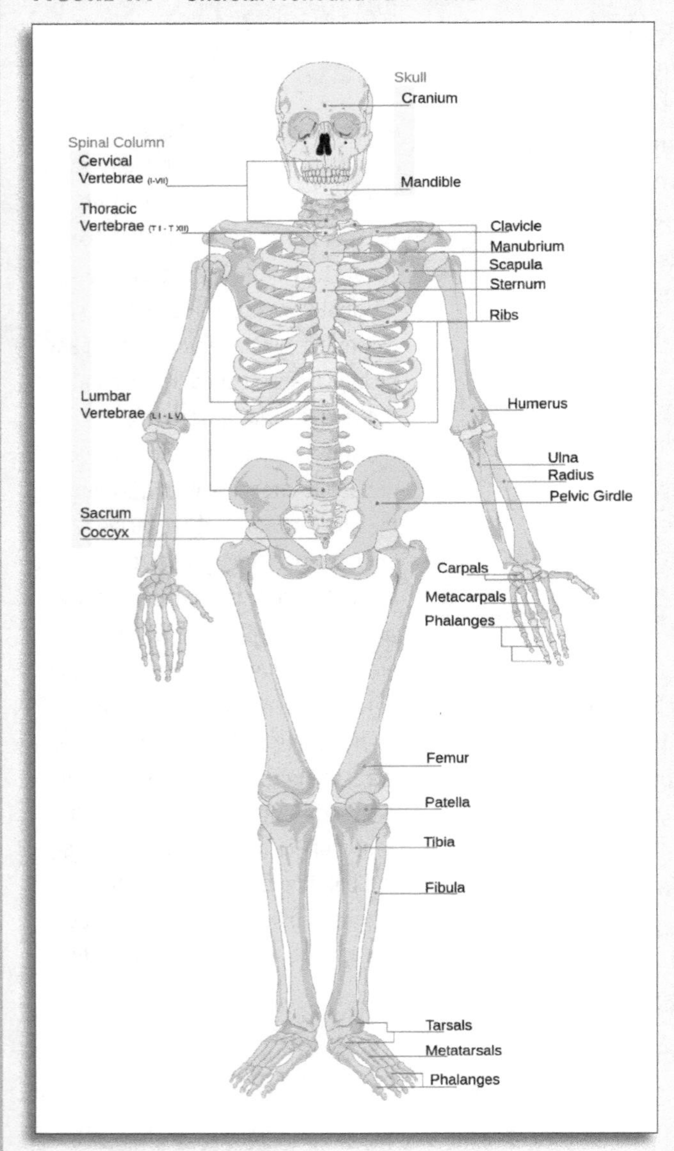

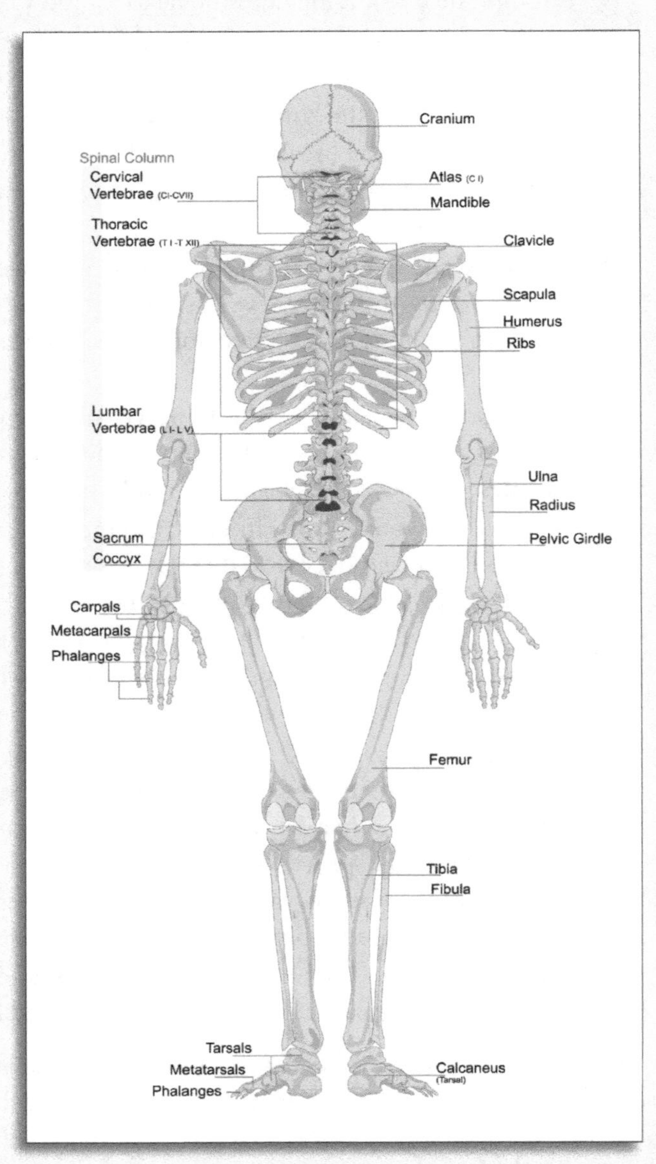

Joints are classified according to the type of movement they allow. In a hinge joint—such as an elbow or a knee joint—the bones are connected in a way that allows movement in one plane only (flexion and extension). But in a ball-and-socket joint—such as a shoulder or a hip joint—the round head of one bone is held in the cup-like cavity of another bone, allowing movement in all directions. Figure 4.2 shows the different kinds of joints in the human body.

tendon
fibrous tissue that connects muscles to bones

We would not be able to move our bones if not for our muscles, which stretch across joints and attach bone to bone, and **tendons**, the tough cords of tissue that attach our muscles to our bones. However, our muscles do not only allow us to move. They are constantly working to hold us up, to stabilize our joints, and to provide other involuntary movements. Humans have three types of muscle tissue, each with a specific function:

FIGURE 4.2 Types of Synovial Joint

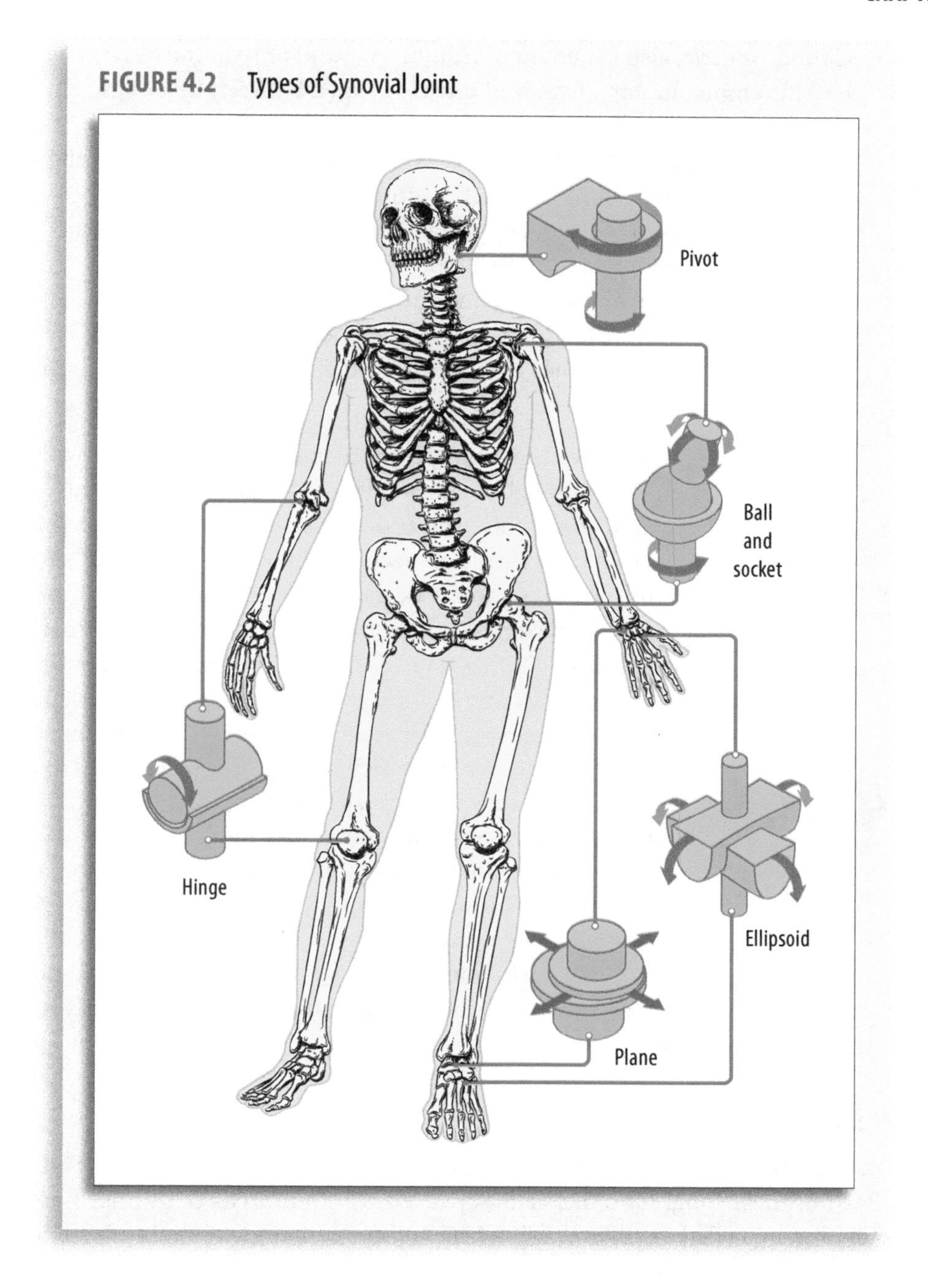

1. *Skeletal muscle* is controlled voluntarily by the nervous system and the brain. It is what allows us to move, and it is the kind of muscle we are usually referring to when we say "muscle." It is extremely sensitive tissue that is quick to adapt. We will discuss skeletal muscle in detail in the following pages.
2. *Smooth muscle* is an involuntary muscle that is controlled automatically by signals from the brain and body. Smooth muscle plays a key role in functions that happen without our thinking about them, such as breathing, digestion, and blood flow. Almost every organ contains smooth muscle, and most smooth muscle is found around the body's organs, such as the digestive tract and the circulatory and excretory systems.

3. *Cardiac muscle*, also called myocardium, is found only in the heart. The heart is an involuntary, fist-sized muscle located between the lungs, behind the breastbone, that pumps blood through a network of blood vessels called arteries. Myocardium allows the heart to contract continuously without tiring, in response to nerve signals from the brain. When the heart contracts, it forces blood into two main arteries, the pulmonary artery and the aorta, from which it is transported to the rest of the body. When the heart relaxes, blood that has circulated through the body can move back into the heart.

FIGURE 4.3 Tendons and Ligaments

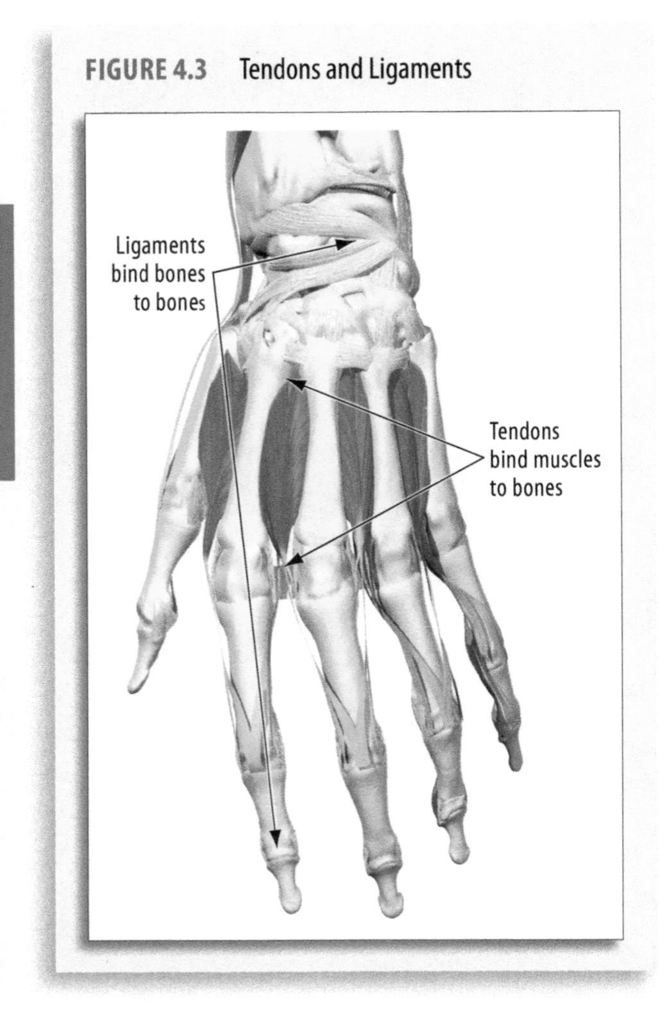

We have approximately 640 muscles in our bodies, which can make up half of our weight. Like our bones, our muscles come in different sizes and shapes, which determine their functions. You do not need to know the names of all of them, but you should be familiar with the major muscle *groups*. The exercises described in this text, and in the accompanying *Fit for Duty, Fit for Life Training Guide*, refer to these larger groups to indicate which muscles a particular exercise is training. For example, the two major muscle groups in the upper leg, which we refer to as the hamstrings and the quadriceps, are actually made up of three and four muscles, respectively. The individual muscles within these groups work together to carry out their group's function.

Figure 4.3 shows tendons and ligaments; Figure 4.4 shows the major muscle groups.

Turn to **assignment 4.1** (in the appendix) and see how many of the body's bones and muscles you can identify and name.

How Do Muscles Work?

Our skeletal muscles are composed of bundles of cells called *muscle fibres* (Figure 4.5). Each of these long, tube-like cells is packed with hundreds of thinner fibres, made of protein, called *myofibrils.* Myofibrils in turn contain two kinds of *myofilaments*: thin filaments, made of actin proteins, and thick filaments, made of myosin proteins. The thick and thin filaments are organized into bundles called *sarcomeres.*

When a muscle is relaxed, the thick and thin filaments within a sarcomere overlap each other slightly. When a nerve impulse tells a muscle fibre to contract, the thick and thin filaments slide past each other until they overlap, shortening the sarcomere (Figure 4.6). The same action happens to every sarcomere within a muscle fibre, causing the muscle fibre to contract. As the load increases, more muscle fibres are recruited by the central nervous system and a stronger force is generated by the muscle.

Conversely, when a muscle stretches, the overlap of the actin and myosin filaments decreases, allowing the muscle fibre to elongate. Once the muscle fibres reach their maximum length, the surrounding connective tissue is stretched. The more fibres that are stretched, the greater the length developed by the stretched muscle.

FIGURE 4.4 The Major Muscle Groups

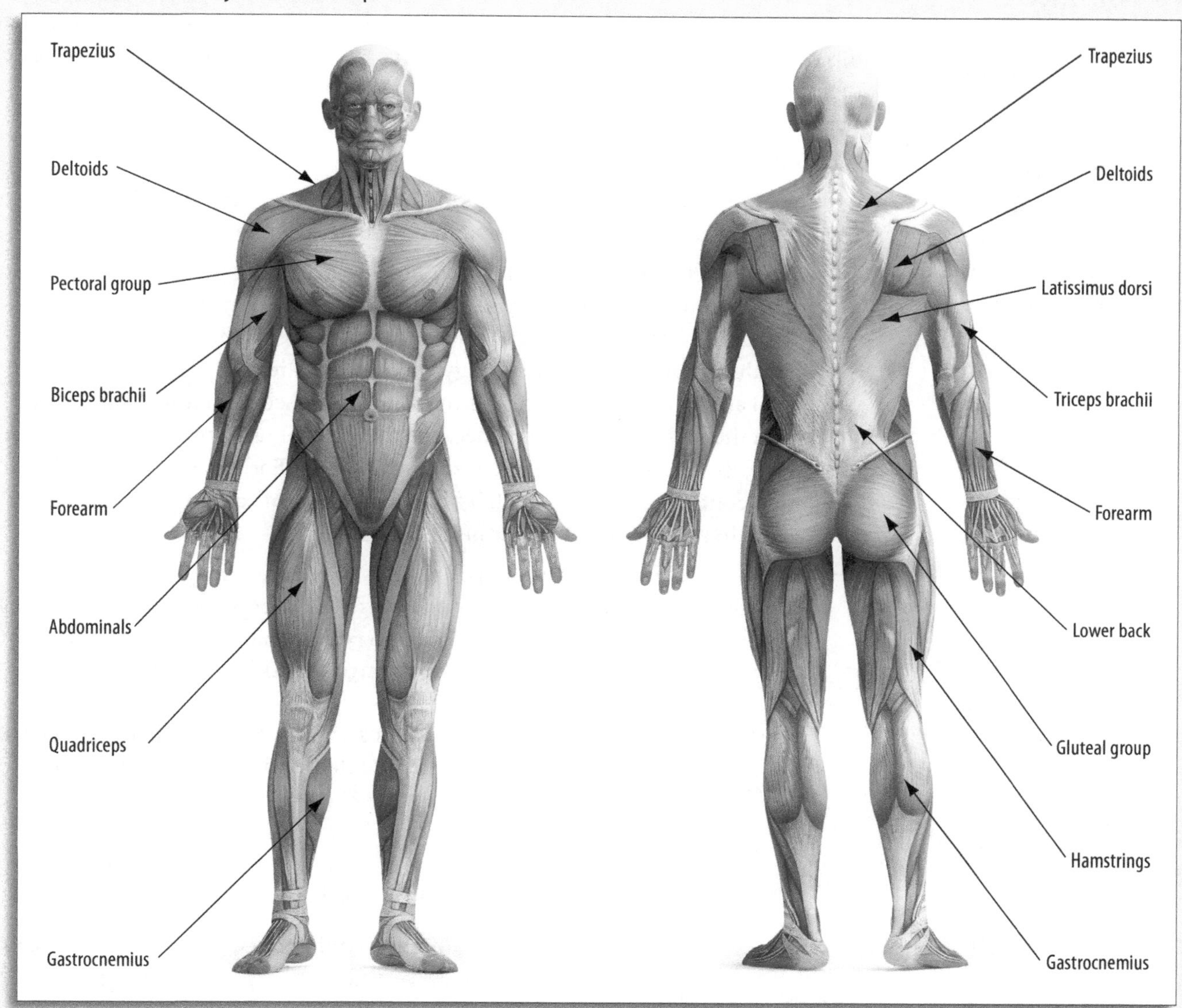

FYI

Strains Versus Sprains

Strains and sprains are two common injuries, but they are not the same thing.

A strain refers to a muscle that has been stretched too far by applying too much tension or pressure. Strains cause pain in the muscle, tenderness, and sometimes swelling and bruising as a result of torn muscles. Warming up properly, which increases blood circulation to the muscles, can prevent strains.

A sprain is an injury in which ligaments are either overstretched or torn. Sprains can be mild, moderate, or severe. Ankles and wrists can be sprained. Because sprains swell and appear bruised, they can be confused with broken bones.

You will learn more about both these common injuries in Chapter 14.

DID YOU KNOW?

In order to contract, our muscles need energy. Structures in our cells called mitochondria use glucose and oxygen to produce a compound known as ATP, or adenosine triphosphate. When ATP breaks down, it creates energy. The more mitochondria in a muscle fibre, the more energy it can produce.

Because muscle fibres work as a result of electrical impulses, our muscles need to be insulated from one another to prevent the activation of one fibre from activating others—for example, so that we can contract our quadriceps without contracting our glutes. A connective tissue wrapping around individual muscles isolates them from others.

Types of Muscle Fibres

Our muscles contain two different kinds of fibres: fast-twitch and slow-twitch. Most of the muscles in our body contain both types of fibres.

- *Fast-twitch fibres* can contract very quickly, providing powerful acceleration. They build force rapidly but also use up oxygen and muscular energy rapidly (usually in less than 60 seconds, or 1–3 reps). This means they can produce small amounts of energy very fast but are easily fatigued.

  Fast-twitch fibres are bigger in diameter and contain fewer mitochondria than slow-twitch fibres. Because they do not use oxygen to produce energy, they do not require a rich supply of blood. For this reason, muscles that contain a lot of fast-twitch fibres are lighter in colour than muscles that contain a lot of slow-twitch muscle fibres.
- *Slow-twitch fibres* produce large amounts of energy slowly. They build force slowly, consume less energy, and use muscular energy more gradually. They are more resistant to fatigue than fast-twitch fibres, so they can work for longer periods without becoming tired.

  Slow-twitch fibres are smaller in diameter than fast-twitch fibres. They contain more mitochondria and require a rich supply of oxygenated blood to produce the energy they need for muscle contraction. Muscles that contain a lot of slow-twitch fibres are red because of the many blood vessels they contain.

FIGURE 4.5 Muscle Fibre

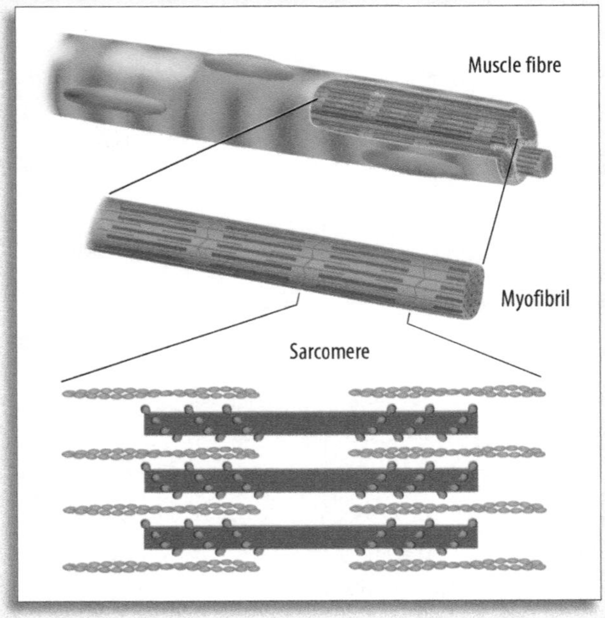

Muscle fibre

Myofibril

Sarcomere

Because of these differences, fast-twitch and slow-twitch fibres serve different purposes in the body and are useful for different kinds of activities. Fast-twitch fibres are good for sprinting and for quick movements, like jumping. These kinds of fibres make up the muscles that move the eyes, and are found in large numbers in the muscles of the arms. Slow-twitch fibres, by contrast, are useful in helping maintain posture and in activities that require endurance, like long distance running. The soleus (a muscle in the calf) is made up mainly of slow-twitch fibres, as are the muscles in the back that help keep the spine upright and those in the neck that keep the head upright.

How Muscles Cooperate with Each Other

Our muscles work both as movers *and* as stabilizers. Certain muscles work primarily as movers (for example, the biceps muscle), while others serve primarily to give

FIGURE 4.6 Relaxed and Contracted Muscle Fibre

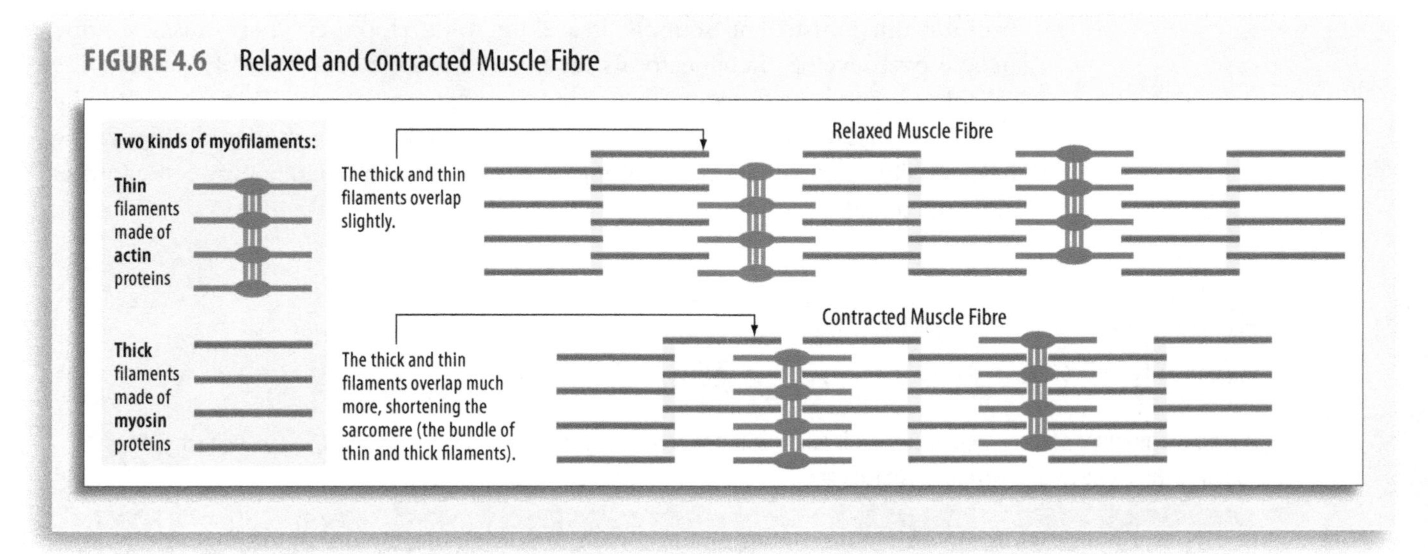

stability to the joints (for example, the multifidus, one of the muscles in the back). Depending on the movement involved, many muscles can function as movers *or* stabilizers.

Our muscles move our bones by contracting and relaxing. They are arranged around joints in pairs known as agonists and antagonists (see below). When muscles cause a limb to move through the joint's range of motion, they usually act in cooperating groups composed of the following:

- **Agonists** are muscles that move a bone in one direction. They contract to move a limb through a normal range of motion. Agonists are known as prime movers because they generate movement.
- **Antagonists** are muscles that move a bone in the direction opposite to that of the agonist. They return the limb to the original position. They also stabilize our joints.
- **Synergists** are muscles that assist the agonists indirectly in producing a joint's movement. Because synergists play various roles, several terms are used to describe them, including stabilizer, neutralizer, and fixator.
- **Fixators** are the muscles that provide the support to hold the rest of the body in place while movement occurs.

agonist
a muscle that causes specific movement by contracting

antagonist
a muscle that acts in opposition to the movement caused by the agonist, returning a limb to its initial position

synergist
a muscle that assist an agonist indirectly in producing a joint's movement

fixator
a muscle that provides support while movement occurs

Muscles are not agonists, antagonists, synergists, or fixators in isolation; they act as such specifically in the context of particular movements. For example, the biceps muscle is not always an agonist, but it is an agonist in elbow flexion, which moves the lower arm toward the shoulder.

Some common agonist/antagonist muscle pairs include:

- biceps/triceps
- quadriceps/hamstrings
- pectorals/latissimus dorsi
- abdominals/spinal erectors

Many people focus on agonists in training sessions, sometimes causing imbalance and dysfunction when these muscles are overtrained at the expense of undertraining antagonists. For example, in seeking to develop their chest muscles, some people overdevelop their pectorals (agonists) but do not adequately develop the rhomboids and mid-/lower trapezius in the back (antagonists). This can eventually pull the scapulae out of alignment, causing the shoulders to round forward. For the best possible performance, it is important to achieve a balance between agonists and antagonists.

FYI

Describing Body Positions and Movements

There are a number of terms you should be familiar with that relate to the body and its movements, as you will encounter them in the names and descriptions of exercises.

CATEGORY	TERM	DEFINITION
POSITIONS	***Supine***	The position of lying face up (for example, when doing crunches)
	Prone	The position of lying face down (for example, when beginning a push-up)
MOVEMENTS *Note that the following terms always refer to the joints involved in an action, as this is where movement occurs.*	***Extension***	Any movement that moves a limb or body part from a bent to a straight position or opens a joint (for example, a backbend or extending your arm or leg behind the midline of your body).
	Flexion	Any movement that bends a limb or a joint, or brings the bones closer together (for example, elbow flexion occurs in a bicep curl).
	Adduction	This refers to the arms, legs, fingers, or toes moving toward the midline of the body (for example, if you are standing with your legs hip-width apart, adduction at the hip joint will bring your feet closer together; if your arms are above your head, adduction of the shoulder joints will bring them back down to your sides).
	Abduction	This refers to the arms, legs, fingers, or toes moving away from the midline of the body (for example, abduction of the joints at the base of your knuckles will spread your fingers apart; if your arms are down at your sides, abducting the shoulder joints will raise your arms).
	Medial (internal) rotation	This action, which occurs at the shoulder and hip joints, turns a limb in toward the midline of the body (for example, medial or internal rotation of the hip joint occurs when you turn your left leg so that your left toes are pointing toward the right).
	Lateral (external) rotation	This action, which occurs at the shoulder and hip joints, turns a limb away from the midline of the body (for example, if your feet are together, opening your toes out so that your feet form a "V").
	Rotation	This refers to the spinal column and neck twisting either to the right or the left (for example, turning your head to look over your shoulder).
	Circumduction	This action occurs at the shoulder and hip joints and combines flexion, extension, adduction, and abduction to create a circular movement (for example, the action in your shoulder joint when swimming the backstroke).

Muscular Contractions

When we speak of a muscle "contracting," this does not imply that the muscle shortens. Instead, it means only that tension has been generated. Muscles can contract in the following ways:

- In an **isotonic contraction**, a muscle contracts in response to a constant force or load that is applied to it. There are two types of isotonic contractions:
  - *Concentric contractions* take place when the muscle actively shortens against the opposing load and the ends of the muscle are drawn closer together. A biceps curl on the way up is an example of an exercise that produces a concentric contraction.
  - *Eccentric contractions* take place when the muscle actively lengthens as it resists the load and the ends of the muscle are pulled farther apart. A biceps curl on the way down is an example of an exercise that produces an eccentric contraction.

  Eccentric contractions are much stronger than concentric contractions and therefore can produce greater exercise benefits. However, eccentric contractions cause more muscle soreness and increase the risk of soft tissue damage.
- In an **isometric contraction**, the muscle is activated but does not lengthen or shorten. There is no movement, and the muscle remains at a fixed length. This kind of muscular action occurs when muscles attempt to push or pull an immovable object—for example, if you were to stand facing a wall, extend your arms out at a 90-degree angle, and push against the wall.
- In an **isokinetic contraction**, the muscle length changes to contract maximally throughout the full range of movement. Various isokinetic exercise machines are available, which generally involve the use of a wheel, lever, crank, or similar device. The most popular, called the isokinetic dynamometer, provides resistance that matches that of the user as it measures the strength and power of various muscle groups.

isotonic contraction contraction of a muscle in response to a load applied to it; includes concentric and eccentric contractions

isometric contraction occurs when muscle length remains constant, or when contractile force equals resistive force

isokinetic contraction occurs when muscle length changes, contracting maximally throughout the full range of movement

Figure 4.7 illustrates the difference between isotonic and isometric contractions.

Concentric repetitions in weight training cause muscles to shorten in length. Over time, your muscles can shorten to the point where their range of motion becomes restricted. This can result in a decrease in the amount of force you can generate in the muscle. However, stretching can counter the effects of concentric repetitions so that your elongated muscle can generate more force.

FIGURE 4.7 Difference Between Isotonic and Isometric Contractions

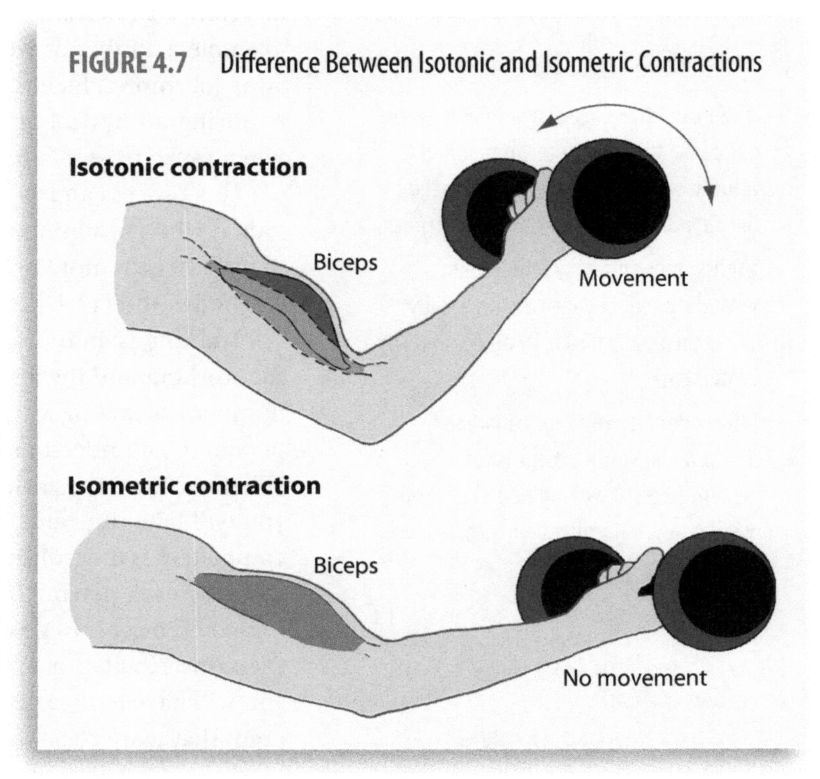

FYI

"No Pain, No Gain"?

It is common to feel varying degrees of soreness in the muscles both during and sometimes for several days following strenuous exercise. The two kinds of pain have different causes.

When we exercise vigorously, we may feel soreness or a burning feeling in an active muscle—for example, during sprints. This soreness results from a buildup of lactic acid, which occurs whenever the muscles are active for more than a minute or two and become fatigued. This usually encourages us to stop the activity. Within a few hours to a day, the lactic acid is cleared away by the body and the burning disappears.

In addition to soreness during strenuous activity, we may also experience delayed-onset muscle soreness (DOMS), particularly after trying a new exercise or suddenly increasing the length or intensity of our workout. DOMS is characterized by severe muscle tenderness, stiffness, decreased strength, and decreased range of motion that usually peaks between 24 and 72 hours after a hard workout. Placing new demands or stresses on a particular muscle can cause microscopic tears in the muscle fibres, which can cause soreness, swelling, and inflammation as the muscle repairs itself. After the rebuilding process—which is one reason why you must give your body sufficient time to recover following a hard workout—the muscle is stronger than before. This means that the next time you do the activity that caused the DOMS, you will likely experience less soreness. To cause the same amount of micro-damage to the muscle fibre the next time, you would need to add more stress to those muscles. This is the principle behind building muscle mass.

Research has shown that eccentric contractions result in more muscle cell damage than concentric contractions, so exercises involving these kinds of contractions—such as downhill running—will result in increased soreness in the days following the exercise.

FACTS ABOUT...

Canadian Youth and Physical Activity

- Four out of five Canadian adolescents do not participate in the recommended volume of physical activity suggested by the *Canadian Physical Activity Guidelines*.
- Slightly more primary school than secondary school youth are physically active on a daily basis (19 percent versus 17 percent).
- Total sedentary time for Canadian children and youth accounts for 62 percent (6 of 10 waking hours) of their waking day, with girls being less active than boys.

SOURCES: CSEP, 2011; Canadian Adolescents at Risk Research Network, 2004; Colley, Garriguet, Janssen, Craig, Clarke, et al., 2011.

What Is Training?

In the simplest terms, training refers to making your body more efficient. If you can train your body through general fitness activities (for example, running or weight training), you will be able to do parts of your job more efficiently (for example, chasing potential criminals, enduring a physical altercation, or being able to function at 4 a.m. when asked to search for a lost person).

This process and the changes that take place depend on the individual who is training and the goals that he or she has set. The goal may be to gain more muscle, to reduce body fat, to have the best time on the 1.5-mile (2.4-km) run, or to reduce stress.

Training is an individual process. It depends on the objectives of the workout and the attributes of the individual involved. There are a number of ways in which to modify your body's attributes, and each person must understand that there may be a variety of options available to achieve those changes. Finding out which way works best for you will take time and effort. Human performance results cannot be completely standardized. In other words, no one program works the same for each person. It is impossible to expect that a fitness instructor would be able to give your entire class the same program and have the same results for everyone by the end of the course. Ultimately, you will have to do a great deal of training on your own to find a program that works best for you.

Health-Related Fitness

The Police Fitness Personnel of Ontario (PFPO) has advocated the importance of health-related fitness in policing for over 25 years. It compiles evidence to support the fact that officers who are fit will be able to do their jobs more effectively and safely, and has promoted a lapel-pin fitness award.

The five components of health-related fitness are cardiorespiratory endurance, muscular strength, muscular endurance, flexibility, and a healthy body composition. Regular physical activity leads to improvements in all five areas.

cardiorespiratory endurance
heart and respiratory system endurance; the ability to perform prolonged large-muscle activities at moderate to high intensity

muscular strength
the amount of force a muscle can produce with a single maximum effort

Cardiorespiratory Endurance

Cardiorespiratory endurance (heart and respiratory system endurance) is the ability of the heart to pump blood throughout the body efficiently. This means your body can perform prolonged large-muscle activities, such as swimming or jogging, at moderate to high intensity. It is probably the most important component of fitness. When you regularly engage in activities that improve cardiorespiratory endurance, you enhance your body's ability to regulate blood flow and use oxygen and other fuels. As a result, you lower your resting heart rate and blood pressure, and your ability to dissipate heat increases. Having the stamina for a foot chase is one example of how cardiorespiratory endurance is important in law enforcement.

Cardiorespiratory endurance is dealt with in greater detail in Chapter 5.

Muscular Strength

Muscular strength is the amount of force a muscle can produce with a single maximum effort. Strong muscles are important for daily activities such as lifting and pulling heavy objects, climbing stairs, vacuuming, and carrying groceries. Abundant musculature provides good structural support for the back and helps prevent back and leg pain. It enhances recreational activities—for example, by helping a player jump higher in volleyball, hit a tennis ball harder, and kick a soccer ball farther.

Muscular strength is also important for overall health. A greater muscle mass increases the body's metabolic rate (the rate at which the body breaks down food, producing energy). Strength training is vital to prevent diseases such as osteoporosis. Muscular strength can be developed by training with weights or by doing calisthenics, which do not require special equipment.

Muscular strength is dealt with in greater detail in Chapter 6 and in the *Fit for Duty, Fit for Life Training Guide* that accompanies this textbook.

FYI

Aerobic Versus Anaerobic Exercise

The two basic categories of exercise are aerobic and anaerobic. It is helpful to understand the differences between them, because both should be incorporated into any fitness routine to produce the greatest benefit.

The word "aerobic" means "with oxygen." As the name implies, aerobic exercise uses oxygen to produce the energy necessary for muscle movement, by burning fats and carbohydrates. Aerobic exercise is usually called "cardiovascular exercise," or just "cardio." It includes activities that work large muscle groups and increase the heart rate and respiration during and shortly following the exercise—for example, walking, cycling, swimming, jumping rope, and running. Aerobic exercise builds endurance and strengthens the major muscles, the lungs, and the heart. Among its many benefits are a lower resting heart rate and lower blood pressure, a decreased risk of heart disease, and improved lung function.

In contrast to "aerobic," the term "anaerobic" means "without oxygen." As the name implies, this kind of exercise does not require oxygen to produce energy, and only carbohydrates are burned. When we exercise anaerobically for longer periods of time, lactic acid accumulates and we experience muscle fatigue. Examples of anaerobic exercise include high-intensity activities that expend energy in short bursts, such as weight lifting, push-ups and sit-ups, and the shuttle run. Anaerobic exercise helps increase muscle mass and strength.

Muscular Endurance

muscular endurance
the ability of a muscle to sustain a prolonged contraction or to contract over and over again

Muscular endurance is the ability of a muscle to sustain a prolonged contraction or to contract over and over again. Muscular endurance is important for injury prevention and proper posture. Without a strong back and strong abdominal muscles, a person's spine is subjected to stress that can result in lower-back pain. For law enforcement officers, who must wear an equipment belt weighing 7 to 9 kilograms, abdominal strength is important. Muscular endurance exercises involve applying a force to the muscle that is greater than what the muscle is used to. Muscular endurance can be achieved by exercising with weight-training equipment. In these exercises, light weights are combined with many repetitions.

Flexibility

flexibility
the ability to move the joints freely through their full range of motion

Flexibility is the ability to move the joints freely through their full range of motion. As a person ages, lack of flexibility can create poor posture and be debilitating. Stiff joints and a restricted range of motion can lead to lower-back problems, an issue that we will look at in Chapter 11. Without flexibility, it is easier to get hurt when reaching or twisting inappropriately. In particular, lower-back and hamstring inflexibility can be issues when getting in and out of a police cruiser. Greater flexibility leads to muscles that are more supple and less prone to injury. Flexibility can be maintained by following a regular fitness program.

You will read more about flexibility later in this chapter.

Body Composition

body composition
the proportion of lean tissue to fat in the body

Body composition (discussed in greater detail in Chapter 7) refers to the proportion of lean tissue (muscle and bone) to fat in the body. A healthy body composition requires a large proportion of lean tissue and a small proportion of fat. Fat is important for organ protection, for control of heat production and heat loss, and as a source of energy that the body can use. However, people with excessive fat risk joint problems, back pain, heart disease, high blood pressure, stroke, gallbladder disease, cancer, and other illnesses. The healthiest way to lose fat is to exercise and to adhere to a sensible diet recommended by your doctor. Weight training is the best way to increase lean tissue mass.

Performance/Skill-Related Fitness

The six components of performance/skill-related fitness are speed, coordination, reaction time, agility, balance, and power. These are greatly enhanced when you exercise regularly. Although not considered essential for a healthy life, the six components are especially important in law enforcement—for example, if you are involved in a foot chase, a physical altercation, or a rescue. All of these situations require you to be in top physical condition and be able to respond to trouble quickly and appropriately. Both health-related and performance/skill-related fitness are evaluated by the Physical Readiness Evaluation for Policing (PREP) test, the Physical Ability Requirement Evaluation (PARE) test, and the Police Officer Physical Abilities Test (POPAT). (The POPAT was developed for police in British Columbia and has been modified to create the PARE test based on the analysis of specific demands for RCMP and Corrections Canada jobs.) These tests will be discussed in detail in Chapter 15.

Speed

Speed is the ability to move quickly. During a foot chase, for example, a law enforcement officer requires leg and foot speed.

Coordination

Coordination involves the mind and body working together to perform motor tasks smoothly and accurately. Good coordination is needed, for example, to jump over obstacles, kick a soccer ball, and hit a golf ball. Using firearms also requires good coordination. Without it, hitting a target is almost impossible.

Reaction Time

Reaction time is the time that elapses between stimulation and the beginning of a person's reaction to the stimulus. For a law enforcement officer, being able to react quickly to a volatile situation can mean the difference between success and failure and even between staying alive and getting killed.

Agility

Agility is the ability to rapidly and accurately change the body's direction of movement. Skiing, mountain biking, and self-defence are examples of activities that require agility.

Balance

Balance refers to the body's ability to maintain equilibrium while stationary or moving. Walking across a support beam, performing on a balance beam, and self-defence are activities that require good balance.

Power

Power is the ability to transform energy into force at a rapid rate. Power is necessary in sports such as discus throwing and the shot put. In law enforcement, power is necessary to move a person out of the way, scale a wall, or jump a railing.

The Health Benefits of Physical Activity

Before reading any further, go to **assignment 4.2** (in the appendix) and see if you can list some of the health benefits of physical activity.

Regular physical activity produces long-term improvements in body function. These benefits are both physical and psychological.

FYI

Blood Pressure and Resting Heart Rate

Among the many benefits of physical activity are lower blood pressure and a lower resting heart rate:

- As blood travels though the body, it exerts a force against the blood vessels. The force is called blood pressure, and it changes over the course of a day. When blood pressure stays high for a longer period of time, it is called high blood pressure, or hypertension, and it poses health risks. Hypertension makes the heart work harder and can cause the walls of the arteries to harden (called arteriosclerosis). Among other medical problems, this increases the risk of heart disease and stroke.
- Our resting heart rate is influenced by factors including our genes, age, and fitness level, as well as medical conditions, medication, and stress. A higher resting heart rate is a risk factor for heart disease, and is correlated with an increased risk for high blood pressure and atherosclerosis. In addition to exercise, you can lower your resting heart rate by using stress-reducing techniques to reduce stress, avoiding tobacco products, and losing weight.

Physical Benefits

The health of Canadians has been a huge issue with researchers. Many papers and research grants have addressed this issue in hopes of providing a business case for governments to initiate programs to improve health status. These studies have pointed out the key benefits of physical activity (MHLTC, 2011):

- maintenance of healthy weight
- improved digestion
- improved posture and balance
- stronger muscles and bones
- increased bone density
- better circulation
- strengthened heart and lungs
- strengthened immune system
- prolonged good health in seniors
- reduced risk of premature death from heart disease, stroke, and certain types of cancer
- reduced risk of developing high blood pressure; lower total blood cholesterol and triglycerides and increased high-density lipoproteins (HDL or "good" cholesterol)

Psychological Benefits

A regular fitness program offers not only physical but also psychological benefits. Some of the psychological benefits are as follows (MHLTC, 2011):

- reduced stress levels
- relief from symptoms of depression and anxiety
- increased energy
- improved sleep
- improved posture and balance
- more confidence and a more positive outlook on life
- improved mood
- prolonged independence in seniors
- better quality of life

Turn to **assignment 4.3** (in the appendix) and list the physical and psychological benefits of physical activity that are most important to you.

Physical activity is very important. Although Canadians are now more active in their leisure time than they were two decades ago (see Figure 4.8), a recent study found that only 15 percent of Canadian adults move enough to get substantial health benefits; among 6- to 19-year-olds, the number drops to 7 percent (CBC News, 2011).

Overweight children, in particular, experience physical and psychological health problems. They are at increased risk of developing chronic diseases later in life, because they are more likely to become overweight adults (Perez, 2003; Janssen & LeBlanc, 2010). The most profound concern has been a progressive increase in

DID YOU KNOW?

By 2007–2008, 48 percent of Canadians aged 20+ years were at least moderately active (≥1.5 MET-hours daily, equivalent to at least 30 minutes of moderate to vigorous activity).

SOURCE: Health Canada, 2008

FIGURE 4.8 Physical Activity in Canada, 1995, 2005, and 2010

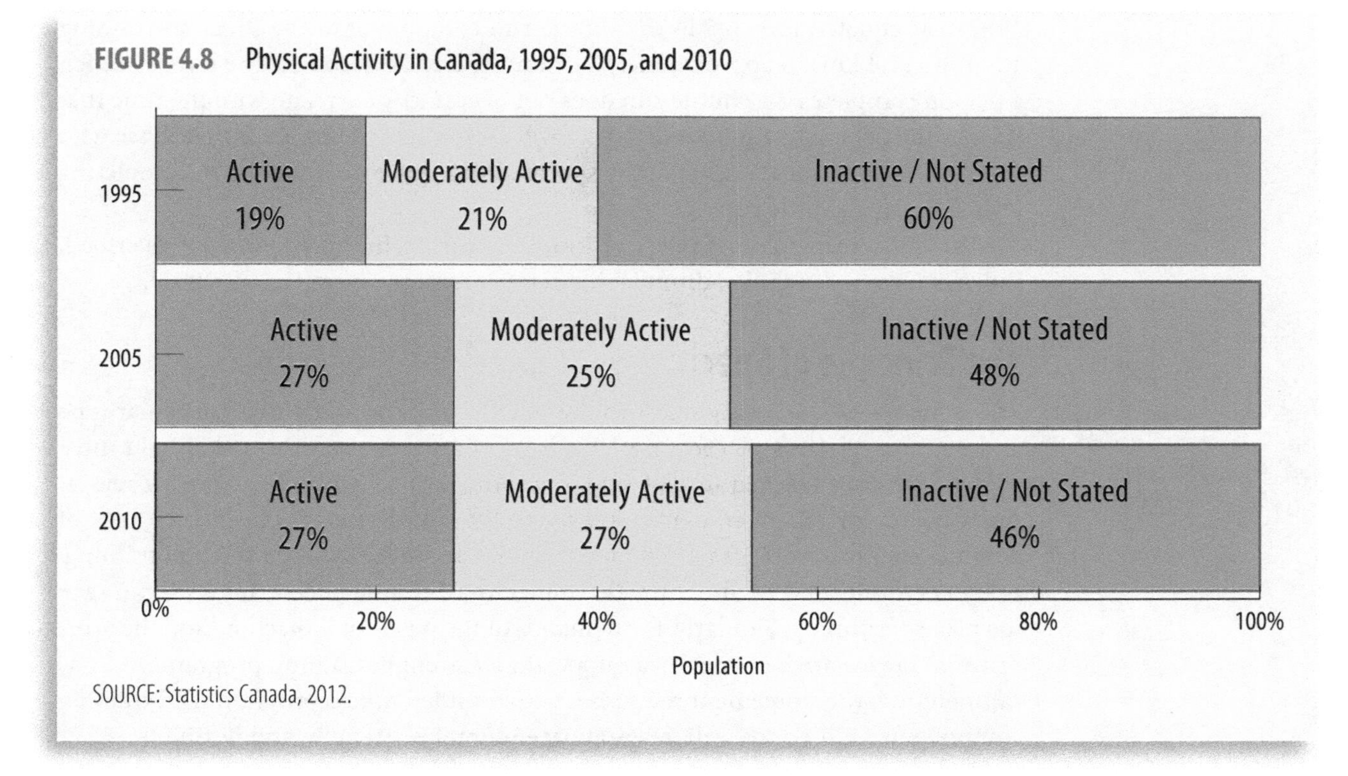

SOURCE: Statistics Canada, 2012.

the body mass index (BMI) of Canadian youth (aged 7 to 13) noted from 1981 to 1996, with the prevalence of obesity in this age group more than doubling over this period (Tremblay & Willms, 2000). As of 2009, 25 percent of children and youth were overweight or obese (Tremblay, Shields, Laviolette, Craig, Janssen, et al., 2010). Physical activity levels among children and youth are low, with 62 percent of waking hours—or 8.6 hours every day—devoted to sedentary activities (CBC News, 2011). Inactive time increases with age: the same study found that adults were sedentary for 69 percent of their waking hours, or 9.5 hours per day.

The implications of health-related diseases associated with physical inactivity can be reversed if individuals are willing to take ownership of their physical well-being. As you research the components of physical training, remember the goals you set in Chapter 2. They will assist you in determining which goals may be most important.

The Principles of Exercise

The goal of exercise is to bring about some of the physical and psychological benefits discussed above and to improve the body's functioning. Although there is inevitably a limit to the level of fitness and performance you can attain—a limit that varies from person to person—training gives everyone the chance to experience at least some of the physical and psychological benefits of exercise.

Particular fitness outcomes require particular exercises. For example, to conform to the aerobic component of the Bona Fide Occupational Requirement (BFOR) (discussed as part of the PARE test in Chapter 15), you have to be willing to devote some time to running. Léger (1985; Léger & Lambert,

FYI

Costs of Physical Inactivity

Physical inactivity costs the Canadian health-care system at least $2.1 billion annually (Katzmarzyk, Gledhill, & Shephard, 2000) in direct health-care costs, and the estimated total annual economic burden is approximately $53 billion (Katzmarzyk & Janssen, 2004). The Canadian government has undertaken the development of a healthy living strategy with an emphasis on physical activity, where areas such as healthy body weight, mental health, and injury prevention will be identified (Ministry of Health, 2005).

1982) has equated level 6.5 in the shuttle run component of the PREP to running 1.5 miles (2.4 km) in approximately 11 minutes and 30 seconds. The level at which a person completes the shuttle run does not necessarily correlate with the time that it takes the person to run that distance, although results do indicate that those who can successfully run 1.5 miles in the specified time have no difficulty in completing level 6.5 in the shuttle run.

The basic principles of physical training are specificity, progressive overload, individuality, reversibility, diminishing returns, and recovery (CSEP, 2003).

The Principle of Specificity

principle of specificity refers to the ability of the body to adapt to a particular type and amount of stress placed on it

The **principle of specificity** refers to the body's ability to adapt to a particular type and amount of stress placed on it. To develop a particular fitness skill, you must choose exercises tailored to that skill. Over the past 15 years, the primary reason many law enforcement students have failed the shuttle run has been their lack of commitment to aerobic training—specifically, running. Although interval training, weight training, and cycling provide some cross-training effects, nothing can take the place of running. Similarly, the demands of the push–pull machine and the arm-restraint device are best met by an upper-body strength training program. A commitment to law enforcement requires a well-rounded fitness program with training components tailored to cardiorespiratory endurance, strength, and flexibility.

The specificity principle is sometimes referred to as the SAID (specific adaptation to imposed demand) principle. Muscle adaptation will occur when you place a specific demand for improvement on a specific skill. It is important, then, to train to a high aerobic level to be successful in aerobic training. It is also important to train anaerobically to manoeuvre easily up and down the stairs on the PREP and PARE BFORs. And it is imperative that you have leg strength to use the push–pull machine easily.

The Principle of Progressive Overload

Progressive overload refers to placing a greater stress or load on the body than it is used to. The body needs to be subjected to increasing gradual demands in order to produce continual improvements. If the body is not worked hard enough or, on the other hand, is worked too hard, physical training will not produce benefits. Excessive exercise may in fact cause detraining and injuries.

principle of progressive overload refers to training and overloading the muscles that help the body to adapt to more and more stress

The **principle of progressive overload** takes into account that both the skeletal and cardiac muscles adapt to the overloading. This means that the body becomes more efficient and able to handle greater loads. For example, in order to complete a 1.5-mile run easily, your training has to go from a jog to a run, from running for 20 minutes to 40 minutes, and increasing your pace from about 9 to 12 kilometres per hour. If you decrease your levels of exercise, the gains that you achieved will start to disappear.

Progressive overload is accomplished by gradually increasing these criteria, which together are known as the FITT (frequency, intensity, time, type) principle:

- *Frequency* Most objectives require a training level of three to five times a week. People whose fitness level is low should begin with three times a week, and then gradually build up to five. Once your goals are reached, physical activity two or three times a week is needed to maintain your fitness level.

- *Intensity* To benefit from an exercise, you need to increase the intensity of the exercise gradually over the course of your training program—for example, by slowly increasing the weight pushed or pulled for strength training, gradually raising jogging speed to increase cardiorespiratory intensity, or stretching muscles more and more with each workout to increase flexibility. But increasing the intensity of a workout must be done in small steps to avoid injuries. Also, for beginners, intensity is less important than frequency and duration.
- *Time* (duration) Exercise produces benefits only if your exercise sessions last for extended periods of time. As you progress, you should increase the duration of the sessions. A runner who wants to increase cardiorespiratory endurance, for example, may begin with 20-minute sessions and slowly move up to 60-minute sessions (20–60 minutes is typical for endurance training).
- *Type of exercise* The exercises relate to the specific program you are involved in. In aerobic training, they include activities that work large-muscle groups and that can be done in a rhythmic fashion, such as brisk walking, cycling, swimming, and running. In weight training, they include activities that focus on the muscles that you want to strengthen or increase. Bodybuilders tend to isolate a muscle group and work it to exhaustion. Athletes in sports, on the other hand, train movements rather than muscles. It is important to divide your time and energy among various types of movements—endurance, strength and power, speed and agility, and tactical—that mirror the BFOR tests, taking into account the importance of recovery time (see The Principle of Recovery, below).

The Principle of Individuality

Each body's response to exercise is different. Several factors come into play, including physical and psychological makeup, age, gender, the ability to recover after a workout, and susceptibility to injury. These all play a part in designing a program. For example, in weight training, individuals must either change the number of repetitions or sets they are performing, or for a few weeks change their entire program, in order to confuse the muscles into having to work in a different way and cause changes at the cellular level.

The Principle of Reversibility

According to the **principle of reversibility**, all the benefits of exercise are lost if you stop training. Atrophy occurs when muscles undergo periods of complete or near-complete inactivity. In fact, up to 20 percent of exercise benefits can be lost in the first two weeks of not training, and as much as 50 percent can be lost in less than two months. Not only do muscles lose strength with disuse, but they also decrease in size. *Detraining* is the term used to describe the time period in which someone who has undergone a significant amount of training either stops completely or to a large extent. This happens for a number of reasons, including the inability to train because of an injury, the lack of an available open gym when an individual is off-shift, a lack of motivation, or the need for family time. One way to prevent much of this loss is to maintain the intensity of your workouts, even if you cannot maintain the frequency and duration.

principle of reversibility refers to all the benefits of exercise that are lost if you stop training

The Principle of Diminishing Returns

The principle of diminishing returns is based on the fact that a person's training gains will reflect his or her prior level of training. People who have had little training make significant gains both in terms of strength and aerobic capacity. Those who are highly trained make relatively small gains. For example, those who start running at the beginning of a course for the first time are able to see significant decreases in their times (sometimes by as much as 3–4 minutes), while those who run regularly usually see only small gains (their time for their run decreases by less than one-half minute). It becomes very important to try new training methods or different equipment in order to see further gains.

Devising an exercise program that is most suited to you depends on your goals, the requirements of the law enforcement community, and your fitness level. Depending on your size, you may have to spend substantially more time in a program to meet the demands of the BFOR standards and prepare for the demands of the job.

The Principle of Recovery

principle of recovery refers to the recuperation time or amount of rest required after a workout

The **principle of recovery** is tied to the recuperation time or amount of rest required after a workout. Torn muscle tissue needs time to repair. In cardiorespiratory training, beginners should exercise at least five times a week and leave at least a day to rest. Similarly, in weight training, beginners should allow a day's rest between each day of training. In strength training, beginners may need 48 hours or more between workouts. Also, be aware that more demanding exercise programs typically require more rest between training sessions.

People who do not feel a small increase in strength after each workout, or who experience pain with each workout, may need to reduce the frequency with which they train.

Turn to **assignment 4.4** (in the appendix) and review your fitness training goals.

Training Methods

When training for the BFOR tests, it becomes necessary to focus on increasing your speed, endurance, strength, agility, and flexibility. To achieve these goals, a number of training methods have been devised to provide variety and challenge, including periodization, concurrent training, interval training, high-intensity interval training (HIIT), fartlek training, resistance training, and plyometric training.

Periodization

periodization overall training plan where an individual maximizes performances at peak times

Periodization refers to an overall training plan in which an individual maximizes performances at peak times. This approach reduces the risk of injury and mental burnout. In sports, training periods are separated into off-season, pre-season, and in-season. There is a distinct period during which athletes learn necessary skills and motor development, and then gradually improve in skill, strength, and endurance while competing in their sport. Some of you may want to consider this as a method for reaching your goals.

In order to pass fitness standards, individuals need to set up programs. These should include a brief period in which to become familiar with the BFOR equipment. The preparation period that follows should include a high-volume, low-intensity training program in order to learn the routine. In the preparation period, it is important to ensure that you work on both agonist and antagonist muscle groups, as well as smaller muscle groups to ensure musculoskeletal balance. This should be followed by a strength phase, in which strength is built up to perform a task with ease, and a power phase to address the fact that training intensity increases while volume may be decreasing. Hypertrophy (increased muscle size) and maximal strength usually occur midway through this phase. The competitive or in-season stage usually combines shorter periods of training in specific skills at more intense levels, with tapering or complete rest just prior to a competition.

In terms of meeting BFOR standards, this means that individuals need to train generally toward increasing their level of fitness. Then they are required to train on the equipment needed to practise the push–pull, arm-restraint, shuttle run, and victim relocation components, as well as jumping over objects and interval training on stairs. The final stage is meant to ensure that the individual can easily attain level 6.5 on the shuttle run, do the equipment movements with ease, and be able to complete the circuit in the required time frame prior to testing. He or she would have maximum strength and power in this maintenance phase. Less time is required to maintain strength, while more emphasis is placed on tactical and skill-based training.

Concurrent Training

Concurrent training refers to the principle that you train for either strength or power at the same time you train for endurance. Those who train more generally have leaner muscle mass and lower body-fat composition, which makes the tasks of the job easier to do. This means you are doing your cardiovascular and resistance training workouts during the same training session, or within one hour of each other. The advantage of the concurrent approach is the parallel development of all qualities. The disadvantage is the risk of overtraining and the consequent limits on training effects. Depending on the intensity of the cardiovascular training, there may be some reduction in performance. For example, while doing leg presses after a cycling class, you may see some reduction in strength. For this reason, some individuals train for strength before working the cardiovascular system. The reverse approach is used when weight loss and endurance gains are a priority.

concurrent training
training for either strength or power at the same time as training for endurance

Interval Training

Interval training is based on the concept that the body's energy systems can make both aerobic and anaerobic gains by training with relatively intense exercises followed by a period of recovery. Intensity and recovery times depend on the individual's level of fitness. Usually, this approach means alternating short, high-intensity bursts of speed with slower recovery phases throughout a single workout. For example, runners will do intervals of 400 metres to train for 1.5-mile (2.4-km) runs with a rest period of walking 50–100 metres and then repeating the 400-metre run. By attempting to increase the number of repetitions and varying the speed, many runners are able to reduce their time on the run.

interval training
training that is based on the concept that the body's energy systems can make both aerobic and anaerobic gains by training with relatively intense exercises followed by a period of recovery

High-Intensity Interval Training

high-intensity interval training (HIIT)
a form of training designed to increase aerobic performance

High-intensity interval training (HIIT) is a type of interval training that mixes high-intensity bursts of exercise with moderate-intensity recovery periods. It can be exhausting but has considerable advantages. It can be the quickest way to lose fat, become fit, and increase sports performance. The goal is to increase your anaerobic threshold. This is the point during the anaerobic exercise when lactic acid starts to build up at a rate greater than it can be removed from the muscle. Based on the individual's speed, anaerobic threshold training typically lasts 20 minutes; the threshold is reached when an athlete attains between 50 and 85 percent of maximum aerobic capacity (the more fit the athlete, the higher the percentage). An example for beginners would be six sets of five to six all-out, 30-second sprints, with a four-minute rest between each set. Because this type of training completely exhausts your muscles of energy, it is important to have a day or two between such workouts. You must warm up and cool down to prime your muscles properly, and then cool down and stretch after the workout.

Fartlek Training

fartlek training
interval training of running distances at intense levels followed by recovery periods at predetermined intervals

Fartlek training (derived from the Swedish term for "speed play") refers to a type of high-intensity interval training of running distances at intense levels followed by recovery periods at predetermined intervals. Fartlek provides an excellent endurance and strength session and also helps to improve speed and race awareness. It is known to stress both the aerobic and anaerobic energy pathways. The theory behind it is to run at a set pace, take a break, and begin again. This becomes a very structured interval training program for runners, cyclists, and swimmers. Fartlek has grown into a popular method of training used by runners to provide an enjoyable and constructive alternative to simply pounding the streets with no purpose or plan (for example, run 200 metres, walk 100 metres, and repeat). It is freer in form and is done over a variety of terrains (for example, hills and sandy beaches).

Resistance Training

resistance training
the most common form of weight training which incorporates exercises that result in gains to muscle mass and strength as well as the potential for improved flexibility and range of motion

The most common form of weight training is **resistance training**. This approach increases muscle mass and strength, as well as potential for improved flexibility and range of motion. Resistance training is usually associated with a reduced number of injuries. Benefits depend on the number of repetitions and sets, the length of rest periods between exercises, and the intensity and volume of workouts. Individuals can use dumbbells, exercise balls, bands, or machines.

Pilates programs have become a very popular resistance workout. The Pilates system focuses on increasing flexibility and strength without building bulk by doing a series of controlled movements. These are isometric exercises that are held for six to ten seconds and repeated five to ten times. As a result, they are not recommended for people with high blood pressure or heart disease, because the contractions cause blood pressure to rise.

Plyometric Training

plyometric training
a form of resistance training that works on developing strength and power

Plyometric training is a form of resistance training that works on developing strength and power. Through a series of drills that usually use one's own body weight or medicine balls, exercise bands, stability balls, or weighted vests, individuals develop programs that include exercises that feature explosive movements through counter-movements to build muscular energy and power. These exercises focus not only on the contraction of the muscle but also on how fast it can contract. Examples include squat-jumps, box drills, hopping, jump-rope, and ballistic medicine ball drills. Individuals have to be highly motivated to do this kind of training.

Flexibility and Stretching

Flexibility—the ability to move the joints freely through their full range of motion—is determined by the type of joint being used. The range of motion of most joints can be maintained or increased with proper training, but can decline quickly with disuse.

Flexibility is an important component of a balanced fitness program, but one that is often neglected. It is achieved by incorporating stretching exercises into your fitness program. In this section, we will look at the benefits of stretching and describe a number of stretching techniques. The *Fit for Duty, Fit for Life Training Guide* that accompanies this textbook includes descriptions and photographs of recommended upper- and lower-body stretching exercises.

The Benefits of Stretching

There are a number of reasons for incorporating stretching into your fitness program:

- Stretching enhances your body's ability to perform the exercises in your program.
- Stretching hamstrings, quadriceps, hip flexors, and low-back muscles regularly will help reduce the strain on the back. Flexibility training will improve your posture and help prevent low-back pain.
- Stretching reduces the risk of injury from exercising.
- Stretching increases your range of motion and helps to keep your body feeling loose and agile.
- Stretching promotes relaxation and helps reduce stress.

Plowman and Smith (1997) identify other possible benefits of stretching:

- It can enhance physical fitness.
- It can reduce muscle tension.
- It can reduce the risk of joint sprains and muscle strains.
- It increases blood supply and nutrients to joint structures.
- It can reduce the severity of painful menstruation (dysmenorrhea).
- It can reduce resistance and tension in muscles.
- It can optimize the learning, practice, and performance of many types of skilled movements.
- It can promote the development of body awareness.

Furthermore, according to one study (Trehearn & Buresh, 2009), stretching helps our muscles and tendons work more efficiently when we run.

DID YOU KNOW?

In general, women tend to be more flexible than men throughout the lifespan. However, a regular, properly designed stretching program can help to close the "gender gap."

SOURCE: Peterson, 2011.

Stretching not only helps prevent injury and reduce low-back pain, but it may also help you recover from injury faster (Carragee, 2005). It does *not*, however, reduce the risk of injury or muscle soreness (Herbert & Gabriel, 2002), and debate continues regarding the best time to stretch—for example, before, during, or after a workout. According to Shrier (2004), stretching can reduce the risks of sport or workout injury, but it may slow performance if done just prior to the activity.

As noted, muscle tissue is broken down during any weight-bearing activities. Under stress, tiny micro-tears develop in the muscle fibres. This contributes to muscle soreness that often accompanies a strenuous workout. Because stretching brings nutrients to the musculoskeletal system, it can help repair fibres and speed up the healing process. As a result, there is less muscle soreness, so you can come back stronger for your next workout.

Stretching Techniques

There are four stretching techniques: static stretching, dynamic stretching, ballistic stretching, and proprioceptive neuromuscular facilitation (PNF).

Static Stretching

static stretching
a stretching technique that involves bringing a muscle to a maximum or near-maximum stretch by contracting the opposing muscle and holding the stretch for 20–30 seconds without pain

Static stretching is an effective technique for improving flexibility. It is done prior to exercise, and involves bringing a muscle to a controlled maximum or near-maximum stretch by contracting the opposing muscle and holding the stretch for at least 20–30 seconds (without pain). Each stretch is repeated two or three times. Because static stretching is performed slowly, the strong reflex action that characterizes ballistic stretching (see below) does not occur.

Static stretching was developed to prevent injury, increase flexibility, and enhance performance. Athletes whose sports require an increased range of motion, such as gymnastics, are believed to benefit from static stretching, although some research has questioned this. It also relieves muscle soreness and helps prevent muscle imbalance, knots, and tightness. There is concern that static stretching may be detrimental to performance and may not decrease the incidence of injury.

Dynamic Stretching

dynamic stretching
a stretching technique that involves performing movements within the full range of motion of the joint; it gradually increases reach and range of motion while the limbs are moving

Dynamic stretching, or functional stretching, consists of exercises that use the specific movements of the tasks or skills you are doing to prepare the body for movement. It involves moving your body and gradually increasing your reach, speed, or both. Dynamic stretching consists of controlled leg and arm swings that gently move you through your range of motion. Kicking an imaginary soccer ball is a dynamic stretch for the hamstrings and groin muscles. Twisting from side to side is a dynamic stretch for the trunk.

Some of the benefits of dynamic exercises include developing balance, "waking up" the muscles by increasing blood flow and nutrients to the tissue, providing specific movements commonly used in a particular skill or sport (Hendrick, 2000), and enhanced performance (Needham, Morse, & Degens, 2009). Dynamic stretching does not seem to elicit the performance reduction effects that static and PNF stretching (see below) do in runners.

Ballistic Stretching

Ballistic stretching promotes the stretch reflex but increases the risk of injury to muscles and tendons. It usually involves quick, well-coordinated action–reaction movements using the momentum of a moving limb to stretch the muscles beyond their normal range of motion, sometimes involving bouncing during a stretch. For this reason it is not recommended, and many textbooks avoid discussing it (Ethyre & Lee, 1987). An example in law enforcement would be when you are throwing a punch and the elbow joint goes beyond the normal range of motion. Recent research has shown that although ballistic stretching produces less stretch than static stretching, fewer individuals suffer injuries or complications from bouncing to stretch past their normal range of motion than was previously believed (Covert, Alexander, Petronis, & Davis, 2010). Other research has shown some effect in increasing power, suggesting that dynamic stretching may be more productive (Samuel, Holcomb, Guadagnoli, Rubley, & Wallmann, 2008). More research is required before ballistic stretching is adopted for particular activities.

ballistic stretching
a stretching technique that promotes the stretch reflex but increases the risk of injury to muscles and tendons; it requires quick, well-coordinated action–reaction movements that stretch the muscles beyond their normal range of motion

Proprioceptive Neuromuscular Facilitation

Proprioceptive neuromuscular facilitation (PNF) involves contracting and relaxing the muscles before stretching. Usually, the exercises require the assistance of a partner. Originally used in physiotherapy, this type of stretching has gained acceptance in the general fitness community. The two common types of PNF are:

- *Contract–relax (C–R) stretching* The muscle you want to stretch is contracted and then relaxed passively first. The now-relaxed muscle is then slowly actively stretched isometrically. This technique requires equipment (a towel or skipping rope) or a partner's assistance.
- *Contract–relax–antagonist–contract (CRAC) stretching* Begin by contracting and relaxing the muscle opposite to the one to be stretched (for example, while grasping a towel under your foot to draw your toes toward your head, first contract the gastrocnemius, then relax and pull on the towel to stretch the gastrocnemius further). Follow this by contracting the muscle to be stretched. The final action is the stretch itself. Contracting the opposite muscle promotes a reflex relaxation of the muscle to be stretched. This technique requires the assistance of a well-trained partner.

proprioceptive neuromuscular facilitation (PNF)
a stretching technique that involves contracting and relaxing the muscles before stretching

PNF is believed to be the most effective way of enhancing active flexibility, which is the active contraction and relaxation of the muscles that are being stretched (Alter, 1990, p. 10). By relaxing the muscle, PNF allows it to be stretched farther, but PNF presents a higher risk of injury than static stretching and can increase blood pressure to dangerous levels (Alter, 1990). It also has the disadvantage of often requiring a knowledgeable partner's assistance to avoid injury from overstretching.

Based on studies by McNair, Dombroski, Hewson, and Stanley (2000), and Knudson, Bennett, Corn, Leich, and Smith (2001), dynamic stretches involving slow, controlled movements through the full range of motion are considered more appropriate for a warm-up, while static stretches are more appropriate in a cool-down. You will have to decide based on trial and error which helps you more while preventing injury.

Guidelines for Safe and Effective Stretching

It is important that your warm-up begin not with stretching but with large-muscle activities such as walking or jogging, which facilitate safe stretching by increasing muscle temperature. A pre-exercise warm-up should consist of at least 5–15 minutes of light aerobic exercise followed by stretching exercises for all the major muscle groups. Examples appear in the *Fit for Duty, Fit for Life Training Guide* that accompanies this textbook. Performing stretching exercises at the end of your workout will increase your flexibility. Whether the workout is aimed at cardiorespiratory or resistance training, your body temperature will be raised, making stretching easier.

The FITT formula introduced earlier in this chapter provides a template for you to devise a stretching routine that meets your needs:

- *Frequency* Daily stretching is the best. You need to stretch before and after a workout. Regular stretching can help prevent tightness, muscle imbalance, and soreness. Stretching after exercises can help return muscles to their normal length, remove waste products that have built up from the workout, and reduce stiffness.
- *Intensity* Stretch to your limit, but avoid painful stretching, holding at least 20–30 seconds, and repeating the stretch 2–4 times. In dynamic stretching, you should do the exercises at a lower intensity than your workout, repeating 4–5 times over an 8- to 10-minute period. A cardiovascular exercise routine should involve at least 8–10 minutes of stretching at a low intensity (50–60 percent maximum heart rate). Before resistance training, you should do a set of exercises for large- and then small-muscle groups, using lighter weights to warm up.
- *Time* Stretch at least 8–10 minutes as part of your warm-up and cool-down (some athletes stretch for as long as an hour).
- *Type* Static and dynamic stretching and possibly PNF are good choices. **Assignment 4.5** (in the appendix) will help you assess your flexibility and then choose specific exercises tailored to your goals.

TOP TIPS ...

For Safe and Effective Stretching

- Complete a range of stretching exercises for all the different muscle groups. Pay attention to the muscle groups that are involved most in any sport you participate in.
- Proceed slowly and avoid ballistic stretching by not bouncing.
- Breathe out as you stretch and continue to breathe as you hold the stretch.
- Use the proper movements for each exercise.
- Stretch individual muscle groups one at a time.
- Don't strain to compete with the person next to you.
- When working with a partner, ensure that he or she knows your limits.
- Stop the stretch if you begin to feel pain.

Guidelines for Starting a Fitness Program

To ensure that you enjoy exercising and do so safely, here are some guidelines for starting a fitness program:

- *Start slowly* When you begin your program, remember that duration and frequency should take precedence over intensity. If you are experiencing muscle soreness 48 hours after your workout, or are experiencing a lack of energy or decreased physical performance, you are probably suffering from overtraining and are at risk of injury. Remember that you are making a lifelong commitment to fitness, so it is not important to get in shape as fast as possible. Instead, gradually build up to your desired fitness level, and then work on maintaining that level.
- *Train specifically to meet the job demands of law enforcement* Your body will adapt to the demands that you place on it. You need to focus on upper-body strength, cardiorespiratory endurance, and flexibility training to stay as healthy as you can throughout your career.
- *A proper warm-up and cool-down are essential* A warm-up should gradually warm up the muscles, including the heart, so that they can respond to the demands of your physical activity. A warm-up should include exercises that increase your heart rate as well as stretch all muscle groups, and include low-intensity movements similar to the exercises you will be doing. A cool-down should bring the body back to normal through the use of slow and gradual movements to prevent the pooling of blood.
- *Think about the order in which you do your exercises* Start with the large muscle groups and work your way down to the smaller ones. Training large muscle groups (such as thighs, chest, and back) will take most of your energy; therefore, you need to do them when you are at your strongest. Smaller muscles (such as biceps, triceps, and forearms) should be trained after larger muscles because they do not require as much energy to train.
- *Get enough fluids into your system* Two hours before a workout you should have at least half a litre of a cool drink. During a workout, you should have 150–225 millilitres of fluid every 15 minutes. After a workout, you should drink about 1 litre for every kilogram of body weight lost. You can determine how much body weight you lose during a workout by weighing yourself before and after the workout. Drinking water is a good way to replenish your fluids. Sports drinks, which help to replace electrolytes lost through sweating, are also acceptable, although many people find them too hard on the digestive system and need to dilute them.
- *Train regularly* Remember that you need a regular workout routine. Three to five times a week is necessary to see results from endurance training and to maintain those results. Intersperse your sessions with weight training or interval training on the other days. People who exceed the recommended number of workouts risk injury.
- *Try one of the different fitness classes offered through your school* You do not have to make a long-term commitment, but you might find them challenging and outside your normal workout practices, which can help improve your skills and level of fitness.

- *Train with a partner* The motivation and encouragement that you get from a fitness partner will help you through the hard times when your fitness routine does not seem to be producing results. A partner is also invaluable in weight training as a spotter and generally to ensure that you are adhering to the proper techniques.
- *Remember that everyone has a unique physical makeup* Everyone progresses at a different rate or experiences different improvements. Fitness is a very personal thing. If you compare yourself to others, you may set yourself up for failure, especially if the others are already at a higher fitness level.

Remember, too, that in order for your exercise program to work effectively, you must make it fit your needs.

In the balance of Part 2 of this book, Chapter 5 will give you more specifics relating to cardiovascular training, while Chapter 6 focuses on weight training.

> "There are really only two requirements when it comes to exercise. One is that you do it. The other is that you continue to do it."
>
> —*The New Glucose Revolution for Diabetes*
> by Jennie Brand-Miller, Kaye Foster-Powell, Stephen Colagiuri, and Alan W. Barclay

KEY TERMS

agonist, 67
anatomy, 60
antagonist, 67
ballistic stretching, 83
body composition, 72
cardiorespiratory endurance, 71
concurrent training, 79
dynamic stretching, 82
fartlek training, 80
fixator, 67
flexibility, 72
high-intensity interval training (HIIT), 80
interval training, 79
isokinetic contraction, 69
isometric contraction , 69
isotonic contraction, 69
ligament, 61
muscular endurance, 72
muscular strength, 71
periodization, 78
physiology, 60
plyometric training, 80
principle of progressive overload, 76
principle of recovery, 78
principle of reversibility, 77
principle of specificity, 76
proprioceptive neuromuscular facilitation (PNF), 83
range of motion, 61
resistance training, 80
static stretching, 82
synergist, 67
tendon, 62

EXERCISES

Multiple Choice

1. The four basic kinds of human tissue include
   a. ligaments, tendons, bones, and muscles
   b. skeletal, smooth, connective, and epithelial
   c. agonists, antagonists, synergists, and fixators
   d. epithelial, connective, muscle, and nerve
   e. bones, muscles, nerves, and organs
2. During which of the following contractions does muscle length remain constant?
   a. concentric
   b. eccentric
   c. isometric
   d. isokinetic
   e. isotonic
3. The warm-up and cool-down components of your workout should each last ____________.
   a. 5 minutes
   b. 5–15 minutes
   c. 10–25 minutes
   d. 25–40 minutes
   e. don't need these
4. Which best describes the "F" in the FITT formula?
   a. 1–3 days per week
   b. 3–5 days per week
   c. 2–3 days per week
   d. 5–7 days per week
   e. none of these
5. Intensity, type of exercise, ____________, and ____________ are the four factors involved in fitness development.
   a. time, speed
   b. frequency, distance
   c. frequency, time
   d. distance, time
   e. none of these
6. The purpose of a warm-up is
   a. to avoid tearing large-muscle groups
   b. to prepare for the workout psychologically
   c. to increase heart rate
   d. to increase internal temperature
   e. all of these
7. The most important health-related component of physical fitness is
   a. body composition
   b. cardiorespiratory endurance
   c. muscular strength
   d. muscular endurance
   e. flexibility
8. The best indicator for measuring the intensity of your workout is
   a. the total time you take to work out
   b. rapid breathing
   c. the amount you sweat
   d. your heart rate
   e. your fatigue level

9. Skill-related fitness components include
- **a.** aerobic and strength training
- **b.** speed and endurance training
- **c.** speed and agility
- **d.** flexibility and hand–eye coordination
- **e.** body composition and aerobic training

10. Which of the following terms refers to the ability of a muscle to exert force for only one maximum effort?
- **a.** muscular atrophy
- **b.** muscular hypertrophy
- **c.** muscular overload
- **d.** muscular strength
- **e.** muscular endurance

11. The maintenance of equilibrium while stationary or while moving is termed
- **a.** agility
- **b.** balance
- **c.** coordination
- **d.** poise
- **e.** reaction time

12. Which should be the primary advantage of good health-related physical fitness?
- **a.** improved work efficiency
- **b.** excellence in sports
- **c.** enjoyment of leisure
- **d.** prevention of disease
- **e.** a good appearance

13. "Speed play," known as ____________ training, refers to interval training of distances at intense levels followed by recovery periods at predetermined intervals.
- **a.** periodization
- **b.** concurrent
- **c.** fartlek
- **d.** interval
- **e.** plyometric

14. The ____________ training technique involves training for power or strength at the same time as endurance training.
- **a.** periodization
- **b.** concurrent
- **c.** fartlek
- **d.** interval
- **e.** plyometric

15. Using your body weight and minimal equipment, ____________ training involves a series of drills that involve explosive movements through counter-movements to build muscular energy and power.
- **a.** periodization
- **b.** concurrent
- **c.** resistance
- **d.** interval
- **e.** plyometric

16. ____________ training is based on the concept that the body's energy systems can make both aerobic and anaerobic gains by training with relatively intense exercises followed by a period of recovery.
- **a.** periodization
- **b.** concurrent
- **c.** resistance
- **d.** interval
- **e.** plyometric

17. The disadvantage of concurrent training is
- **a.** you see gains in all areas that you work
- **b.** you see more gains in aerobic over strength
- **c.** you see more gains in strength over aerobic
- **d.** you risk overtraining and limit the gains that can be seen
- **e.** there are no disadvantages

18. Stretching for flexibility is most effective during which of the following?
- **a.** the warm-up
- **b.** the workout
- **c.** endurance training
- **d.** the cool-down
- **e.** doesn't really matter when

19. Dynamic stretching involves
- **a.** quickly moving a limb to its limits
- **b.** the full range of motion achieved in a slow, controlled stretch
- **c.** a natural response that causes a stretched muscle to contract
- **d.** a stretch–contract–stretch partner-assisted flexibility program
- **e.** alternating between a slow, controlled stretch and then a few quick stretches

20. Proprioceptive neuromuscular facilitation (PNF) involves
    a. quickly moving a limb to its limits
    b. the full range of motion achieved in a slow, controlled stretch
    c. a natural response that causes a stretched muscle to contract
    d. a stretch–contract–stretch partner-assisted flexibility program
    e. alternating between a slow, controlled stretch and then a few quick stretches

21. Which of the following involves quick, coordinated movements that stretch the muscles while you are moving and incorporates the stretch reflex?
    a. PNF stretching
    b. ballistic stretching
    c. static stretching
    d. concentric stretching
    e. eccentric stretching

Short Answer

1. Describe how isotonic and isometric contractions differ.

2. Identify and distinguish between the two types of muscle fibre.

3. What are the components of health-related fitness?

4. What are the components of performance/skill-related fitness?

5. What are some of the physical benefits of participating in a fitness program?

6. What are some of the psychological benefits of participating in a fitness program?

7. Identify and explain the five principles of physical training.

8. What guidelines should you be aware of when beginning a fitness program?

9. Describe the principle of specificity and give an example.

10. How do you apply the principle of overload? Give an example.

11. How do you counter the principle of reversibility? Give an example.

12. How would you use periodization training to prepare for the shuttle run?

13. Describe fartlek training and how it can apply to training for the BFORs.

14. Describe interval training and how it can improve your 1.5-mile (2.4-km) run.

15. Using the plyometric training technique, describe how you could train for the various components of the PREP or PARE BFORs.

16. What are some of the benefits of stretching?

17. Why is flexibility so important for those in law enforcement?

REFERENCES

Alter, M.J. (1990). *Sport stretch.* Champaign, IL: Human Kinetics.

Brand-Miller, J., Foster-Powell, K., Colagiuri, S., & Barclay, A.W. (2007). *The new glucose revolution for diabetes.* Cambridge, MA: Da Capo Press.

Canadian Adolescents at Risk Research Network. (2004, February). *Physical activity patterns in Canadian adolescents.* Kingston, ON: Queen's University.

Canadian Society for Exercise Physiology (CSEP). (2003). *The Canadian physical activity, fitness and lifestyle appraisal: CSEP's guide to healthy living.* Ottawa: Author.

Canadian Society for Exercise Physiology (CSEP). (2011). *Canadian physical activity guidelines.* http://www.csep.ca/english/view.asp?x=1.

Carragee, E.J. (2005). Persistent low back pain. *New England Journal of Medicine, 352*(18), 1891–1898.

CBC News. (2011, January 19). Canadian youth woefully inactive: Report. http://www.cbc.ca/news/health/story/2011/01/19/fitness-canadians-health.html.

Coalition for Active Living. (2004, January). Physical activity community not surprised by troubling physical activity trends published today. Press release. http://www.activeliving.ca/English/index.cfm?fa=MediaRoom.PressReleases.

Colley, R.C., Garriguet, D., Janssen, I., Craig, C.L., Clarke, J., & Tremblay, M.S. (2011, March). Physical activity levels of Canadian children and youth. Research article. *Health Reports, 22*(1). Catalogue no. 82-003-XPE. Ottawa: Statistics Canada.

Covert, C.A., Alexander, M.P., Petronis, J.J., & Davis, D.S. (2010). Comparison of ballistic and static stretching on hamstring muscle length using an equal stretching dose. *Journal of Strength & Conditioning Research, 24*(11), 3008–3014.

Ethyre, B.R., & Lee, E.J. (1987). Comments on proprioceptive neuromuscular facilitation stretching techniques. *Research Quarterly for Exercise and Sport, 58*, 184–188.

Health Canada. (2008). *Healthy Canadians: A federal report on comparable health indicators 2008.* Publication no. H21-206/2008E-pdf. http://publications.gc.ca/site/eng/412048/publication.html.

Hendrick, A.N. (2000). Dynamic flexibility training. *Strength and Conditioning Journal, 22*(5), 33–38.

Herbert, R.D., & Gabriel, M. (2002). Effects of stretching before and after exercise on muscle soreness and risk of injury: Systematic review. *British Medical Journal, 325*, 468–470.

Janssen, I., & LeBlanc, A.G. (2010). Systematic review of the health benefits of physical activity and fitness in school-aged children and youth. *International Journal of Behavioural Nutrition and Physical Activity, 7*, 40.

Katzmarzyk, P.T., Gledhill, N., & Shephard, R.J. (2000). The economic burden of physical inactivity in Canada. *Canadian Medical Association Journal, 163*(11), 1435–1440.

Katzmarzyk, P.T., & Janssen, I. (2004). The economic cost of physical inactivity and obesity in Canada: An update. *Canadian Journal of Applied Physiology, 29*, 90–115.

Knudson, D., Bennett, K., Corn, R., Leich, D., & Smith, C. (2001). Acute effects of stretching are not evident in kinematics of the vertical jump. *Journal of Strength & Conditioning Research, 15*(1), 98–101.

Léger, L. (1985). SportMed Technology fitness appraisal kit: 20-metre shuttle run test with one-minute stages. Montreal: SportMed Technology.

Léger, L.A., & Lambert, J. (1982). A maximal multistage 20-m shuttle run test to predict VO_2 max. *European Journal of Applied Physiology, 49*, 1–5.

McNair, P., Dombroski, E., Hewson, D., & Stanley, S. (2000). Stretching at the ankle joint: Viscolelastic responses to holds and continuous passive motion. *Medicine & Science in Sports & Exercise, 33*, 354–358.

Ministry of Health. (2005). *The Integrated Pan-Canadian Healthy Living Strategy.* The Secretariat for the Intersectional Healthy Living Network, the F/T/P Healthy Living Task Group, and the F/T/P Advisory Committee on Population Health and Health Security. Catalogue no. HP10-1/2005.

Ministry of Health and Long-Term Care (MHLTC). (2011, October 21). Why exercise is vital to health. http://www.mhp.gov.on.ca/en/active-living/exercise.asp.

Needham, R.A., Morse, C.I., & Degens, H. (2009). The acute effect of different warm-up protocols on anaerobic performance in elite youth soccer players. *Journal of Strength & Conditioning Research, 23*(9), 2614–2620.

Perez, C. (2003). Children who become active. *Health Reports (Suppl.), 14*, 17–28.

Peterson, J.A. 2011. "Nice-to-Know Facts About Flexibility and Stretching." http://www.fitness.com/articles/1354/nice_to_know_facts_about_flexibility_and_stretching.php.

Plotnikoff, R., Bercovitz, K., & Loucaides, C.A. (2004, December). Physical activity, smoking and obesity among Canadian school youth. *Canadian Journal of Public Health, 95*(6), 413–418.

Plowman, S.A., & Smith, D.L. (1997). *Exercise physiology for health, fitness, and performance.* Needham Heights, MA: Allyn and Bacon.

Samuel, M.N., Holcomb, W.R., Guadagnoli, M.A., Rubley, M.D., & Wallmann, H. (2008). Acute effects of static and ballistic stretching on measures of strength and power. *Journal of Strength & Conditioning Research, 22*(5), 1422–1428.

Shrier, I. (2004). Does stretching improve performance? A systematic and critical review of the literature. *Clinical Journal of Sports Medicine, 14*(5), 267–273.

Statistics Canada. (2012). Health indicator profile, age-standardized rates annual estimates, by sex, Canada, provinces and territories (CANSIM Table 105-0503). Ottawa: Author.

Trehearn, T.L., & Buresh, R.J. (2009). Sit and reach flexibility and running economy of men and women collegiate distance runners. *Journal of Strength & Conditioning Research, 23*(1), 158–162.

Tremblay, M.S., Shields, M., Laviolette, M., Craig, C.L., Janssen, I., & Connor Gorber, S. (2010). Fitness of Canadian children and youth: Results from the 2007–2009 Canadian Health Measures Survey. *Health Reports, 21*, 1–14. Statistics Canada Catalogue no. 82-003. http://www.statcan.gc.ca/pub/82-003-x/2010001/article/11065-eng.pdf.

Tremblay, M.S., & Willms, J.D. (2000, November 28). Secular trends in the body mass index of Canadian children. *Canadian Medical Association Journal, 163*(11). http://www.ecmaj.ca/content/163/11/1429.full.

5

Cardiorespiratory Fitness

LEARNING OBJECTIVES

After completing this chapter, you should be able to:

- Explain why cardiorespiratory fitness is important in law enforcement.
- Understand and monitor your heart rate at rest and during exercise.
- Determine your target heart rate zone for exercise.
- Determine how high-intensity interval training (HIIT) can fit into your cardiorespiratory program to assist you in successfully completing BFOR testing.
- Set up a cardiorespiratory fitness program that is most suited to you.

OVERVIEW

Cardiorespiratory fitness (endurance), probably the most important component of fitness, is the ability to perform prolonged large-muscle activities at moderate to high intensity. This chapter will examine the importance of cardiorespiratory fitness in law enforcement and provide advice on creating a cardiorespiratory fitness program that will help you meet law enforcement requirements.

The Importance of Cardiorespiratory Fitness in Law Enforcement

Cardiorespiratory fitness makes your body more efficient and helps you cope with the physical demands of your job and everyday life. The key to cardiorespiratory fitness is aerobic exercise—prolonged, rhythmic exercise that uses large-muscle groups. Emergency services, including those in law enforcement, experience higher physical demands than workers in more sedentary occupations (Anderson, Plecas, & Segger, 2001). Examples of aerobic exercise include swimming, running, and cycling. Research by the Ontario government and the RCMP (Ontario, 1997) has demonstrated the importance of aerobic conditioning in law enforcement. The researchers found that aerobic conditioning not only facilitated foot chases but also helped officers cope with long shifts and the changing demands of the job. Both the Ontario government and the RCMP stress the importance of aerobic conditioning by incorporating a cardiorespiratory component into their physical readiness evaluations (PREP and PARE, respectively; see Chapter 15).

The Benefits of Cardiorespiratory Fitness

As you have read in Chapter 4, exercise has many benefits. The following are some of the benefits of cardiorespiratory fitness:

- improved cardiorespiratory functioning, which allows the heart to meet the demands of everyday life more efficiently (blood pressure and the risk of heart disease are also reduced) (Marcus, 1998; Elley & Arroll, 2002)
- reduced levels of cholesterol, triglycerides, and other potentially harmful substances in the blood, which in turn reduces the risk of heart disease (US Department of Health and Human Services, 1996; Varady & Jones, 2005)
- improved metabolism (metabolism is, among other things, the process by which the body converts food into energy) (Bouchard, Shephard, Stephens, Sutton, & McPherson, 1990; Hassinen, Lakka, Hakola, Savonen, Komulainen, et al., 2010)
- increased bone density, which reduces the risk of osteoporosis and improves posture, balance, and coordination, and can help reduce the risk of falls (Arnold & Faulkner, 2010; Warburton, Gledhill, & Quinney, 2001a, 2001b)
- improved immune system (excessive training, however, can depress the immune system) (Bouchard et al., 1990; Nieman, Henson, Austin, & Brown, 2005)
- reduced risk of developing diabetes mellitus and its associated risks (in conjunction with resistance exercise) (Sigal, Kenny, Boulé, Wells,

Prud'homme, et al., 2007; Larose, Sigal, Khandwala, Prud'homme, Boulé, et al., 2011)

- reduced risk of some cancers, including those of the colon, breast, and female reproductive organs (Vainio & Bianchini, 2002; Irwin, Smith, McTiernan, Ballard-Barbash, Cronin, et al., 2008)
- increased energy, stamina, and resistance to physical fatigue (Bouchard et al., 1990; Gibala, Little, van Essen, Wilkin, Burgomaster, et al., 2006)
- ability to fall asleep faster and deeper; improved concentration, productivity, and mood (Buman & King, 2010)
- improved psychological and emotional well-being resulting from improved appearance, enhanced self-image and self-confidence, and decreased stress, anxiety, and depression (Papousek & Schulter, 2008; Shephard, 1997)

DID YOU KNOW?

Besides its cardiorespiratory benefits, physical activity delivers oxygen and nutrients to your tissues to help you work more efficiently and have energy to do other things that you enjoy. It also stimulates various brain chemicals that leave you feeling happier and more relaxed than you were before your workout.

Assessing Cardiorespiratory Fitness

Your cardiorespiratory fitness affects your body's ability to maintain a level of exertion (exercise) for an extended period of time. The ability to supply energy for activities lasting more than 30 seconds depends on the consumption and use of oxygen (O_2). Most physical activities in daily life and athletics take more than 90 seconds; most BFOR tests last 2–5 minutes and may include a maximal aerobic assessment (shuttle run), so O_2 consumption is critical for survival as well as performance.

Aerobic fitness consists of two main components. The first is central cardiorespiratory fitness (heart and lungs). The second, peripheral component is the specific muscles involved in the movement.

Central Cardiorespiratory Fitness

The central cardiorespiratory system will improve as long as you stress your cardiac function and ventilation system. Your improvement is limited by three factors:

1. cardiac output: the amount of blood pumped per minute, which is a function of stroke volume (blood pumped per heartbeat and heart rate [beats/minute])
2. blood volume: dehydration or other factors affecting volume reduce the effectiveness of the cardiovascular system
3. red blood cell count and O_2 carrying capacity

Peripheral Cardiorespiratory Fitness

The peripheral component of aerobic fitness requires specific training to cause the muscles to adapt to the specific task (that's why cross-training on a bike will help your running but will not replace the need to run). The two biggest limiting factors in peripheral aerobic fitness are:

1. the ability of the muscles to remove and use O_2 from the blood
2. the ability of the muscles to maintain a balanced pH (specifically, minimizing the buildup of lactic acid, thus delaying the onset of fatigue)

Maximum Aerobic Capacity

maximum aerobic capacity (VO_2 max or MVO_2)
a measure of cardiorespiratory fitness; estimated as the point at which oxygen uptake plateaus and does not increase with further increases in workload

A person's **maximum aerobic capacity (VO_2 max or MVO_2)** is a measure of his or her cardiorespiratory fitness. VO_2 max is the volume of oxygen consumed per minute. It is estimated as the point at which O_2 uptake plateaus and does not increase with further increases in workload. Once people reach their maximum aerobic capacity, they cannot continue to work at that intensity for more than a minute or two because their demand for oxygen exceeds their ability to supply it.

Proper testing of a person's VO_2 max is costly and requires a controlled laboratory environment. The test is onerous and time-consuming, and therefore demands a highly motivated subject if an accurate assessment is to be obtained. As a result, simpler tests have been developed. For example, in the late 1970s the Ontario Police College, adopting the standards set by Dr. Kenneth Cooper (1982), implemented a 1.5-mile (2.4-km) run as an indirect measure of cardiorespiratory fitness (see Chapter 15 for further details). When the Physical Readiness Evaluation for Policing (PREP) was implemented, the 20-metre shuttle run replaced the run. Other tests of cardiorespiratory fitness include the Astrand-Rhyming bicycle ergometer test, the YMCA bicycle ergometer test, the Rockport Fitness Walking Test, the Ebbeling treadmill test, and the Canadian Physical Fitness and Lifestyle Appraisal (CPFLA) step test (to find out more information about these tests, research them on the Internet).

For law enforcement applicants who do not run on a regular basis, or who are obese or otherwise in poor condition, cardiorespiratory training is of the utmost importance. You need to be physically fit to meet the demands of the PREP and PARE BFOR tests and other tests of occupational skills administered to law enforcement applicants. Conditioning your cardiorespiratory system will help you work toward your goals.

A word of caution: those who do not engage in regular physical activity and have joint or obesity problems or high blood pressure (144/94 or 140/90, depending on the test protocol) may require medical clearance before taking a cardiorespiratory test. Be sure to fill out the Physical Activity Readiness Questionnaire (PAR-Q) in **assignment 1.1** and talk to your fitness instructor before taking any cardiorespiratory test.

Go to **assignment 5.1** (in the appendix) and assess your readiness for participating in cardiorespiratory training.

Getting Started on Cardiorespiratory Training

Before you begin cardiorespiratory training, consider the frequency, intensity, duration, and type of your aerobic exercise sessions. These considerations are addressed by the FITT (frequency, intensity, time, and type) formula (Table 5.1).

Although all four variables in the FITT formula are important, intensity is the key variable. The Canadian Society for Exercise Physiology (2003) identifies three techniques that effectively allow you to judge the intensity of your workout: heart rate monitoring, the Borg scale, and the talk test. Intensity can be checked during and at the end of the workout to determine whether you are at the required target heart rate.

TABLE 5.1 The FITT Formula

FITT	HEALTH-RELATED BENEFITS	PERFORMANCE-RELATED BENEFITS	HIGH-PERFORMANCE-RELATED BENEFITS
Frequency (days/wk)	3	3–4	5+
Intensity (% of MHR)	50–60	60–85	70–90*
Time (min/day)	5–20	20–60	30–60
Type	Any rhythmic activity, including walking, cycling, jogging, swimming, and using a stairmill machine		

* At this intensity, there may be a risk of overtraining, which can lead to injuries and anorexia.

Understanding Heart Rates

The first heart rate (HR) that you should be aware of is your **resting heart rate**, which you experience during sleep or prior to getting out of bed in the morning. With exercise, you can decrease your HR as your heart and lungs become stronger. The heart is then able to pump more blood (increase *stroke volume* [SV]) throughout the body with less effort. The lungs are able to take in more oxygen (increase *maximum oxygen uptake* [VO_2 max or MVO_2]) with less effort, which means more blood and oxygen will reach the working muscles. Having enough oxygen going into the blood keeps the lactic acid out (removes the hydrogen ions) so that you can sustain a prolonged aerobic workout.

resting heart rate
your heart rate when you are in a resting state such as sleep

Resting heart rates vary between 40 and 100 beats per minute (bpm), with 70 bpm being the average. As your cardiorespiratory system improves, your resting heart rate decreases.

The **maximal heart rate (MHR)** is the rate at which your heart beats at maximum effort during a sustained aerobic activity. You will normally never work at 100 percent of your maximum unless you are doing a specific program or test in a supervised setting (for example, a maximal treadmill test).

maximal heart rate (MHR)
your heart rate when your heart beats at maximal effort during a sustained aerobic activity

The **exercising heart rate** is the rate at which your body is in motion during sustained exercise. The goal is to stay within your target heart rate range, which is normally between 70 and 85 percent of maximal heart rate for someone who is fit.

exercising heart rate
your heart rate when your body is in motion during sustained exercise

Heart Rate Monitoring

Heart rate monitoring—the most common technique—is easily learned. You put your index and middle fingers over either the radial artery (located on the wrist just below the base of the thumb) or the carotid artery (located on the left and right sides of the neck). Do not press too hard on the carotid artery, as this may trigger a reflex that slows the heart rate. During exercise, the heart rate is determined by counting the beats for 10 seconds and then multiplying by 6 to get beats per minute. When you are at rest, you should count the beats for 15 seconds and then multiply by 4.

Determining Your Target Heart Rate Zone

To judge whether you are exercising at a benefit-producing intensity, you must determine your **target heart rate (THR) zone**. First, determine your maximal heart

target heart rate (THR) zone
the zone that a person's heart rate must reach during exercise to improve or maintain aerobic fitness

rate by subtracting your age from 220. This gives you your MHR in beats per minute. Next, multiply your MHR by 60 percent and 85 percent. The resulting numbers are the lower and upper limits, respectively, of your THR zone.

To benefit from exercise, you must exercise at an intensity that raises your heart rate into the THR zone for 30–60 minutes 3–5 times a week. Unfit people who exercise at an intensity just short of the lower limit of their THR zone will obtain some health benefits but will not improve or maintain aerobic fitness. Physical activity should include moderate activity (such as brisk walking, skating, and bike riding) with vigorous activities (such as running and playing soccer). In fact, Health Canada is encouraging all Canadians to be physically active by increasing their awareness and understanding of the benefits of physical activity and the range of opportunities to be physically active in daily life (Healthy Living Unit, 2008).

Here's how to determine the THR for a 25-year-old:

MHR	=	220 − 25	=	195 bpm
THR zone lower limit	=	0.60 × 195	=	117 bpm
THR zone upper limit	=	0.85 × 195	=	166 bpm

Figure 5.1 shows the THR zone for ages 20 to 70. This chart is often posted on gym walls. Table 5.2 lists the effects of training at the various target heart rate zones.

FYI

Exercise Intensity and Maximum Heart Rate

If you are not as fit as you could be, then starting at a lighter intensity and working up to a higher intensity is prudent. Here is how exercise intensity relates to the maximum heart rate:

- Light exercise intensity:
  40–60 percent of your maximum heart rate
- Moderate exercise intensity:
  60–85 percent of your maximum heart rate
- Vigorous exercise intensity:
  80–90 percent of your maximum heart rate

FIGURE 5.1 Target Heart Rate (THR) Zone

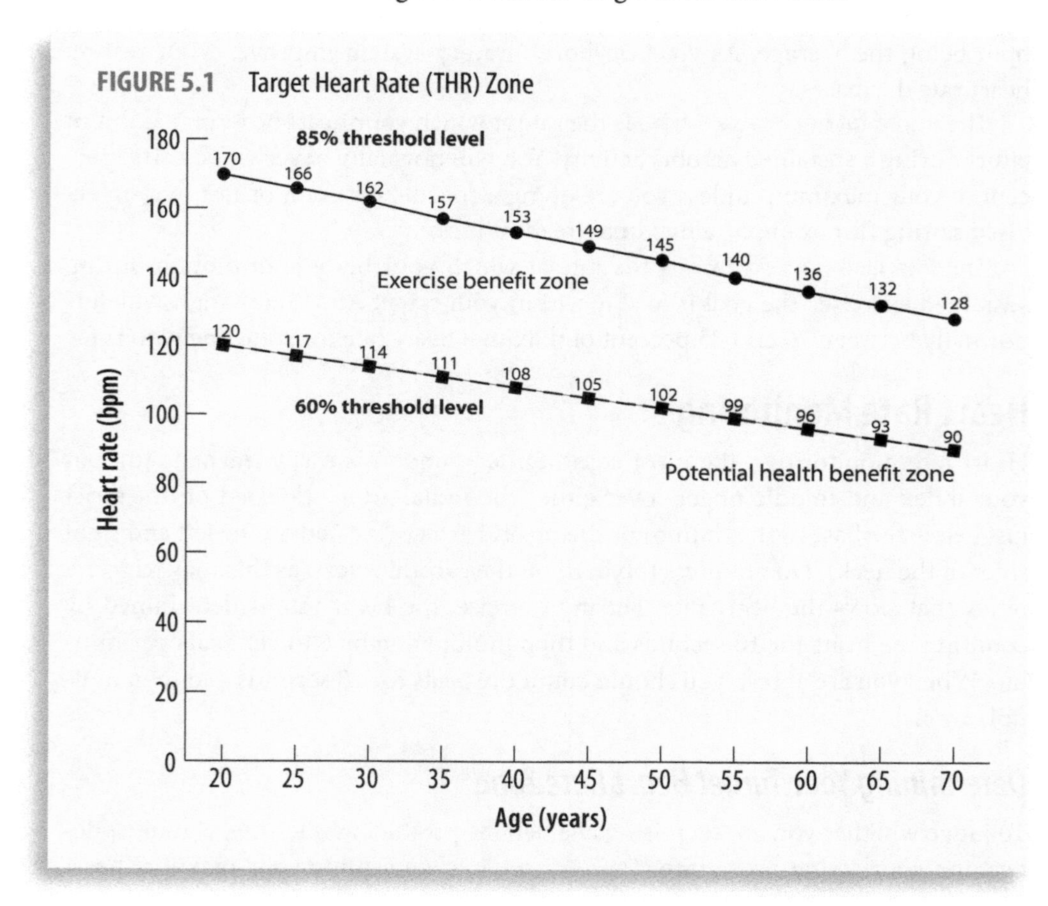

TABLE 5.2 Effects of Training at Various Target Heart Rate Zones

TARGET HEART RATE ZONE	EFFECT: WORKING AT THIS TARGET HEART RATE ZONE . . .
50–60%	• keeps health risks to a minimum • does not produce visible gains, but maintains cardiovascular capacity for daily activities
65–75%	• is the level used by novices starting out and as a warm-up and cool-down for advanced individuals • builds a proper cardiorespiratory base • improves transport of nutrients and oxygen throughout the body • can be sustained for long periods of time
80–85%	• works both aerobic and anaerobic energy systems • burns significant numbers of calories • is used not only to build cardiorespiratory endurance (improving heart and lung capacity) but improving leg strength • can be sustained for long periods of time
85–90%	• is used only for interval training • is extremely intense and should be used only by highly conditioned individuals; novices need to develop a solid cardiorespiratory base first • is important for improving power (maximal muscular contraction in an explosive movement), speed (how fast you can go), and quickness (ability to change direction very rapidly) • uses only the anaerobic energy system and thus cannot be sustained for long periods

Go to **assignment 5.2** (in the appendix) and determine your resting heart rate and target heart rate.

The Borg Scale

Developed by Gunnar A. Borg (1998), a Swedish psychologist, the **Borg scale** method does not involve counting the number of heartbeats, which can be difficult for some people while they are exercising. The Borg rating of perceived exertion (RPE) is based on how hard you feel your body is working during exercise. It is based on the physical sensations a person experiences during physical activity, including increased heart rate, increased respiration or breathing rate, increased sweating, and muscle fatigue. Although this is a subjective measure, a person's exertion rating may provide a fairly good estimate of the actual heart rate during physical activity (Borg, 1998). There is a high correlation between a person's perceived exertion rating times 10 and the actual heart rate during physical activity. For example, if a person's RPE is 12, then 12 × 10 = 120; if the person's heart rate were measured, it should be approximately 120 beats per minute. Note that this calculation is only an approximation of heart rate, and the actual heart rate can vary quite a bit depending on age and physical condition.

Borg scale
a method for determining the intensity of exercise, used as an alternative to heart rate monitoring

FIGURE 5.2
The Borg RPE* Scale®

6	No exertion at all
7	Extremely light
8	
9	Very light
10	
11	Light
12	
13	Somewhat hard
14	
15	Hard (heavy)
16	
17	Very hard
18	
19	Extremely hard
20	Maximal exertion

* RPE = Rating of Perceived Exertion

SOURCE:
Adapted from Borg, 1982.

With experience of monitoring how your body feels, it will become easier to know when to adjust your intensity. For example, a walker who wants to engage in moderate-intensity activity would aim for a Borg scale level of "somewhat hard" (12–14). If that person describes his or her muscle fatigue and breathing as "very light" (9 on the Borg scale), then he or she would want to increase intensity. On the other hand, if the walker felt the exertion was "extremely hard" (19 on the Borg scale), he or she would need to slow down to achieve a moderate-intensity range. (See Figure 5.2.)

The disadvantage of using the Borg scale is that some people underestimate or overestimate their level of exertion. It is important to monitor your heart rate regularly to ensure that your perceived exertion corresponds with the level of intensity you are trying to achieve.

To determine whether your perception is close to your actual heart rate, multiply the number that corresponds to your perception by 10. Because people just starting an exercise program may not be able to tie their intensity to a subjective perception of exertion, it is important for them to check their heart rate regularly to determine whether they are within their THR zone.

The Talk Test

The **talk test** is a handy guide for beginners who are concerned about their exercise intensity. A person who is active at a light intensity level should be able to sing while doing the activity. One who is active at a moderately intense level should be able to carry on a conversation comfortably while engaging in the activity. If a person becomes winded or too out of breath to carry on a conversation, then the activity can be considered vigorous and the person may find it too hard to continue.

talk test
a method for determining the intensity of exercise, used as an alternative to heart rate monitoring; if a person is breathless and cannot carry on a conversation while exercising, he or she is working too hard

Creating a Cardiorespiratory Fitness Program

Individuals who are enrolled in the Police Foundations Program are expected to meet certain aerobic requirements. The colleges have included only one to three hours a week of fitness training to bring their students up to police standards. This may mean that you need to put in an additional two or three hours a week, but it is likely that you will be looking at putting in more hours outside of class time to achieve the goals you have set. If your fitness program offers you one hour a week of aerobic training, then, depending on your fitness level, you will have to add two to four hours of aerobic training to your weekly schedule on your own. If your fitness facility offers cycling classes, aerobics, or interval training classes, take advantage of them. Not only will they likely help to push you more, you'll have other people there to help motivate you and encourage you to test to your limits.

So what program should you follow? Your instructor may have already established a regime that he or she expects you to follow. If not, the following pages offer some simple guidelines for a training program lasting 16 weeks, which is a little longer than the length of a semester at most Ontario community colleges. The guidelines are designed for people whose fitness level is either average to good or very good to excellent. If your fitness level is poor to fair, ask your instructor to help you establish a program that is safe and effective for you and that he or she can monitor. For those who have already reached an excellent level of fitness, all that is required is maintenance.

Remember that an exercise program can be affected by conditions in the environment in which you exercise. For example, a run may involve one or more of the following factors:

- topographical features such as hills and sand, or wet surfaces that make for slippery conditions
- obstacles such as ditches, fences, and underbrush
- meteorological and air-quality factors such as heat, humidity, cold, snow, wind, pollution, and thin air at higher altitudes
- bulky clothing or equipment that obstructs movement

You may need to adjust your running program to compensate for these variables.

Your fitness program must also take seasonal factors into account.

Your Winter Fitness Program

Staying active during the winter can be enjoyable. Whether you head out for a run, a walk, or a day of skiing, dressing for comfort will increase your enjoyment. A career in law enforcement also means that you will have to experience the outdoors throughout the year.

See the box below for some guidelines for fitness training during Canadian winters.

FYI

How to Dress for Winter Running

The best way to stay warm is to dress in layers:

- The first layer, or base layer, is next to your skin; it is the most important. It should fit snugly against the skin and should never be made of cotton, which absorbs water readily and takes a long time to dry. Once this layer becomes damp, it actually accelerates heat loss. Synthetic underwear, such as polypropylene or wicking polyesters, is more appropriate. These fabrics wick—pull moisture away from the skin—and dry quickly, often with one's own body heat, making them more comfortable.
- The second layer, or insulation layer, provides warmth. The amount of insulation you need will depend on the temperature and your workout. This layer is designed to trap warm air surrounding your body. Low exertion and colder weather call for a bulkier layer than high exertion and colder weather. It is extremely important not to overheat, as this increases the moisture that leaves the body. A body in motion does not need as much insulation as a body at rest. This middle layer must still wick moisture, should fit loosely over the first layer, and should be easy to remove so you can adjust to conditions.
- The final layer, sometimes called the element layer (the layer exposed to the elements), prevents heat loss. There are three ways a body can lose heat:
    1. through *convective heat loss*, which occurs when the wind strips away the thin layer of body-temperature air surrounding us, forcing the body to expend precious energy to rewarm this lost air;
    2. through *conductive heat loss*, which occurs when there is contact between the body and any object cooler than itself (for example, rain or wet cotton); and

continued . . .

FYI *continued*

3. through *evaporative heat loss*, which occurs when anything we are wearing is drying out. The element layer is very important because it can prevent all three heat-loss processes by keeping heat in. An outer layer should provide a combination of wind resistance, water resistance, and breathability.

Lower temperatures cause blood to be shunted away from the hands and feet to the centre of the body to keep the internal organs warm and protected. Remember that heat loss from your head alone can be as much as 50 percent at the freezing mark, so make sure you wear a hat or at least earmuffs and mittens. Superficial warming of the hands will return blood flow to prevent tissue damage. Blood flow will not return to the feet unless the temperature of the torso is normal or slightly higher (less than 1°C above normal). To keep your feet warm, you must also keep the rest of your body warm at all times.

Always check the air temperature and wind chill factor (combined effect of temperature and wind) before exercising in the cold. Data from the National Safety Council (www.nsc.org) suggest little danger to properly clothed individuals with skin exposed at –7 °C, even with a 50-km/h wind. A danger does exist for individuals with exposed skin when the wind chill factor falls below –29 °C. That condition can be achieved by any combination of temperatures below –7 °C with a wind of 65 km/h, and temperatures below –29 °C with no wind. If you are exercising near the danger zone for skin exposure, it also is advisable to warm the air being inhaled by wearing a scarf or mask over your nose and mouth. Check with weather sites like The Weather Network (www.theweathernetwork.com) before going out.

The telltale sign of frostbite is a patch of skin that turns hard, pale, and cold. Burning, tingling, stinging, or numbing sensations may be present. An affected person may appear to be clumsy, which can result from impaired motor control. When the affected body part is rewarmed, a throbbing or burning pain may result. Frostbite, like burns, is classified according to the degree of tissue injury. Some minor injuries result in swelling, redness, loss of sensation, and white plaque on the skin. With more severe lesions there can be blisters that may become filled with blood. In the most extreme cases, full-thickness freezing damages bones and muscles, resulting in tissue death and loss of the affected area.

Sunny days are most enjoyable for everyone, but remember to protect your eyes. In winter your eyes are exposed to light from above and from below as well, when it is reflected off snow. The reflection doubles the intensity of ultraviolet (UV) rays. Prolonged exposure can actually burn your eyes and eventually cause snow blindness. Symptoms can include pain in the eyes and extreme sensitivity to light. If you ever experience snow blindness, you should go inside to a dark or dimly lit room and apply cool compresses to your eyes until the pain subsides and tolerance to light returns. Protect your eyes from both sun and wind with sunglasses. Sunglasses should block UVA and UVB rays between 290 and 400 nm (The Weather Network, 2007). It is also important to use sunblock, which can prevent sunburn and reduce your risk of skin cancer. Use at least SPF (sun protection factor) 30; higher doesn't hurt.

Training in Hot Weather

Equally important is to prepare for physical activity in hot weather. Here are some things to consider:

- Any shirt is better than going bare-chested or running in just a sports bra. A shirt will protect you from the sun, but if it is not UVA/UVB-protected, you can wash it in a special detergent such as SunGuard™ to provide added protection.
- A hat, sunglasses, and sunscreen are important to protect your eyes, face, and body from developing atypical moles, which are a possible precursor to melanoma.
- Stay hydrated to prevent heat exhaustion, heat stress, and heat stroke. When the weather is both hot and humid, and your workout is intense, your sweat may not evaporate, causing your core body temperature to soar. High core temperature may result in reduced sweating, fever, unusual fatigue, headache, sleep loss, or the sensation that you are "coming down" with something. In extreme cases, individuals can suffer seizures or death from heat stroke.
- Run at the coolest time of the day, usually in the morning around sunrise. Run in the shade, under trees, or through trails to avoid solar radiation. Run a shorter distance, or run slower, than you would in cooler weather.

Play it smart with the heat. Allow yourself up to two weeks to acclimatize to hot weather. And remember to hydrate appropriately before, during, and after a run.

Whatever season you begin running, according to the American College of Sports Science (2009), it may take up to six months to reach the maintenance phase. If you experience any discomfort or pain, inform your instructor and consult your doctor. You may have to modify your program.

Choosing the Proper Footwear

Determining the right running shoe is very personal. What you need to start running is the right shoe, not the right price. And with all the high-tech shoes out there, choosing the most appropriate model becomes difficult. Here are some factors you need to consider:

- *Understand pronation* In biomechanics, pronation is rolling from your heel to toe through the foot strike, placing stress on the median (middle) of the foot. A proper neutral motion is to strike with the outside of the heel, with the foot rolling inward about 15 percent until the weight is distributed up to the ball of your foot evenly across the front. *Supination* or *underpronation* puts most of the pressure along the outside of the foot, where the force is concentrated; it causes you to use your smaller toes to push off. *Pronation* rolls from the outside to the inside of your foot. The arch flexes too far inward or stays collapsed, putting pressure on the inside of the foot. This means the foot and ankle have problems stabilizing the body and you do not absorb the shock as efficiently. You end up pushing off with your big toe and second toe. (See Figure 5.3.) Both under- and overpronation can cause imbalances in the ankles, knees, and hips, leading to gait injuries. If you cannot determine the type of foot motion that you have, ask the salesperson to help you.

FIGURE 5.3 Underpronation and Overpronation

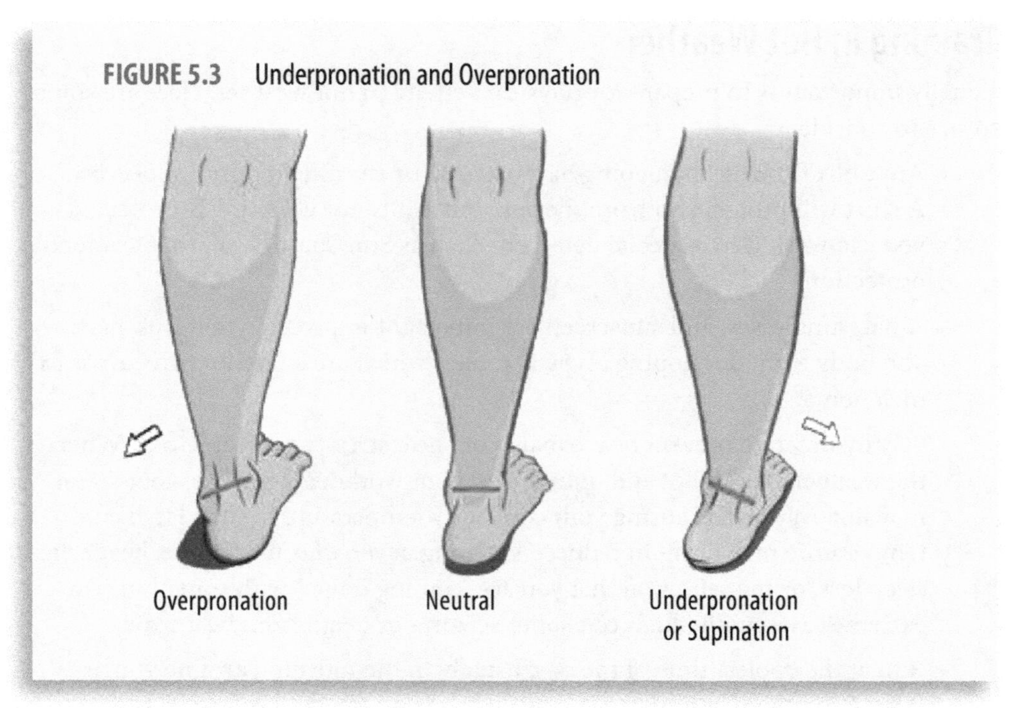

- *Determine your foot type* Look at the arch of your foot. If you have a low arch, you have "flat feet" and uderpronate or supinate, which can lead to overuse injuries. In this case, you need to look at shoes that offer motion control. If you have a high arch, you are more likely to be walking on the outside of your foot and need to choose cushioned running shoes. If you have a neutral arch, then you will want to look at stability running shoes. (See Figure 5.4.)
- *Wear pattern and foot strike* Foot strike refers to how you land. Most runners are heel strikers, who land on the outside of the heel and then roll up to push off the ball of the foot and toes. This produces a wear pattern around the ball of the foot. Such people may need more cushioning at the forefoot. A few runners are forefoot strikers who land more on the ball of the foot. These people may need more cushioning in the heel.

FIGURE 5.4 Flat to High-Arch Foot Types

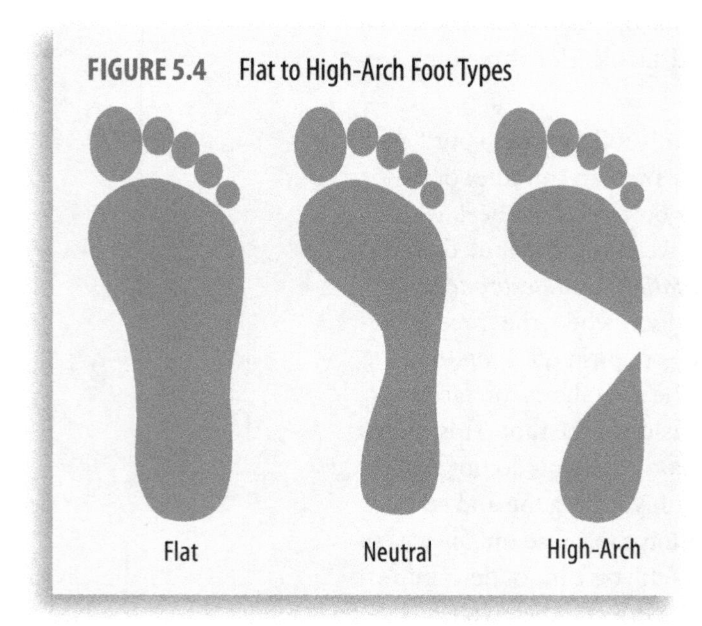

The FYI box on the next page offers some guidelines to ensure a good fit.

Guidelines for Cardiorespiratory Fitness Training

This section offers guidelines to help you set up your fitness program. There are separate guidelines for people whose fitness level is average to good and for those whose fitness level is very good to excellent. If you feel that your fitness level is below average, consult with your instructor.

FYI

If the Shoe Fits . . .

When trying on a shoe for proper fit, here are some guidelines:

- Make sure the salesperson measures your foot while you are standing so that your foot is spread out when weight is distributed on it.
- If you use orthotics or insoles, bring them with you to ensure a good fit.
- Check to make sure you have adequate room in the toebox by pressing your thumb into the shoe above your largest toe. You should be able to fit your thumb between the toe and the shoe's vamp (upper).
- Pick a shoe with the proper width for your foot. If your foot is narrow, do not let someone talk you into a shoe that causes your foot to slide around.
- The heel of your foot should fit snugly against the back of the shoe without sliding out when you walk.
- The top of the shoe (upper) should fit snugly without pressing or irritating the top of your foot.
- Run in your shoes in the store to ensure they fit well, feel comfortable, and provide arch support where needed. Some stores will let you try them on indoor treadmills for a week to see if they are right for you and do not cause blisters or foot pain. Ask the salesperson about the store's return or exchange policies.
- Shop around to ensure that you get the best shoe for you. Don't be persuaded into taking something else because the store doesn't have the right size.

Average to Good Fitness Level

1. Make sure you answered "no" to all the questions on the PAR-Q questionnaire (in **assignment 1.1**) or have been cleared by a medical examination. Check with your instructor if you are unsure about your medical suitability to undertake a fitness program at this time.
2. Begin each session with a proper warm-up and end with a cool-down. It is important to do a warm-up that mimics what you are going to be doing. For example, if you are doing a cycling class, then you should be warming up for at least five minutes prior to the start of the class. It is also important to cool down those muscles before you stretch them out.
3. Check the intensity of your exercise by monitoring your heart rate, or use the Borg scale or talk test. If you experience aches or pains or suffer an injury, stop exercising or reduce the intensity of your exercise until you are fit to continue or have seen a doctor. Be sure to advise your instructor of the problem.

Very Good to Excellent Fitness Level

1. These guidelines apply to people who exercise at an intensity level at the upper limit of their THR zone and have been involved in high-intensity aerobic activities, including running, for a number of years. Make sure you have answered "no" to all the questions on the PAR-Q questionnaire (in **assignment 1.1**) and have been cleared by a medical examination to participate in vigorous activities.
2. Begin each session with a proper warm-up and end with a cool-down.

TABLE 5.3 Training Guidelines for People of Average to Good Fitness

WEEK NO.	DURATION (MIN/DAY)	INTENSITY (% OF MHR)	FREQUENCY (DAYS/WK)
1	15–20	65–70	3
2	15–20	65–70	3
3	20	70	3
4	20	70	3
5	25	70	4
6	25	75	4
7	25	75	4
8	30	75	4
9	30	75	4
10	35	75	5
11	35	75	5
12	40	75	5
13	40	75	5
14	40	80	5
15	40	80	5
16	40	80	5

3. Check the intensity of your exercise by monitoring your heart rate, or use the Borg scale or talk test. If you experience aches or pains or suffer an injury, reduce the intensity of your exercise, substitute a lower-impact activity, or stop exercising until you are fit to continue or have seen a doctor. Be sure to advise your instructor of the problem.

Training to Your Upper Limit

When you work at the upper limit and over the percentages in Tables 5.3 and 5.4, if you are not in great shape, you go into what is termed an *anaerobic threshold*. That is, if you push too hard, your body no longer meets its demand for oxygen. You start feeling exhausted, you hyperventilate from excess amounts of lactic acid in your body, and your heart can no longer provide enough oxygen to your working muscles to sustain the demands of the task. At this point, you are typically able to continue for only a short period of time, 30 seconds to 1 minute. However, as you become more fit, you can push the range higher. As well, by training your anaerobic system, you can push the threshold through shorter- and faster-interval activities and thereby increase your aerobic capacity. By resting between these high-intensity interval training (HIIT) anaerobic sessions, you enable the oxygen-rich blood to help clean out the lactic acid from your muscles and you can catch your breath before the next set.

TABLE 5.4 Training Guidelines for People of Very Good to Excellent Fitness

WEEK NO.	DURATION (MIN/DAY)	INTENSITY (% OF MHR)	FREQUENCY (DAYS/WK)
1	15–20	65–70	4
2	20	70–75	4
3	25	75	4
4	30	75	4
5	35	75	5
6	40	75	5
7	40	75	5
8	40	75	5
9	40	80	5
10	40	80	5
11	40	80	5
12	40	80–85	5
13	40	80–85	5
14	40	80–85	5
15	30	80–85	5
16	30	80–85	5

NOTE: Weeks 15 and 16 become the maintenance phase for your aerobic conditioning.

Training for the Shuttle Run

The best way to train for the 20-metre shuttle run is to practise, practise, practise. *To train to meet an acceptable level (6.5), an individual must perform aerobic activity 3–5 times per week for at least 20–30 minutes, working at an intensity of 75–85 percent of his or her maximum heart rate.*

Once you have established a solid cardiovascular base, you can train on a treadmill following the guidelines in Table 5.5 to help build up the endurance required to meet the standards set out in the PREP.

Remember that you are increasing intensity to prepare your body for what it will be like when doing the shuttle run. Be aware that the treadmill is not the same as running in the gym or outdoors. In running, you must absorb the pounding of each step at the same time that you propel your body forward. There is also an energy cost for accelerating and decelerating the body at each end of the 20 metres. Ultimately, you cannot expect to succeed by practising only on a treadmill.

When you are having difficulty reaching the upper stages of the shuttle run, keep walking in your lane for about one minute, and then attempt to run the length every other beep. If you are fit enough, you may be able to keep up with the stages. This way, you will have a better understanding of the speed that you must work toward and will have a goal. These training effects will help your cardiorespiratory

TABLE 5.5 Training Guidelines to Build Endurance

TIME FRAME (NUMBER OF MINUTES)	STAGE (MILES PER HOUR)
0–1	4.5
1–2	4.5
2–3	5.0
3–4	5.5
4–5	6.0
5–6	6.5
6–7	7.0
7–8	7.5
8–9	8.0
9–10	8.5
10–11	9.0
11–12	9.5
12–13	10.0
13–14	10.5
14–15	11.0
15–16	11.5

NOTE: In the 20-m shuttle run, it takes 6 minutes and 30 seconds to reach stage 6.5; it takes 7 minutes and 30 seconds to reach stage 7.5. Stage 6.5 is equivalent to 11 minutes and 30 seconds in the 1.5-mile (2.4-km) run. It is important to push yourself further. Set goals for yourself to try to stay on the treadmill one stage longer.

TOP TIPS . . .

For Reluctant Runners

For those people who do not like running, here are a few tips to help you stay on track.

- Go as long as you can keep up the pace without holding on to the treadmill. Get off the treadmill, do your workout, and then return to the treadmill to see how far you can go on the second run.
- Another approach is to go as long as you can and then reduce the treadmill speed to 5; catch your breath and then increase the speed until you need to hang on to the treadmill.
- For those who are just starting to run and who prefer resistance training to cardio training: Get on the treadmill for one minute at the highest speed you can, then stop and do three sets (whether it is three sets of one exercise or one set of three exercises). Then, return to the treadmill for another minute. Over the period of an hour, you should be able to do at least 12 minutes of cardio. This approach will get you ready for longer runs on the treadmill.
- Finally, do the shuttle run outside of class time. Get a group of people together and practise the test in a gym, or set up cones 20 metres apart outdoors and run back and forth to build up your endurance.

system prepare for the demands of the tests. The physiological changes that occur as you train will prepare you to meet the demands of the different BFORs.

Many people use aerobic training to help reduce weight. Most research acknowledges that a conventional way to burn body fat effectively is to choose a particular modality (type of cardiorespiratory exercise) and perform it for at least 20–30 minutes at a moderate level of intensity.

Often individuals feel that this effort is enough. However, working at a higher intensity level will burn more calories in less time. In order for this approach to be effective, the overloading process has to be progressive, which means that you need to start at an appropriate level and build from there. Once a baseline has been established, you should gradually increase speed, incline, resistance, and/or time as you become better conditioned. The body has the ability to adapt to any stressor (exercise) placed on it, which means you have to overload progressively in order to continue to see gains. A beginner who runs on a treadmill at 4.5 mph (the first stage of the shuttle run) for 30 minutes will see caloric expenditure, cardiorespiratory conditioning, and burning of body fat at first. Over time, the intensity or time (30–40 minutes) will have to increase if continued results are to be achieved.

The goal of HIIT training is to keep your heart rate at a higher percentage of your maximal predicted heart rate (85–95 percent MHR). Because you cannot maintain that rate for long, you have to build recovery stages into your workout (you cannot run full-out the entire time). The time frames are usually done minute by minute, while adjusting speed, incline, or both to affect heart rate and the rating of perceived exertion on the Borg scale. This type of training is geared to those who are in advanced cardiorespiratory shape and do not have any pre-existing conditions that limit their ability to exercise safely as outlined in Chapter 1.

The suggested training regime for the shuttle run (Table 5.6) is an example of continuous increases in intensity. This example of a high-intensity workout includes changes in incline and speed to challenge your cardiorespiratory system, and to push those who are fitter a little further.

The idea is to increase your capacity to do work or increase your expenditure of calories. Conditioning in this fashion can be done using treadmills, stationary bikes, elliptical machines, stair steppers, stairmills, student residence stairs, and hills.

Effective cardiorespiratory exercise is not related to calories burned during a session, but to the effect the exercise has on your body during and after the session. High-intensity cardio exercise stimulates your metabolism to run at a higher-level intensity for longer duration. Your metabolism will stay elevated for a longer period of time so that it burns a greater percentage of calories during the day. Change the program to suit your skills and interests.

Some students do not see aerobic training as a priority, or they find it a frustrating experience. They may prefer to focus more on strength training than on aerobics. Based on research from McMaster University (Gibala et al., 2006), sprint training can provide a time-efficient way to induce rapid physiological adaptation similar to traditional long-term endurance training, which can result in improvements in both anaerobic and aerobic performance. Examples include running full-out at your maximum aerobic capacity for one- to two-minute intervals on a treadmill, bike, or elliptical machine after completing two or three weight exercises, and then going back to do two more exercises and repeating the anaerobic interval training. This approach will not replace running for an extended period of time; however, it will increase your aerobic capacity as you work toward meeting the requirements for the aerobic tests (1.5-mile run, shuttle run, and so on).

Turn to **assignment 5.3** (in the appendix) and design your own cardiorespiratory training program.

TABLE 5.6 Suggested Training Regime for the PREP Shuttle Run

TIME (MIN)	SPEED (MPH)	INCLINE	RPE (1–20)*
1	4	1	2
2	4.5	1	2
3	5	1	3
4	5.5	2	4
5	6	2	5
6	6.5	2.5	6
7	7	3	8
8	7.5	3	10
9	8	3.5	12
10	8.5	3	14
11	9	1	16
12	5	4	12
13	5	6	14
14	6	8	16
15	6	10	20
16	6	4	14
17	5	3	10
18	5	3	8
19	4	2	6
20	4	1	4

* RPE = Rating of Perceived Exertion

KEY TERMS

Borg scale, 101
exercising heart rate, 99
maximal heart rate (MHR), 99
maximum aerobic capacity (VO_2 max or MVO_2), 98
resting heart rate, 99
talk test, 102
target heart rate (THR) zone, 99

EXERCISES

Multiple Choice

1. The formula for determining your target heart rate zone is
   - **a.** MHR × intensity + resting heart rate
   - **b.** (220 – age)
   - **c.** (220 – resting heart rate) × 60–80%
   - **d.** (220 – age) × 60–80%
   - **e.** none of these
2. One positive effect of cardiorespiratory fitness is
   - **a.** your blood pressure increases
   - **b.** it takes less time to return to pre-exercise resting heart rates
   - **c.** your resting heart rate increases
   - **d.** your heart's ability to pump blood decreases
   - **e.** your resting heart rate stays elevated
3. George has a resting heart rate of 62 beats per minute (bpm) at age 25. What is his estimated maximal heart rate (MHR)?
   - **a.** 202 bpm
   - **b.** 205 bpm
   - **c.** 195 bpm
   - **d.** 190 bpm
   - **e.** 200 bpm
4. What is George's estimated target heart rate?
   - **a.** 100–120 bpm
   - **b.** 120–140 bpm
   - **c.** 117–156 bpm
   - **d.** 127–176 bpm
   - **e.** 150–195 bpm
5. Which of the following is NOT an aerobic exercise?
   - **a.** jogging
   - **b.** bicycling
   - **c.** fitness walking
   - **d.** tennis
   - **e.** swimming laps
6. The best time to check your heart rate to determine the intensity of your workout is
   - **a.** before beginning your workout
   - **b.** immediately at the end of your warm-up
   - **c.** immediately at the end of your cool-down
   - **d.** immediately at the end of your cardiorespiratory workout
   - **e.** 5 minutes after your cool-down to see whether training effects have occurred
7. Which term describes the greatest amount of oxygen that can be used by your body during intense exercise?
   - **a.** cardiorespiratory endurance
   - **b.** maximum aerobic capacity
   - **c.** cardiorespiratory uptake
   - **d.** maximum endurance
   - **e.** maximum cardiorespiratory uptake
8. Which component of the Physical Readiness Evaluation for Policing addresses cardiorespiratory fitness?
   - **a.** pursuit and restraint
   - **b.** victim relocation
   - **c.** arm restraint combined with the push–pull machine
   - **d.** shuttle run
   - **e.** running up and down stairs
9. The best example of a situation requiring aerobic fitness in law enforcement is
   - **a.** handcuffing a passive person
   - **b.** chasing down someone who is resisting arrest
   - **c.** following a vehicle in your cruiser
   - **d.** running a 4-km run at lunch break
   - **e.** bench pressing your body weight

10. HIIT stands for
    a. high-interval intensity training
    b. heavy intense interval testing
    c. high-intensity interval training
    d. high intensity indicator testing
    e. health indicator intensity test
11. You should take your resting heart rate
    a. before you write a test
    b. after you drive to school
    c. after you finish a timed run
    d. just before you go to bed at night
    e. when you first wake up but before you get out of bed in the morning
12. Exercising heart rate can be taken
    a. while you are running
    b. before you go for a run
    c. after completing your cool-down
    d. after completing your warm-up
    e. after completing 30 curl-ups
13. Maximal heart rate refers to
    a. what your heart rate gets to every time you run
    b. the rate at which you push your heart rate during a leisure run
    c. the maximal rate your heart can pump
    d. what your heart rate is at maximal effort during a sustained aerobic activity
    e. what your heart rate is at the end of a proper warm-up
14. By resting between HIIT anaerobic sessions, you
    a. enable the oxygen-deprived blood to help clean out the lactic acid from the muscles
    b. enable the oxygen-rich blood to help clean out the lactic acid from your muscles
    c. can catch your breath before the next set
    d. a and c
    e. b and c
15. When preparing for the shuttle run on the treadmill, the starting stage is
    a. 4 mph
    b. 4.5 mph
    c. 5 mph
    d. 5.5 mph
    e. 6 mph

Short Answer

1. Why is cardiorespiratory fitness important in law enforcement?

2. Identify some of the benefits of cardiorespiratory fitness.

3. Define maximum aerobic capacity (VO_2 max or MVO_2).

4. Explain why it is important to know your target heart rate (THR) zone.

5. Identify some of the conditions in the environment that can affect an exercise program.

6. What are some ways to keep warm when running in the winter?

7. What are three ways in which the body can lose heat?

8. List four signs of heat stress.

REFERENCES

American College of Sports Science. (2009). *Guidelines for graded exercise testing and exercise prescription* (8th ed.). Philadelphia: Lea and Febiger.

Anderson, G.S., Plecas, D., & Segger, T. (2001). Police officer physical ability testing—Re-validating a selection criterion. *Policing: An International Journal of Police Strategies & Management*, *24*(1), 8–31.

Arnold, C.M., & Faulkner, R.A. (2010, July). The effect of aquatic exercise and education on lowering fall risk in older adults with hip osteoarthritis. *Journal of Aging and Physical Activity*, *18*(3), 245–260.

Borg, G. (1998). *Perceived exertion and pain scales.* Champaign, IL: Human Kinetics.

Bouchard, C., Shephard, R.J., Stephens, T., Sutton, J.R., & McPherson, B.D. (Eds.). (1990). *Exercise, fitness, and health: A consensus of current knowledge.* Champaign, IL: Human Kinetics.

Buman, M.P., & King, A.C. (2010, November). Exercise as a treatment to enhance sleep. *American Journal of Lifestyle Medicine*, *4*, 500–514.

Canadian Society for Exercise Physiology (CSEP). (2003). *The Canadian physical activity, fitness and lifestyle appraisal: CSEP's guide to healthy living.* Ottawa: Author.

Cooper, K. (1982). *The aerobics program for total well-being.* New York: M. Evans.

Elley, C.R., & Arroll, B. (2002, April 2). Review: Aerobic exercise reduces systolic and diastolic blood pressure in adults. *Annals of Internal Medicine*, *136*(7), 493–503.

Gibala, M.J., Little, J.P., van Essen, M., Wilkin, G.P., Burgomaster, K.A., Safdar, A., Raha, S., & Tarnopolsky, M.A. (2006). Short-term sprint interval versus traditional endurance training: Similar initial adaptations in human skeletal muscle and exercise performance. *Journal of Applied Physiology*, *575*(3), 901–911.

Hassinen, M., Lakka, T.A., Hakola, L., Savonen, K., Komulainen, P., Litmanen, H., Kiviniemi, V., Kouki, R., Heikkilä, H., & Rauramää, R. (2010, July). Cardiorespiratory fitness and metabolic syndrome in older men and women. *Diabetes Care*, *33*(7), 1655–1657.

Healthy Living Unit. (2008). Public Health Agency of Canada. *The 2008 report on the Integrated Pan-Canadian Healthy Living Strategy.* http://www.phac-aspc.gc.ca/hp-ps/hl-mvs/ipchls-spimmvs/2008/index-eng.php.

Irwin, M.L., Smith, A.W., McTiernan, A., Ballard-Barbash, R., Cronin, K., Gilliland, F.D., Baumgartner, R.N., Baumgartner, K.B., & Bernstein, L. (2008, August 20). Influence of pre- and post-diagnosis physical activity on mortality in breast cancer survivors: The Health, Eating, Activity, and Lifestyle Study. *Clinical Oncology, 26*(24), 3958–3964.

Larose, J., Sigal, R.J., Khandwala, F., Prud'homme, D., Boulé, N.G., & Kenny, G.P. (2011). Associations between physical fitness and HbA_{1c} in type 2 diabetes mellitus. *Diabetologia, 54,* 93–102.

Marcus, B.H. (1998, March). Evaluation of motivationally tailored vs. standard self-help physical activity interventions at the workplace. *American Journal of Health Promotion, 12*(4), 246–253.

Nieman, D.C., Henson, D.A., Austin, M.D., & Brown, V.A. (2005). The immune response to a 30-minute walk. *Medicine and Science in Sports and Exercise, 37,* 57–62.

Ontario. Ministry of the Solicitor General and Correctional Services. (1997). *Fit to serve: Preparation for the PREP—The Physical Readiness Evaluation for Policing.* Toronto: Author.

Papousek, I., & Schulter, G. (2008). Effects of a mood-enhancing intervention on subjective well-being and cardiovascular parameters. *International Journal of Behavioral Medicine, 15*(4), 293–302.

Shephard, R.J. (1997, April). Exercise and relaxation in health promotion. *Sports Medicine, 23*(4), 211–216.

Sigal, R.J., Kenny, G.P., Boulé, N.G., Wells, G.A., Prud'homme, D., Fortier, M., Reid, R.D., Tulloch, H., Coyle, D., Phillips, P., Jennings, A., & Jaffey, J. (2007). Effects of aerobic exercise, resistance exercise, or both on glycemic control in type 2 diabetes: A randomized trial. *Annals of Internal Medicine, 147,* 357–369.

The Weather Network. (2007). TWN on TV—Ski safety tips. http://www.theweathernetwork.com.

US Department of Health and Human Services. (1996). *Physical activity and health: A report of the Surgeon General* (pp. 85–172). Atlanta: Centers for Disease Control and Prevention.

Vainio, H., & Bianchini, F. (2002). Weight control and physical activity. *IARC Handbooks of Cancer Prevention*, volume 6. Lyon: International Agency for Research on Cancer.

Varady, K.A., & Jones, P.J.H. (2005, August 1). Combination diet and exercise interventions for the treatment of dyslipidemia: An effective preliminary strategy to lower cholesterol levels? *JN: The Journal of Nutrition, 135*(8), 1829–1835.

Warburton, D.E., Gledhill, N., & Quinney, A. (2001a). Musculoskeletal fitness and health. *Canadian Journal of Applied Physiology, 26,* 217–237.

Warburton, D.E., Gledhill, N., & Quinney, A. (2001b). The effects of changes in musculoskeletal fitness on health. *Canadian Journal of Applied Physiology, 26,* 161–216.

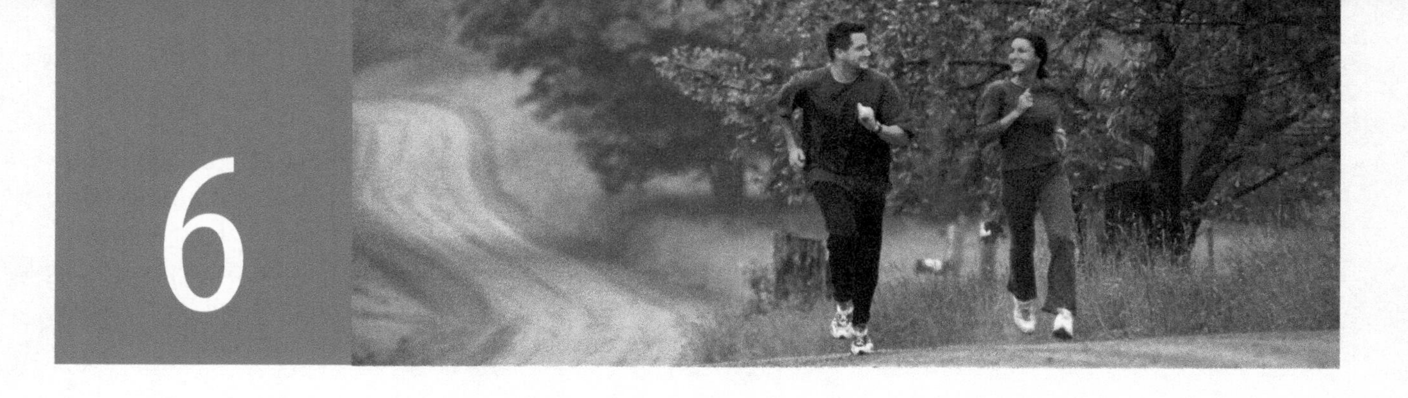

6

Strength, Power, and Endurance Training

LEARNING OBJECTIVES

After completing this chapter, you should be able to:

- Explain the importance of strength, power, and endurance training in policing.
- Explain the benefits of resistance training.
- Understand some of the basic terms and concepts associated with strength, power, and endurance training.
- Design a strength, power, and endurance training program to meet the job-related demands of policing.

OVERVIEW

The health benefits of being physically fit are widely acknowledged. Like cardiorespiratory fitness training, strength, power, and endurance training (also called resistance training) is important for meeting the occupational requirements of law enforcement. In this chapter you will learn basic terms and concepts associated with strength, power, and endurance training. This chapter will also enable you to design a training program for yourself that is effective and safe.

The Importance of Strength, Power, and Endurance Training

Muscle mass, strength, power, and endurance are essential contributing factors to improving musculoskeletal health and maintaining mobility (Marcell, 2003). With a regular training program, you can reduce your body fat, increase your lean muscle mass, and burn calories more efficiently.

Weight training is an important part of an overall fitness program. It can be done using your own body weight and simple, inexpensive equipment (for example, resistance bands), free weights, or machines.

Weight training has always been an integral component of training for specialized units within the emergency services. Strength, speed, quickness, and agility are keys to a successful takedown or rescue. Many students learn the basics of weight training in high school but fail to take them further. Some have no interest in "looking big," many don't have the time to train, and others fail to research and concentrate on proper techniques for developing strength and fitness. Weight training is not just for meeting the physical demands of the job; it is an important part of remaining fit throughout your career and into retirement.

Many services have emergency response teams (ERTs), tactics and rescue units (TRUs), and provincial emergency response teams (PERTs), all of which require cardiorespiratory endurance, muscular strength and endurance, and flexibility to meet the demands of the job on a regular basis. In addition to gruelling physical training, officers must learn rappelling, cover and concealment, tracking and searching, dynamic entry, high-risk vehicle assault, and urban and rural stalking (RCMP, 2001).

The physical demands of defensive tactics and arrest and control require a broad-based, general adaptation. This means that officers must be strong, quick to react, fast, accurate, and flexible in order to do their job. While some cases involve aerobic challenges in chasing a suspect, officers are more likely to face situations that involve altercations, which are shorter, more intense, and more threatening in nature, lasting from seconds to a few minutes. So police training must include workouts that are anaerobic and completely functional, and that work both the lower and upper extremities as well as providing trunk and core movement. As a result, police services in the province of Ontario, as well

DID YOU KNOW?

After the age of 50, sedentary people may begin to lose muscle mass and strength at the rate of approximately 1–2 percent per year (Marcell, 2003). This condition is called *sarcopenia*. It contributes to fractures and falls, with the consequent loss of independence, and also decreases metabolic rate and maximum aerobic capacity.

Bona Fide Occupational Requirements (BFORs)

Since the late 1990s, Bona Fide Occupational Requirements (BFORs) have been the standard for assessing applicants in most of the police services in Ontario. Covering elements of the job that require endurance, strength, and stamina, these assessments have combined these components to create various BFORs that are used by policing. The upper-body strength to restrain and move people is a necessary part of law enforcement (Gledhill & Shaw, 1995; Farenholtz, 1995). For this reason, upper-body strength is one of the fitness components tested by law enforcement organizations. Candidates for law enforcement positions are subjected, for example, to upper-body strength/power tests involving the push–pull machine, the arm-restraint device, an 80-lb (36-kg) bag carry, and a 150-lb (68-kg) body drag.

as the RCMP, have specific BFOR tests that assess one's functional abilities. Some of the assessments last up to 30 minutes and include wearing over 50 pounds (23 kg) of equipment; involve walking, running, and crawling; and require enough upper-body strength to do single chin-ups and negotiate five- to six-foot (2-m) high walls.

Upper-body strength is a special concern for women entering law enforcement, many of whom fail to meet testing standards without appropriate training. Female—and male—candidates must realize that passing the tests may require a greater than usual commitment of time to training. But with the proper training, everyone has the potential to succeed.

Although strength, power, and endurance training are important from a career perspective, they are also important for your overall well-being. Such training gives you more strength and energy to perform everyday tasks, bigger muscles and better muscle coordination, and a higher proportion of lean muscle to body fat. This training also contributes to better flexibility, helps avoid low-back problems, and can prevent falls.

The Benefits of Resistance Training

In the first two to three weeks of an exercise program, muscles begin to gain strength due to the recruitment of more muscle fibres at the same time. Later, after four to six weeks, the muscle fibres increase in size. This is known as **hypertrophy**. Additional physiological benefits from resistance training include:

hypertrophy
the process characterized by high training volume with moderate training intensity in order to build muscle mass

- increased bone mineral density (Nelson, Fiatarone, Morganti, Trice, Geenberg, et al., 1994; Engelke, Kemmler, Lauber, Beeskow, Pintag, et al., 2006)
- higher resting metabolic rate (Pratley, Nicklas, Rubin, Miller, Smith, et al., 1994)
- positive body composition changes (Fiatarone, O'Neill, Ryan, Clements, Solares, et al., 1994; Kerksick, Wismann-Bunn, Fogt, Thomas, Taylor, et al., 2010)
- reduction in the risk of developing metabolic syndrome (Jurca, LaMonte, Church, Earnest, Fitzgerald, et al., 2004; Stensvold, Tjonna, Skaug, Aspenses, Stolen, et al., 2010)
- reduction of back pain (Risch, Newell, Pollock, Risch, Langer, et al., 1993)
- improved glucose utilization, which is important for preventing or controlling diabetes (Miller, Pratley, Goldberg, Gordon, Rubin, et al., 1994; Boulé, Haddad, Kenny, Wells, & Sigal, 2001)

The Basics of Strength, Power, and Endurance Training

Strength, power, and endurance training includes any type of exercise that requires the muscles to move, or attempt to move, against an opposing force. It encompasses weight training but also a much wider range of training activities, such as push-ups and curl-ups. Most training programs are designed to increase muscular strength or muscular endurance, to alter body composition by increasing muscle size and decreasing the percentage of fat in the body, or for both purposes.

Athletes train for a variety of reasons. When training for *absolute strength*, athletes create a force irrespective of body weight (that is, lifting the heaviest possible load). When training for *relative strength* (force generated relative to body weight), athletes consider how strong they are per kilogram of body weight. When an athlete trains for *endurance*, he or she creates a force such as sustained (isometric) or repeated (isotonic) muscular actions against a submaximal resistance (for example, bicep curls).

Strength, power, and endurance training trains two components of the body: the muscles and the central nervous system (CNS), which causes the muscles to fire and thus to contract. It has been well documented that gains experienced during the first six weeks of training stem primarily from CNS adaptation—the muscles learning to synchronize better with one another. Gains arising from muscular adaptation (improved muscle coordination and movement) occur later (Faulkner & White, 1990; Koutedakis, Stavropoulos-Kalinoglou, & Metsios, 2005).

Basic Principles of Weight Training

The Overload Principle

To build muscle mass, a greater than normal load must stress the muscle. This is called the **overload principle**. The process of rebuilding and repairing stressed soft muscle tissue causes the tissue to adapt to the new level of stress. Once the tissue has adapted to the new level, additional stress must be placed on it to spur further improvement. Individuals must be cautious in increasing their training load because an abrupt increase in load may go beyond the muscle's ability to adapt, causing injury.

overload principle
the principle that muscle mass can be built up only if the muscle is subjected to a greater than normal load

Research published by the American College of Sports Medicine (ACSM, 2002) suggests that relatively heavy loads equal to or above 80 percent of one maximal repetition (**1RM**, or "one rep max") are required to achieve optimal strength gains.

1RM
one maximal repetition of weight; the maximal amount of weight that can be lifted through the full range of motion, for one repetition, with proper form

General Adaptation

The **general adaptation** phase prepares your muscles, joints, tendons, and ligaments for intense training. It is characterized by higher repetitions, lower intensities, and short rest periods, which help the neuromuscular components synchronize so that gains can be seen.

general adaptation
the process of preparing muscles, joints, tendons, and ligaments for intense training by educating the neuromuscular component so that gains can be seen; characterized by higher repetitions, lower intensities, and short rest periods

Muscular Strength, Power, and Muscular Endurance

Muscular strength training is characterized by lower training volume—that is, fewer repetitions—and higher training intensity. The goal of strength training is to stress the muscular and neuromuscular systems through heavy resistance training to adapt to heavy loads. Dynamic strength training is characterized by different movement patterns at different speeds involving concentric, eccentric, and plyometric actions.

Muscular power is increased when the same amount of work is done in a shorter period or when a greater amount of work is done during the same period. Power is a function of force and time. Power is required in the movements of daily living, work, and sport.

Muscular endurance training develops athletes' capacity to maintain the quality of their muscles' contractile force (strength) over a long period of time. Athletes who have good endurance levels will have the capacity to maintain productivity and speed over a longer period of time. This is important for police officers, especially those on a canine unit, who may become involved in lengthy foot pursuits. It is also important for those officers on tactical units who must respond quickly and maintain speed while wearing approximately 50 pounds (23 kg) of gear and equipment.

Repetitions

A **repetition (rep)** is one complete movement of an exercise.

repetition (rep)
one complete movement of an exercise

Sets

A **set** is a group of repetitions. For example, "2 sets of 10 reps" means two groups of ten repetitions each, with a rest period between each group.

set
a group of repetitions

Hypertrophy

Hypertrophy is the process characterized by high training volume with moderate training intensity. The goal is to build muscle mass. When you increase muscle size, the muscle has a greater potential of force. Usually, hypertrophy combined with motor neuron activation—in which the brain recruits more motor units to "fire"—produces greater strength gains.

Power Training

Power training is the process through which an athlete works to build overall body explosiveness and reactive ability. The objective is to take the strength gained in the strength phase and convert it to activity-specific power. This phase is characterized by low volume and high intensities, using Olympic and explosive lifts, as well as sport-specific plyometric exercises. High muscular power output is an indication of the ability to perform a high level of (muscle) work in a short period of time. Exercises such as heavy squats and dead lifts that target the very large, powerful muscles of the legs (quadriceps and hamstrings), the buttocks (gluteal muscles), and back (erector spinae) are examples of power exercises.

power training
the process where an athlete works to build overall body explosiveness and reactive ability by taking the strength gained in the strength phase and converting it to activity-specific power

Repetition Maximum Loading

Repetition maximum loading is based on the principle that progressive resistance training uses a load that is heavy enough to result in "task failure" (muscular exhaustion on the tenth repetition). The concern with this method is that an athlete who works to the point of failure has a slower recovery time and less energy for subsequent training.

repetition maximum loading
progressive resistance training using a load that is heavy enough to result in "task failure" (muscular exhaustion on the tenth repetition)

Plyometrics

Plyometrics is based on the principle that the combination of speed and strength is power. It is a method of training that enhances an individual's explosive reaction by means of rapid and powerful muscular contractions through stretch-shortening cycles. The maximum force that a muscle can develop is attained during a rapid *eccentric contraction* (lengthening; for example, a biceps curl on the way down).

plyometrics
a method of training that enhances an individual's "explosive" reaction through rapid and powerful muscular contractions through stretch-shortening cycles; a concentric action immediately preceded by an eccentric action

Our muscles seldom perform only one type of contraction. When a *concentric contraction* (shortening; for example, a biceps curl on the way up) follows an eccentric contraction, the force generated can be dramatically increased. (See Chapter 4 for more about eccentric and concentric contractions.)

At a more cellular level, if a muscle is stretched, most of the energy used to stretch it is lost in the form of heat. There is some leftover energy stored in the elastic components of the muscle. If the stored energy is then used by an opposing contraction (that is, a concentric contraction following an eccentric contraction), then a greater force is generated in those muscles (Bompa, 1999). For the most effective gains, weight training prior to plyometric training is essential to gain the greatest generation of force.

A note of caution: heavy-load explosive resistance exercise training places muscles and joints at increased risk of injury because of the force used to move and accelerate loads at high speeds. For this reason, when beginning, fewer repetitions is a safer approach.

Between-Set Rest Periods

It is important to rest between each set of a specific exercise. Too-short rest periods are the second most frequent error in exercise program design. Proper rest periods can affect metabolic, hormonal, and cardiorespiratory responses to strength training. When you are doing structural and multi-joint exercises, you should rest 2–4 minutes between sets. When you are isolating muscle groups or doing single-joint exercises, you should rest 1–2 minutes. Athletes whose sport demands 1–3 minutes of all-out effort with little or no rest may benefit from a work–rest ratio of 1:1 or slightly higher.

Because chasing and arresting individuals requires you to perform moderate- to high-intensity effort, interval training is important to help improve your anaerobic fitness while working on strength and endurance. This means alternating fast running (80–90 percent of maximum speed, 5–10 intervals, up to 10 seconds) with active recovery (light jogging, up to 30 seconds) along with mixing muscles of the arms, shoulders, back and abdomen (core), and legs to ensure that your body adapts in preparation for those times when it is overloaded.

Basic Guidelines for Strength, Power, and Endurance Training

As in cardiorespiratory training, you need to adhere to certain guidelines to make resistance training effective, safe, and enjoyable.

Starting Out: The First Two to Three Weeks

During your first two to three weeks of training, keep these points in mind:

- For each exercise, you should do only 1–2 sets of 12–15 repetitions. After three weeks, you can gradually increase to 2–3 sets and decrease the number of repetitions to 8–12. If you are a beginner, you need to pick a weight that is comfortable, with the last two or three reps becoming hard but not impossible to lift.

- Your workouts should include a total of no more than 20–25 sets when first starting out. More is counterproductive, and you risk overtraining! Once you can lift your set number of reps comfortably, increase the weight slightly while reducing the number of reps.
- During your workouts, exercise the large-muscle groups first so that the small muscles (which are not fatigued) can support the large muscles. Because small muscles act as stabilizers for larger muscles, it is important first to do the exercises that focus on the large muscle-groups, followed by the small-muscle groups, to get the most out of your workout. Small muscles, such as forearm flexors, recover faster than larger muscles, such as the pectoralis major, and therefore can tolerate more sets without risking soreness or overtraining.
- You can exercise each muscle group a minimum of 2–3 times per week (CSEP, 2011), but remember to leave at least 48 hours between workouts involving the same muscle group. Those who are in advanced training can do 4–5 days per week without an issue as long as they limit each muscle group to two times per week (ACSM, 2002).
- Do high-intensity exercises before lower-intensity exercises.
- Do multiple-joint exercises before single-joint exercises, because the former use more muscle groups and better reflect daily activities. Multiple-joint exercises use more than one joint when performing a movement. Although the focus is on one particular muscle group, there are many other muscles that act as stabilizers. Examples include squats, deadlifts, bench presses, military presses, rowing, and chin-ups. Single-joint exercises, also known as isolation exercises, engage single-muscle groups. Examples include leg curls, biceps curls, quadriceps extensions, lateral raises, and shoulder shrugs.
- When you weight train, always try to use the full range of motion, but don't lock your knees or arms because this can put stress on the joints. Using the full range of motion will help you develop strength and maintain flexibility.
- Try to ensure that you exercise all the major muscle groups. Also, try to achieve a balance between exercising agonists (muscles that move a joint in the desired direction) and antagonists (muscles that simultaneously resist that movement). This will help you maintain flexibility and prevent joint or soft tissue damage. For example, alternate pushing and pulling exercises, especially in split routines (for example, presses then flies). Similarly, alternating upper- and lower-body exercises will give muscle groups time to rest and recover.
- Breathe out during the last two-thirds of the exertion phase of an exercise. Holding your breath can dangerously increase your blood pressure, which can have possibly life-threatening health effects.
- Don't try to lift more than you are able to. There is less chance of injury lifting a lighter weight in a slow, controlled action than lifting a heavier weight in a fast, uncontrolled, "ballistic" action. If you are tired, stop.

- Some people feel slightly dizzy when working the large-muscle groups in the lower body, because blood is diverted to this area. If you feel this way, you should lie down with your feet raised. Do not carry on if you still feel dizzy after a few minutes or if you have a further dizzy spell.
- Modify your workout every three weeks or so; otherwise, the muscles will adapt and your gains will level off. You can modify your workout by altering intensity (recall the FITT formula in Chapter 5), the number of sets, the type and speed of muscular action, the type of exercise, and the length of rest periods between sets and workouts.
- Setting goals is a good way to stay motivated. Make sure that your goals are realistic. Remember that results take time and are sometimes very gradual. Keeping a log may help you monitor your progress. (The *Fit for Duty, Fit for Life Training Guide* that accompanies this textbook provides a Daily Workout Log that you can use.) Although you will begin to see changes in the first six weeks, it can take at least 16 weeks to see the results you want. If nothing is happening after the first six weeks, you will need to modify your training program (Bickel, Cross, & Bamman, 2011).
- Remember the importance of fuelling your body with adequate nutrients and fluids, especially water. Workouts lasting longer than 90 minutes may require electrolyte replacement.

Frequency of Training

For your training to be effective, you must train regularly. Also, it is important to rest the muscles at least 48 hours after a workout to avoid overtraining and to allow your body to repair torn tissue. There are a number of ways to accomplish these objectives. You will likely use either the three-days-a-week routine or the four-day split routine described later in this chapter. People at an advanced stage of training may wish to use the three-day split-phase routine described by Shipley (1998).

Examples of Different Training Programs

Periodization Training

periodization
an organized approach to training that involves progressive cycling of various aspects of a training program during a specific period of time

Periodization is an organized approach to training that involves progressive cycling of various aspects of a training program during a specific period of time to achieve specific goals (such as losing body fat or enhancing certain aspects of the body). Periodization training is the systematic variation of training specificity, intensity, and/or volume to obtain longer training and performance improvements. The aim is to develop basic hypertrophy; strengthen ligaments, tendons, and connective tissue; and build a base from which you can develop. Depending on goals (such as training for a specific test or sport), individuals will choose different programs to meet their needs or health status.

The strategy is to move from higher-volume and lower-intensity programs to lower-volume and higher-intensity programs through a series of phases. Some individuals will start out in the general conditioning phase and work their way to a maintenance phase. This type of training takes into account a recovery phase, which reduces the likelihood of overtraining. Many websites provide a variation on this theme. You have to decide what you want out of a program and what will work for you. For example, to train for the PREP BFOR, you need to train for the pursuit and restraint phases as well as the cardiovascular component, the shuttle run.

For those starting out, Table 6.1 provides general guidelines regarding sets, reps, intensity, load, and rest intervals. Many people follow these until they are comfortable trying more and then move on to a specific training regime.

TABLE 6.1 Example of Periodization Training

	GENERAL CONDITIONING	STRENGTH	POWER	MAINTENANCE	ACTIVE RECOVERY
Sets	2–3	2–6	3–4	1–2	1
Reps	8–12	1–12	3–5	6–10	10–12
Intensity	Moderate	High	High	Moderate	Low
Novice	20–50% 1RM	40–50% 1RM	40–50% 1RM		
Intermediate	40–60% 1RM	60–70% 1RM for strength 70–85% 1RM for hypertrophy	60–85% 1RM		
Experienced		>80% 1RM	>70% 1RM		
Volume (load)	High	Moderate	Low	Moderate	Moderate
Rest: Between sets	1–2 minutes	3–4 minutes	4–5 minutes	1–2 minutes	1–2 minutes
Rest: Single muscle group	≥48 hours	≥48 hours	≥48 hours	≥48 hours	1–2 minutes

SOURCES: Stone, O'Bryant, & Garhammer, 1981; Stone & O'Bryant, 1987; Bompa, 1999; Garber, Blissmer, Deschenes, Franklin, Lamonte et al., 2009.

FYI

Performance-Enhancing Substances

There are three basic types of performance-enhancing substances associated with weight training. *Nutritional aids* include vitamins and minerals, protein and amino acid supplements, carnitine (a substance in your body that helps turn fat into energy), creatine, and caffeine. *Pharmacological aids* include pain-masking drugs, anabolic steroids, prohormones, human growth hormones, and erythropoietin. *Physiological aids* include blood doping and drug masking.

Athletes use amino acids to assist in the repair and building of muscle tissue and the release of growth hormone. Excessive amounts can lead to a toxic effect due to dehydration. See Chapter 8 for further discussion of amino acids.

Anabolic steroids are synthetic derivatives of the male hormone testosterone. They produce retention of phosphate, potassium, and nitrogen; decrease amino acid breakdown; and increase protein synthesis. Most athletes see an increase in their muscle mass and strength, a decrease in body fat, and quicker recovery from training. There has been little consistent evidence in enhanced performance, except in lean body mass. Anabolic steroids have many harmful side effects, including liver damage, increased aggressiveness, acne, stunted growth, gynecomastia (development of breast tissue in males), high blood pressure, and sterility. In women, anabolic steroids may lead to masculinization including excessive facial hair growth, deepening of the voice, and amenorrhea (National Institute on Drug Abuse, 2006). Because the risk factors are great for those who consider steroid use as a means of gaining lean muscle mass, discussing this matter with your physician is very important before deciding to take this pharmacological aid.

Strength Training to Develop Strength and Produce Hypertrophy in Muscles

As your body adapts to a general weight training program, you will begin to see fewer gains. In order to shock your body and begin to see more gains to your large-muscle groups, there are various forms of training that you can undertake to develop those muscles. Here are some suggestions for applying these principles:

- Begin your weight training sessions with 3–4 sets of dead lifts or squats at 85–95 percent of your 1RM; if you don't know your 1RM, aim for 2–6 repetitions (refer to the section "Determining Load," below).
- Rest no longer than 60 seconds between sets.
- Continue to do your traditional combined upper-body/lower-body routine or split routine as normal.
- Drink a carbohydrate beverage during and a carbohydrate/protein beverage after your routine to boost repair and growth of the muscle tissue.

It should be noted that increased muscle bulk from hypertrophy training does not necessarily make you stronger. Contrary to popular belief, increased muscle size does not equate with increased strength. It is the neuromuscular recruitment of the involved muscle fibres that increases strength.

Variations on Training Routines

Because of your time constraints with shiftwork, court time, and family time, you will find that some of these routines will work better than others for you. While at school or in a specialized unit where you must train every day you work, you may be able to get in six days a week of workouts. During other times in your life, you may be restricted to two or three days a week and may have time for only a 40-minute workout. You will have to determine at that point which program will provide you with the most benefits. Here are some examples:

- *Three-days-a-week routine*:
  Train three non-consecutive days a week (for example, Monday, Wednesday, and Friday) and complete all exercises in your workout each time.
- *Three-day split-phase routine*:

Day 1:	Chest, triceps, and abdominals	Day 5:	Repeat day 1
Day 2:	Back and biceps	Day 6:	Repeat day 2
Day 3:	Legs and shoulders	Day 7:	Repeat day 3
Day 4:	Rest	Day 8:	Rest

- *Four-day split routine*:
  This involves training different parts of the body on different days. Ontario Police College (1994) lays out two options (see Table 6.2).

trisets
combining three exercises with little rest in between; can involve working the same muscle group from three different angles, working three different muscle groups, or working different areas of the same muscle from three different angles

Trisets

Trisets are combinations of three exercises done with little rest in between. They can involve working the same muscle group from three different angles, working three different muscle groups, or working different areas of the same muscle from three different angles. Trisets increase training intensity by reducing the average length of rest intervals between sets. Trisets save time and raise the metabolism; however, they are associated with a higher risk of injury. They are done at about 50 percent 1RM with exercises being performed one after the other, then repeated two or three times. Rest periods are from 1–3 minutes. An example of a sequence for the chest and back could be decline dumbbell presses, chin-ups, incline dumbbell flies, and one-arm dumbbell rows.

Split routines can involve working the upper body one day and the lower body another day. This means you can continue to work out on successive days. There are many examples of split routines. See Table 6.3 for a few examples.

TABLE 6.2 Four-Day Split Routine

	OPTION A	OPTION B
Monday and Thursday	Upper body: chest, back, shoulders, and arms	Chest, shoulders, triceps, and abdominals
Tuesday and Friday	Lower body: legs and abdominals	Legs, back, and biceps

SOURCE: Ontario Police College, 1994.

TABLE 6.3 Examples of Trisets

	4-DAY ROUTINE	5-DAY ROUTINE	5-DAY ROUTINE	6-DAY ROUTINE
Monday	Upper	Chest and back	Chest	Upper
Tuesday	Lower	Legs and abs	Shoulders	Lower
Wednesday	Rest	Off	Back	Upper
Thursday	Upper	Arms and shoulders	Rest	Lower
Friday	Lower	Off	Triceps/Biceps	Upper
Saturday	Rest	Start routine over	Leg	Lower
Sunday	Start routine over		Rest	Rest
Special note	Work abdominals each day	Work abdominals each day	Work abdominals and calves each day or minimum three days, but fewer sets	Work abdominals each day

NOTE: Although there are rest days from weight training indicated, you can do cardiorespiratory training and/or play sports on those days.

TABLE 6.4 Training Goals

TRAINING GOAL	NO. OF EXERCISES	NO. OF SETS PER EXERCISE	NO. OF REPETITIONS PER SET	REST PERIOD BETWEEN SETS
Muscular endurance or muscle tone	10–12	2–3	12–18	20–30 seconds
Muscle growth	8–10	3–6	8–12	30–90 seconds
Strength and muscle growth	8–12	3–6	6–12	1–2 minutes
Power (ability to perform quick, explosive exercises)	1–6	3–5	1–5	2–5 minutes

Ultimately, your time constraints, interests, and goals will lead you to choose one or a combination of these programs. An example for the chest and back could be decline dumbbell presses, chin-ups, incline dumbbell flies, and one-arm dumbbell rows. Table 6.4 provides a more specific guideline for beginners, depending on their goals. For each training goal, there are guidelines that help you either to build muscle strength and power or to train your muscles for endurance.

Selecting and Arranging Exercises

A balanced program for beginners should incorporate one to three exercises for each large-muscle group, for a maximum total of 12. The order in which you complete your exercises is also important. Keep the following in mind when you exercise:

1. Do large-muscle group exercises first.
2. Always alternate between an upper-body and a lower-body exercise during your workout.
3. Alternate push exercises with pull exercises.
4. Do high-intensity exercises before lower-intensity exercises.

How you structure your program will affect the intensity of your training, which in turn may affect the rate at which you benefit.

Warming Up

Your workout must always include a proper warm-up (and cool-down). Your warm-up should consist of 5–15 minutes minimum of an aerobic activity such as light jogging or bicycling, followed by stretching. Mimic the types of exercises you will do in your workout, using light weights to prepare the muscles.

Following Correct Form

The correct form in resistance training is a steady, controlled execution of the exercise through the full range of motion. It is important to isolate the muscle group you are exercising. For example, if you are doing biceps curls, you need to concentrate on the biceps and not use your back. You must not bounce any weight you use. When you engage in a controlled movement, you need to take at least as long extending as you do flexing (a count of two on the way up and a count of at least two on the way down). The eccentric contraction will be more effective, and your muscle—not gravity—will do the work.

Proper Breathing Technique

Your blood pressure can increase to dangerous levels if you hold your breath while weight training. It is important to exhale during the lift and continue breathing throughout the exercise to prevent your blood pressure from rising too high.

Determining Load

There is wide agreement that the 1RM (one repetition maximum) is the accepted technique for gauging maximal dynamic muscular strength, and it is widely used at various stages of a training program. 1RM is defined as the maximal amount of weight that can be lifted through the full range of motion, for one repetition, with proper form. Many trainers are hesitant to subject individuals to 1RM tests because of the high risk of injury. To avoid damage to bones, more repetitions are recommended for young athletes during resistance training (American Academy of Pediatrics, 2001).

When starting out, most resistance training programs should aim to maintain a fairly high number of repetitions (10–15 reps) until proper exercise form has been developed (Faigenbaum, 2000). Research has shown that those who have not trained previously will see greater strength increases initially, whereas trained individuals can do more repetitions at given weights. This difference may be due to neural factors, such as increased recruitment and synchronization and metabolic recovery (Brechue & Mayhew, 2009). Ultimately, the number of repetitions that one can complete is affected by the subject's age, sex, training status, size of muscle groups, genetics, use of machines or free weights, and movement biomechanics (ACSM, 2009). Brechue and Mayhew (2009) believe that the best predictions of the level of muscular strength are realized when repetitions are maintained in the 2–5 RM range with loads greater than 85 percent of the 1RM.

You also need to determine the load or weight you will lift. Several methods are available.

Repetition Range Method

This method is appropriate for beginners and for people not involved in lifting maximum or near-maximum loads. It involves the following steps:

1. Determine the number of repetitions necessary for achieving your exercise goal (see Table 6.4).
2. Through trial and error, determine the maximum load that you can lift within this repetitions range. By the third set, you should begin to feel fatigue. If you cannot make it to the third set, lessen the load or do not complete the third set.
3. Work with this load as long as you remain within the desired repetition range through three sets.
4. Increase the load by 5–10 percent once you are able to perform 15 repetitions in the last set during two consecutive workouts.

Percent Maximum Method

This involves determining the maximum load you can lift at a single go. Because lifting maximum loads can cause injury, this method should be used only under the supervision of your instructor or another fitness expert.

Turn to **assignment 6.1** (in the appendix) to determine your workload for your maximum bench press.

Choosing Your Training System

There are several training systems to choose from. Which one you choose depends on your goals and on the amount of time you have to devote to your program.

Circuit Training

In circuit training, you perform a number of exercises in succession at a submaximal level, with little rest in between. This form of conditioning develops strength, endurance (both aerobic and anaerobic), flexibility, and coordination all in one exercise session. It is structured to include a series of exercises or stations to complete in succession, with minimal rest in between. It is a balanced workout that targets all muscle groups while building cardiorespiratory endurance, usually with about 2–3 sets of 10 exercises done for 60 seconds each with 15–30 seconds of rest in between.

Adding a longer cardio component builds in the principles of interval training. By alternating 1 minute of cardio (skipping, steps, sprinting) with ten 1-minute endurance exercises, the athlete pushes the anaerobic system so that the body must adapt to lactic acid fatigue.

Light to Heavy Training

As you progress through the sets, you increase the weight you are working with. This system carries a low risk of injury. The major drawback is that the muscles may tire during the earlier sets, preventing heavier lifting later.

Heavy to Light Training

As you progress through the sets, you decrease the weight you are working with. The advantage is that you may be able to lift heavier weights before the muscles tire. The disadvantage is a high risk of injury if you have not properly warmed up your muscles.

Pyramid Training

pyramid training
a system that combines the light to heavy and heavy to light approaches for weight training

The **pyramid training** system combines the light to heavy and heavy to light approaches. You begin your workout with the light to heavy approach, followed by the heavy to light approach during the second half. This system is good for developing strength. It can cause injury, however, by tempting people to push too hard to finish their sets.

Superset Training

superset training
a system that involves performing two exercises in succession, without rest; often used to exercise opposing muscle groups, it results in increased strength and muscle mass of the targeted muscle group

The **superset training** system involves performing two exercises in succession, without rest. It is often used to exercise opposing muscle groups. It increases strength and muscle mass of the targeted muscle group. Its use is confined to the arms and legs. For example, leg extensions and then squats will increase the size and strength of the quadriceps muscle. In the upper arm, doing a triceps exercise followed by bench press targets the triceps muscle. If the muscle is pre-fatigued, then you will be pushing it beyond comfortable limits. This is where gains or injuries can occur.

Plyometrics

Plyometrics was designed to condition athletes to increase and develop their jumping, sprinting, and explosive power. Owing to the effort required, adequate rest time is needed between exercises to recover. Individuals must be highly motivated to do this type of conditioning. Some guidelines include the following:

- Aim for a 1:5 ratio; for example, 30 seconds flat out with a 2.5-minute rest.
- Always warm up and stretch, especially your legs.
- Use explosive movements to obtain optimal results. Stay focused in order to get the most out of the workout.
- Always use correct foot placement. Aim to land with your ankle fixed.
- Aim to stay on the balls of your feet whenever possible. Avoid landing on your heels or the sides of your feet.
- Do not do circuit training more than twice a week, and remember to allow a minimum of 48 hours' rest between sessions.
- Use only your body weight when performing plyometric exercises.
- Always allow adequate recovery between reps. The importance of recovery cannot be stressed enough.

Examples of exercises include 90-degree jumps, lateral skating, one-leg butt kicks, ski tuck jumps, and two-foot side hops. As you become more advanced, you can try activities like decline hops, two-foot hops off a box, bench jumping, rope jumping, and depth jumps off a box. Alternating between lunges and sprints on a track also constitutes a form of plyometrics.

Designing an Appropriate Program

Comparing absolute fitness levels between males and females has been an issue for years. A high proportion of female applicants fail many entrance tests because of their size, body composition, hemoglobin levels, and muscular strength (Shephard & Bonneau, 2002). BFOR standards have tried to address these issues; however, females, and in some cases smaller males, may still be at a disadvantage if they are not training appropriately. It is important to realize that muscular strength is something that must be continually worked on throughout your career. Statistically, women tend to shy away from strength training. However, in policing it is very important that all officers have the strength when they need it to do the job, whether they are physically restraining an individual, applying handcuffs, or pulling themselves over a wall while wearing a uniform, vest, and belt weighing approximately 25–50 pounds (11–23 kg).

Specialized Programs

There are a number of good programs out there that incorporate a combination of body weight and free-weight equipment such as kettlebells, barbells, bands, and pull-up racks to enhance skill-related physical fitness components while pushing the metabolic pathways both anaerobically and aerobically. These programs are designed to allow anyone to complete the workout regardless of his or her fitness level. Many police officers are either using DVDs or joining gyms that specialize in such programs, and are experiencing significant gains and recognizing the importance of combining endurance training and cardiorespiratory training. Many have turned away from just strength training, which is difficult to maintain throughout an officer's career owing to time commitments and changes in fitness goals.

Table 6.5 lists common exercises that address the specific areas that will help you complete the BFOR police requirements (see also Chapter 15). In addition to having good cardiovascular endurance, you will need to develop upper-body strength to meet the requirements. As you practise for the PREP and PARE, you will come to appreciate that technique plays a role; however, those with good strength are able to get through the protocol without injury. It will be up to you to see that you are able to meet the minimum requirements.

Table 6.6 shows examples of exercises that you can use in designing your own fitness program. Descriptions and photographs of exercises that cover the major muscle groups appear in the *Fit for Duty, Fit for Life Training Guide* that accompanies this textbook.

Most exercises can be easily modified to be done at home if you do not have access to a fitness facility. You will have to determine the starting weight, sets, and repetitions based on the information that you have just read, as well as on your starting fitness level and the goals you want to achieve. Although a basic program could last six to eight weeks, you might become bored after only two weeks. You

TABLE 6.5 Upper Beginner/Lower Intermediate Training Program

	DAY 1 CHEST/TRICEPS	DAY 2 ARMS/SHOULDERS/ABDOMINALS	DAY 3 LEGS/BICEPS	DAY 4 CARDIO/ABDOMINALS
Warm-up	Skipping (3 minutes/no breaks)	Skipping (2 minutes/no breaks)	Skipping (2 minutes/no breaks)	Skipping (2 minutes/no breaks)
	Add light cardio (5 minutes)	Add light cardio (5 minutes)	Add light cardio (5 minutes)	Add light cardio (5 minutes)
	Stretching (min. 10 minutes)	Stretching (min. 10 minutes)	Stretching (min. 10 minutes)	Stretching (min. 10 minutes)
Exercises	Bench press 3 × 15	Bent-over row pronate 2 × 12	Squats 3 × 12	30–45 minutes of continuous CV exercise (65–80% VO_2 Max)
	Incline dumbbell flies 3 × 15	Bent-over row supinate 2 × 12	Leg press 3 × 12	
	Two-handed triceps dumbbell raises 2 × 12	Seated row (bar to belly-button) 3 × 15	Calf raises 3 × 12	
	One-handed triceps raise 2 × 8	Shoulder press, military press, or Arnold press 3 × 15	Leg extensions 3 × 12	
	Push-ups 3 × max	Abdominal curls or side curl-ups 2 × 35–50 (fatigue)	Biceps curl, preacher curl, or easy curl with straight bar 3 × 10	Abdominal curls or side curl-ups 2 × 35–50 (fatigue)
Rest period	30 seconds between sets; CV-based	30 seconds between sets; CV-based	45 seconds between sets	

TABLE 6.6 Examples of Exercises for Designing a Weight Training Program

MAJOR MUSCLE GROUP	ADDITIONAL MUSCLES USED	EXERCISES
Trapezius		Shoulder shrugs
		Lower pulley row to neck
		Dumbbell incline shoulder raise
		Shoulder shrugs
	Biceps, shoulders	Upright row
Deltoid		Barbell incline shoulder raise
	Biceps, latissimus dorsi	Barbell rear deltoid row
		Bent-over dumbbell rear deltoid raise
	Front deltoids, forearms	Dumbbell side lateral raises
	Trapezius	Bent-over low-pulley side lateral
Pectoralis		Around the world
	Triceps, shoulders	Barbell bench press—medium grip
	Triceps, shoulders, latissimus dorsi	Bent-arm barbell pullover
		Butterfly or pec deck fly
	Muscles of the shoulder	Cable crossover
	Muscles of the shoulder	Dumbbell fly
Latissimus dorsi	Biceps, middle back	Close-grip front lats pull-down
	Middle back	Cable rows
		Pull-ups
		Straight-arm pull-down
Triceps brachii	Muscles of the chest and core	Bench dips
		Cable lying triceps extensions
		Cable triceps extension
Biceps brachii	Forearms, latissimus dorsi	Chin-ups
		Concentration curls
		Dumbbell biceps curls
		Barbell curls
Abdominals (rectus abdominis)		Ab crunch machine
		Air bike
		Bent-knee hip raise
		Leg raises
		Cable crunch
		Cross-body crunch
		Crunch—legs on exercise ball
		Incline reverse crunch
		Abdominal ball crunch

continued . . .

TABLE 6.6 Examples of Exercises for Designing a Weight Training Program *continued*

MAJOR MUSCLE GROUP	ADDITIONAL MUSCLES USED	EXERCISES
Rhomboids (strengthens middle back)	Biceps, latissimus dorsi	Bent-over barbell row
	Biceps, latissimus dorsi	Bent-over two-dumbbell row
		Bent-over row with dumbbell
		Incline bench pull
		Lying T-bar row
Erector spinae (lower back)	Hamstrings, gluteals, upper back	Hyperextensions
	Gluteals, obliques, rectus abdominis	Superman
	Gluteals, obliques, rectus abdominis	Knee tucks
Quadriceps		Barbell full squat
	Hamstrings, gluteals, calves	Barbell dead lift
		Cable hip adduction
	Calves, gluteals	Dumbbell rear lunge
		Knee extensions
	Hamstrings, gluteus maximus	Leg press
Gluteals (maximus and medius)		Bridge
		One-legged cable kickback
	Hamstrings	Stiff-legged barbell dead lift
		Glutes kickback
Hamstrings (biceps femoris)	Glutes	Lying leg curls
		Seated leg curls
	Glutes, core	Stability ball leg curls
Brachioradialis (strengthens forearms for baton and firearms)		Wrist curl
		Dumbbell lying supination
		Palms-down dumbbell wrist curl over a bench
		Wrist roller

can then modify your program to fit your specific needs and interests. The available equipment plays a significant role in what changes you can make to your program.

Turn to **assignment 6.2** (in the appendix) to start designing your strength, power, and endurance training program.

Training Programs

You will need to develop your own weight training program. You may want to emphasize endurance, or you may want to include more strength training to meet the demands of the job and BFOR standards to apply for that job. Ultimately, you will determine what works best for you.

Tables 6.7 and 6.8 offer examples of two weight training programs that were developed to show students how a program is organized. The upper beginner/lower intermediate training program is a cardiorespiratory-based program, but it can be used for strength training depending on the weights you incorporate. The intermediate/advanced training program is a strength training program that can incorporate power. An intermediate program should not be tried if you have not done a weight training program before. Because each person has different maximal weights, Table 6.8 is a shell that can be modified and changed to reflect your personal needs and preferences. You can also replace exercises to suit your preference or availability of equipment. Table 6.9 lists optional exercises that you can incorporate into a program.

Many gyms will have exercise instructions posted beside equipment and have qualified personnel who can provide you with instructions and suggestions to suit

TABLE 6.7 Upper Beginner/Lower Intermediate Training Program

	DAY 1 CHEST/TRICEPS	DAY 2 ARMS/SHOULDERS/CORE	DAY 3 LEGS/BICEPS	DAY 4 CARDIO/CORE
Warm-up	• Skipping (3–5 minutes, no breaks) • Add light cardio: Slow jog/cycle/stairmill (5 minutes) • Stretching (min. 10 minutes)	• Skipping (2–3 minutes/no breaks) • Add light cardio: Slow jog/cycle/stairmill (5 minutes) • Stretching (min. 10 minutes)	• Skipping (3–5 minutes/no breaks) • Add light cardio: Slow jog/cycle/stairmill (5 minutes) • Stretching (min. 10 minutes)	• Skipping (3–5 minutes/no breaks) • Add light cardio: Slow jog/cycle/stairmill (5 minutes) • Stretching (min. 10 minutes)
Exercises	*Chest* • Bench press, Dumbbell press, or Incline dumbbell flies: 3 × 15 • Peck deck, Cable press, Cable flies, or Cable crossovers: 3 × 15	*Arms/Shoulders* • Bent-over row pronate: 2 × 12 • Bent-over row supinate: 2 × 12 • Seated row (bar to belly-button, roll shoulders back): 2 × 12 • Shoulder press, Military press, or Arnold press: 3 × 15	*Legs* • Squats: 3 × 12 • Leg press: 3 × 12 • Calf raises: 3 × 12 • Box jump: 3 × 12 • Dumbbell lunges: 3 × 12 • Leg extensions: 3 × 12	*Cardio* • 30–60 minutes of continuous CV exercises (60–85% VO_2 max)
	Triceps • Tricep dips, Lying tricep extensions, Overhead cable or dumbbell extensions, or Tricep kickbacks: 2 × 10 • Push-ups (OPFA standards): 3 × max.	*Core Exercises* • Plank: front, side bridge (work up to 5 minutes) • Stir the pot: 3 × 15 • Jackknife with stability ball: 3 × 15 • Barbell rollout: 3 × 155	*Biceps* • Bicep curls, Preacher curls, or Easy curls with a straight bar: 3 × 12 • Alternate hammer curls or Cable hammer curls: 3 × 12	*Core Exercises* • Plank: front, side bridge) (work up to 5 minutes) • Stir the pot: 3 × 15 • Jackknife with stability ball: 3 × 15 • Barbell rollout: 3 × 15
Rest period	• 30 seconds between sets • CV-based	• 30 seconds between sets • CV-based	• 45 seconds between sets	

TABLE 6.8 Intermediate/Advanced Training Program

		WEEK	1	2	3	4	5	6	7	8
		REPS	6–8	6–8	4–6	10–12	4–6	4–6	10–12	4–6
		% OF MAXIMAL WEIGHT LIFTED	70%	75%	80%	75%	85%	90%	75%	80%
DAY	**EXERCISE**	**SETS**								
1	Bench press	4								
	Fly	3								
	Crossover	2								
	Preacher curl	4								
	Hammer curl	3								
	Concentration biceps curl	2								
	Seated calf	4								
2	Lats pull-down	4								
	Wide-grip chin-up	3								
	Seated rowing	3								
	Back extension	2								
	Triceps dumbbell extension	4								
	Seated row (split rope)[a]	3								
	Close grip bicep bench	2								
3	Squat	4								
	Leg extension	3								
	Leg press	2								
	Reverse curl	3								
	Sevens[b]	3								
	Chest press	3								
	Push-up (fatigue)	3								
4	Military press	4								
	Lateral raise[c]	3								
	Frontal[d]	2								
	Shrug	4								
	Leg curl	4								
	Dip	2								
	Abs (fatigue)	2								

a Seated row (split rope): Pull the split rope straight back to the side, and extend your elbows straight back behind your back.

b Sevens: Biceps curl with easy bar with three positions: (1) start at bottom of extension and go to 90 degrees; (2) start at 90 degrees and bring to full flexion; (3) start at full extension and go to full flexion.

c Lateral raise: Have the dumbbells out to the side with your knees bent, and bring the dumbbells out to the side in a shoulder fly.

d Frontal: Have the dumbbells starting behind the buttocks and raise them to shoulder height out in front.

your program to your needs. Some people rely on free weights only; others incorporate machines with free weights; and others work with what they have at home. You will be the judge of what works best. Your instructor should be able to offer some guidance if you feel that one group of muscles is being worked more than another.

Upper Beginner/Lower Intermediate Program

This program (see Table 6.7), designed for a four-day cycle, is intended to be cardiorespiratory-based. It is not a power-based program, although day 3 works large muscles, which could, depending on the starting weights, be a strength-building component. You must first determine your starting weights so that you can work toward the number of sets and reps indicated.

Intermediate/Advanced Program

This program (see Table 6.8) is for people who have already spent at least 12 weeks in a program and have advanced to being able to lift between 70 and 75 percent of their maximal weight for each exercise, 6–8 reps for three sets. This program addresses gains in strength.

After reviewing this program, turn again to **assignment 6.2** (in the appendix) and add to your strength, power, and endurance program.

TABLE 6.9 Strength, Power, and Endurance Training Program Exercise Options

BODY PART	EQUIPMENT AND EXERCISE		
	No equipment	Exercise ball, bands, tubing, free weights, medicine ball	Machines
Chest	• Push-ups • Dips	• Chest presses • Push-ups • Barbell bench press • Dumbbell chest press on ball • Chest press with tubing • Push-ups with medicine ball	• Bench press • Decline/incline bench press • Cable crossover • Chest fly
Back	• Modified back extensions • Side leg lifts (lower back) • Prone leg lifts (lower back) • Hip extensions (lower back)	• Bent-over rowing (upper body) • Side leg lifts (lower body) • Good mornings • Lats pull-down • Medicine ball twists (upper body)	• Lats pull-downs (upper back) • Lower-back extension (lower back) • Wide pull-downs (upper back) • Seated lats rows (lower back) • Pull-downs (upper back) • Dead lifts (upper back) • Hip extensions (lower back) • Rowing machine (upper and lower back)

continued . . .

TABLE 6.9 Strength, Power, and Endurance Training Program Exercise Options *continued*

BODY PART	EQUIPMENT AND EXERCISE		
	No equipment	**Exercise ball, bands, tubing, free weights, medicine ball**	**Machines**
Legs	• Leg extensions • Leg curls • Squats • Front and side lunges • Stairs • Single and double leg jumps • Vertical jumps	• Seated calf presses • Squats • Wall squats • Front and side lunges • Calf raises • Ball squeeze and lift • Medicine ball lunge • Hamstring rolls • Seated lateral raise with hip flexion • Oblique lift	• Leg extension • Leg curls • Squat • Lunge • Hip extension • Hip abduction • Hip adduction • Standing leg kickback • Seated calf press • Leg press • Hip flexion
Shoulders	• Chin-ups • L-seat dips	• Upright rowing • Shoulder shrugs • Dumbbell press above the head • Upright row • Seated arm raises • Behind-the-head press • Bent-over row	• Rear deltoid rows • Lateral shoulder raise • Seated shoulder press • Front shoulder raise • Shoulder shrug • Reverse fly • Stiff-arm pull-down • Rear deltoid row • Upright rowing • Low-pulley cable cross-raises • Shoulder presses
Arms	• Bicep curls • Tricep curls • Bench dips	• Bicep curls • Tricep curls • Tricep kickbacks • Tricep presses	• Triceps push-down • French press • Triceps extension • Preacher curl • Reverse tricep push-down • Standing biceps curl with pulleys • Tricep kickback • Wrist extension • Wrist curl • Reverse curl • Resisted dip • Hammer grip curls • Overhead extensions
Abdomen	• Curl-ups • Bent-knee side crunches • Crossed-leg oblique crunches • V-sits • Leg lifts • Pelvic tilts • Curl-ups	• Medicine ball crunches • Medicine ball throws to partner	• Reverse crunch • Resisted reverse crunch • Seated (resisted) abdominal crunch • Seated (resisted) oblique abdominal crunch • Ab crunch with attachment • Trunk rotation • Standing oblique crunch

NOTE: Kettlebells have become very popular in the last few years and many of these exercises could use them. However, technique is critical, and therefore having proper instruction to use them is key. Make sure to take lessons to ensure proper posture and technique.

KEY TERMS

1RM, 120
general adaptation, 120
hypertrophy, 119
overload principle, 120
periodization, 124
plyometrics, 121
power training, 121
pyramid training, 130
repetition maximum loading, 121
repetition (rep), 121
set, 121
superset training, 130
trisets, 126

EXERCISES

Multiple Choice

1. Which of the following is a correct safety guideline for weight training?
   a. move joints through the full range of motion
   b. exhale on exertion and inhale on the release
   c. inhale on exertion and exhale on the release
   d. arch your back while lifting heavy weights
   e. arch your back to help you lift your weights
2. During which of the following actions does muscle length remain constant?
   a. plyometrics
   b. overload
   c. isometric
   d. isokinetic
   e. isotonic
3. What is strength, power, and endurance training also known as?
   a. weight training
   b. aerobic training
   c. cardiorespiratory training
   d. resistance training
   e. overload training
4. It is important to rest the muscles for a minimum of how many hours after weight training to avoid overtraining?
   a. 12
   b. 18
   c. 24
   d. 36
   e. 48
5. What is the name of the principle that states that to build muscle mass, the muscle must be subjected to a greater than normal load?
   a. the slow-twitch principle
   b. the isokinetic principle
   c. the recovery principle
   d. the overload principle
   e. the muscle endurance principle
6. What is a group of consecutive repetitions of a resistance exercise called?
   a. a set
   b. a measure
   c. a rep
   d. a sequence
   e. a game
7. Which of the following is poor advice for strength training?
   a. warm up slowly and completely
   b. hold your breath during the lifting phase
   c. select exercises for all major muscle groups
   d. train initially for endurance if you are a beginner
   e. vary the routine to avoid boredom
8. The maximum amount of force that a muscle can generate at one time is called
   a. power
   b. progression
   c. sticking point
   d. muscular endurance
   e. strength

9. The ability of muscle to exert force repeatedly without fatiguing is called
   a. muscular endurance
   b. muscular strength
   c. plyometrics
   d. one repetition maximum
   e. muscle capacity
10. To evaluate dynamic strength, an individual must
   a. perform as many leg press exercises as possible by pressing a heavy weight to exhaustion
   b. do three sets of 20 push-ups within five minutes
   c. perform as many sit-ups as possible in one minute
   d. perform a bench press by lifting the heaviest weight possible
   e. jump repeatedly on and off a box for one minute
11. Overload is defined as
   a. overtraining
   b. working the body harder than accustomed
   c. carbohydrate loading for endurance athletes
   d. periodizing exercises in a program
   e. carrying more weight than is necessary for an exercise
12. Plyometrics training involves
   a. a slow progressive repetition of an exercise
   b. a force exerted by a muscle by maintaining a constant level of resistance
   c. an organized approach to training that involves progressive cycling
   d. an explosive reaction through rapid and powerful muscular contractions
   e. a process characterized by high training volume with moderate training intensity
13. Which of the following factors does NOT put women at a disadvantage in entrance tests?
   a. size
   b. muscular endurance
   c. body composition
   d. hemoglobin levels
   e. muscular strength
14. What is absolute strength?
   a. being able to lift a load once
   b. lifting the greatest load irrespective of your body weight
   c. lifting the greatest load respective to your body weight
   d. lifting the most repetitions irrespective of your body weight
   e. lifting the least repetitions respective to your body weight

Short Answer

1. Define "overload principle."

2. How should you warm up before a workout?

3. What is the difference between pyramid and superset training?

4. What are some of the advantages of circuit training?

5. What are some benefits of interval training?

REFERENCES

American Academy of Pediatrics. (2001). Strength training by children and adolescents. *Pediatrics, 107*, 1470–1472.

American College of Sports Medicine (ACSM). (2002). Progression models in resistance training for healthy adults. *Medicine and Science in Sports and Exercise, 34*, 364–380.

American College of Sports Medicine (ACSM). (2009). Progression models in resistance training for healthy adults. *Medicine and Science in Sports and Exercise, 41*(3), 687–708.

Bickel, C.S., Cross, J.M., & Bamman, M.M. (2011, July). Exercise dosing to retain resistance training adaptations in young and older adults. *Medicine and Science in Sports and Exercise, 43*(7), 1177–1187.

Brechue, W.F., & Mayhew, J.L. (2009). Upper-body work capacity and 1RM prediction are unaltered by increasing muscular strength in college football players. *Journal of Strength and Conditioning Research, 23*(9): 2477–2486.

Bompa, T. (1999). *Periodization: Theory and methodology of training.* Champaign, IL: Human Kinetics.

Boulé, N., Haddad, E., Kenny, G., Wells, G.A., & Sigal, R.J. (2001, September). Effects of exercise on HbA_{IC} and body mass in type 2 diabetes mellitus: A meta-analysis of controlled clinical trials. *Journal of the American Medical Association, 286*(10), 1218–1227.

Canadian Society of Exercise Physiology (CSEP). (2011). *Canadian physical activity guidelines for adults—18–64 years.* http://www.csep.ca/english/view.asp?x=804.

Engelke, K., Kemmler, W., Lauber, D., Beeskow, C., Pintag, R., et al. (2006). Exercise maintains bone density at spine and hip EFOPS: A 3-year longitudinal study in early postmenopausal women. *Osteoporosis International, 17*, 133–142.

Faigenbaum, A.D. (2000). Strength training for children and adolescents. *Clinics in Sports Medicine, 19*, 593–619.

Farenholtz, D. (1995). *Correctional Officer's Physical Abilities Test (COPAT): Physical training, conditioning, and maintenance program.* Ottawa: National Headquarters, Correctional Service of Canada.

Faulkner, J.A., & White, T.P. (1990). Adaptations of skeletal muscle to physical activity. *Proceedings of the International Conference on Exercise, Fitness, and Health* (pp. 265–275). Champaign, IL: Human Kinetics.

Fiatarone, M.A., O'Neill, E.F., Ryan, N.D., Clements, K.M., Solares, G.R., et al. (1994, June 23). Exercise training and nutritional supplementation for physical frailty in very elderly people. *New England Journal of Medicine, 330*, 1769–1775.

Garber, C.E., Blissmer, B., Deschenes, M.R., Franklin, B.A., Lamonte, et al. (2009, March). Quantity and quality of exercise for developing and maintaining cardiorespiratory, musculoskeletal and neuromotor fitness in apparently healthy adults: Guidance for prescribing exercise. Position paper. *Medicine and Science in Sports and Exercise, 41*(3), 687–708.

Gledhill, N., & Shaw, C. (1995, October). Constable Selection Project. Final report: Medical, physical, skills and abilities project. Race Relations and Policing Unit. Toronto: Ministry of the Solicitor General and Correctional Services.

Jurca, R., LaMonte, M.J., Church, T.S., Earnest, C.P., Fitzgerald, et al. (2004). Associations with muscle strength and aerobic fitness with metabolic syndrome in men. *Medicine and Science in Sports and Exercise*, *36*, 1301–1307.

Kerksick, C.M., Wismann-Bunn, J., Fogt, D., Thomas, A.R., Taylor, L., et al. (2010). Changes in weight loss, body composition and cardiovascular disease risk after altering macronutrient distributions during a regular exercise program in obese women. *Nutrition Journal*, *9*, 59–78.

Koutedakis, Y., Stavropoulos-Kalinoglou, A., & Metsios, G. (2005). The significance of muscular strength in dance. *Journal of Dance Medicine and Science*, *9*(1), 29–34.

Marcell, T.J. (2003). Sarcopenia: Causes, consequences and preventions. *Journal of Gerontology*, *58A*(10), 911–916.

Mayhew, J.L., Ball, T.E., Arnold, M.D., & Bowen, J.C. (1992). Prediction of 1RM bench press from relative endurance performance in college males and females. *Journal of Applied Sports Science Research*, *6*, 200–206.

Miller, J.P., Pratley, R.E., Goldberg, A.P., Gordon, P., Rubin, et al. (1994). Strength training increases insulin action in healthy 50- to 65-year-old men. *Journal of Applied Physiology*, *77*, 1122–1127.

National Institute on Drug Abuse. (2006, August). Anabolic steroid abuse. Research Report Series. http://www.drugabuse.gov/PDF/RRSteroids.pdf.

Nelson, M.E., Fiatarone, M.A., Morganti, C.M., Trice, I., Greenberg, R.A., et al. (1994). Effects of high-intensity strength training on multiple risk factors for osteoporotic fractures. *Journal of the American Medical Association*, *272*, 1909–1914.

Pratley, R.B., Nicklas, M., Rubin, J., Miller, A., Smith, M., et al. (1994). Strength training increases resting metabolic rate and norepinephrine levels in healthy 50- to 65-year-old men. *Journal of Applied Physiology*, *76*, 133–137.

Ontario Police College. Physical Training Department. (1994). *Weight training personal program design.* Toronto: Queen's Printer.

Risch, S., Newell, N., Pollock, M., Risch, E., Langer, H., et al. (1993). Lumbar strengthening in chronic low-back pain patients. *Spine*, *18*, 232–238.

Royal Canadian Mounted Police (RCMP). (2001). Emergency response team: Selection criteria. http://www.rcmp-grc.gc.ca/ert/ert2_e.htm.

Shephard, R., & Bonneau, J. (2002). Assuring gender equity in recruitment standards for police officers. *Applied Physiology, Nutrition and Metabolism*, *27*(3), 263–295.

Shipley, P. (1998). *Ontario provincial weight training program.* Toronto: Ontario Provincial Police and Ministry of the Solicitor General and Correctional Services.

Stensvold, D., Tjonna, A.E., Skaug, E., Aspenses, S., Stolen, T., et al. (2010). Strength training versus aerobic interval training to modify risk factors of metabolic syndrome. *Journal of Applied Physiology*, *108*, 804–810.

Stone, M.H., & O'Bryant, H.S. (1987). *Weight training: A scientific approach.* Minneapolis: Burgess.

Stone, M.H., O'Bryant, H.S., & Garhammer, J. (1981). A hypothetical model for strength training. *Journal of Sports Medicine and Physical Fitness*, *21*(336), 342–351.

PART 3

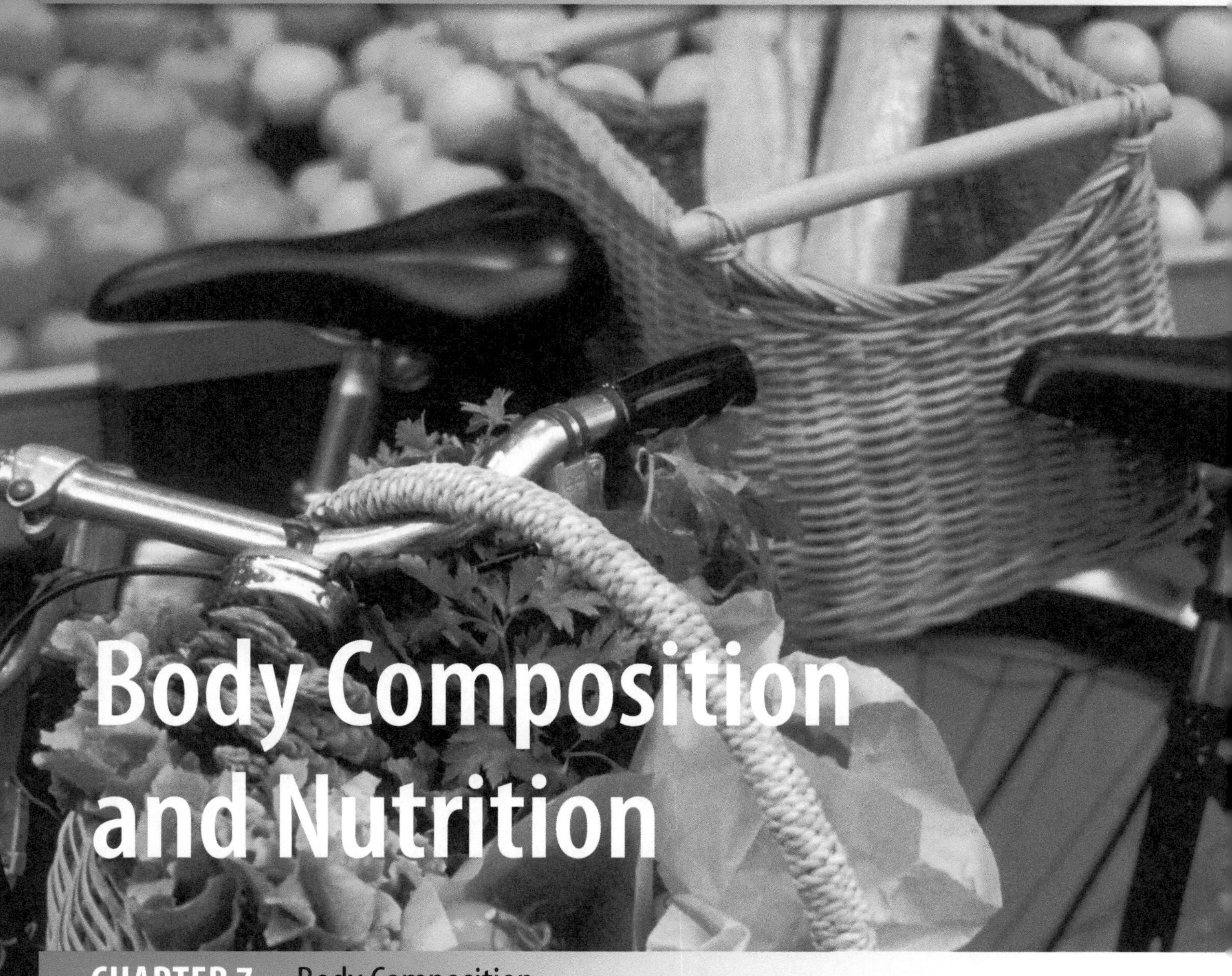

Body Composition and Nutrition

7

Body Composition

LEARNING OBJECTIVES

After completing this chapter, you should be able to:

- Understand the issues surrounding overweight and obesity in Canada.
- Distinguish between the concepts of overfat and overweight.
- Describe the three somatotypes (body types).
- Explain how basal metabolism affects body composition.
- Explain eating disorders, including anorexia nervosa, bulimia nervosa, binge eating disorder (BED), and the female athlete triad.
- Describe several methods for measuring body composition.

OVERVIEW

In Chapter 1 you learned that weight-related problems are a health risk for many Canadians. This chapter examines obesity, eating disorders, and other weight-related issues more closely by delving into the question of what constitutes a healthy body composition.

Misguided Views of the Body

While many Canadians are justly concerned about being overweight, many others who are within a healthy weight range are obsessed with weight loss. The media equate beauty with thinness in women and muscularity in men, ideals that fuel the obsession with weight (CSEP, 1996). Many people compare their bodies to the perfect long limbs and liposuctioned bellies in airbrushed photos. Losing weight isn't simply about fitting into your "skinny jeans." The stress and anxiety caused by unrealistic weight-loss goals can lead to serious eating disorders, such as anorexia, bulimia, and yo-yo dieting.

Recent research suggests that we have nurtured an obesity epidemic (Sharma & Kushner, 2009). With our sedentary work habits and lifestyles, a constant time crunch, and our fast-food culture, we have turned obesity into a chronic disease. People struggle to maintain a healthy body weight. If eating better and exercising more worked for everyone, there would not be so many fad diets on the market. The simplistic lifestyle advice to "eat less—move more" (ELMM) is not very effective—a fact well known to most people who have tried this approach. The reality is that many factors can hinder your ability to lose weight, including mental illness, chronic pain, family or social barriers, and environmental conditions. It is not always easy to make healthy choices. Like smoking cessation, effective obesity prevention may require a multifaceted, long-term approach involving interventions that operate on multiple levels and in complementary ways (PHAC, 2011).

There has been a significant increase in the combined overweight/obesity rate among youth aged 12 to 17 over the past 30 years (Shields, 2005), and almost one-third (32.6 percent) of Canadians over the age of 18 have a **body mass index (BMI)** in the overweight category (Health Canada, 2010).

body mass index (BMI) a method for assessing body composition, based on weight and height

The BMI is a popular method among health-care professionals for determining whether, and to what extent, a person is overweight or obese. It is based on a weight-to-height ratio, and excludes considerations of frame size and muscle mass. Excluding pregnant women and those under age 18, whose rate of growth varies, the BMI puts individuals into four categories: underweight, normal weight, overweight, and obese. The obese category is divided further into three classes.

In Canada in 2009, more adult males (39.1 percent) than females (26 percent) were either overweight or obese (PHAC, 2011). The health consequences of excess weight include increased risk for type 2 diabetes, cardiovascular disease, high blood pressure, osteoarthritis, some cancers, and gallbladder disease.

DID YOU KNOW?

Between 2001 and 2009, the percentage of Canadian adults with a BMI in the overweight category rose from 14.1 percent to 32.6 percent. The BMI in the obese category went from 14.9 percent in 2003 to 17.2 percent in 2009.

SOURCES: Health Canada, 2010; Shields, 2010.

Canadians have been battling the bulge for decades, but despite better food labelling, healthier food options in schools, reduced amounts of trans fats in processed foods, and tax incentives to promote physical activity, the costs of obesity to the Canadian health-care system have risen from nearly $1.6 billion in 2001 to an estimated $4.6 billion (in direct costs) to $7.1 billion (in indirect costs) (Katzmarzyk

& Janssen, 2004; Community Foundation of Canada, 2011). Three factors contribute to this burden: the increase in numbers of individuals who are obese; rising costs of treatments specific to obesity-related illnesses; and a demographic shift, with a general trend for older individuals (our fastest-growing population demographic) to be obese.

In the 1960s and 1970s, insurance companies based their life and health premiums on height–weight tables. The more you weighed within a certain height class, the more you paid. The insurance companies did not take bone size into account, nor did they look at fat as a percentage of body weight. They simply assumed that higher weight equalled higher risk. But research in the 1990s led health experts to the idea that there are many kinds of healthy body shapes and sizes, and to the notion that each person has an "acceptable weight range." We no longer look simply at weight, but now consider the percentages of fat, bone, and muscle in our bodies. Further, being overweight for your height does not necessarily mean that you are unfit.

Although body image is often assumed to be a women's problem, research has revealed that men are increasingly dissatisfied, preoccupied, and impaired by concerns over their appearance. One study found that the percentage of men who are dissatisfied with their overall appearance (43 percent) had nearly tripled over 25 years (Pope, Phillips, & Olivardia, 2000). There is also a growing form of male *body*

FACTS ABOUT ...

Body Weight

Body weight is affected by our genetic makeup, our eating choices, our level of physical activity, and our social, cultural, physical, and economic environments. Where we live, learn, play, and work are all factors that affect our body weight. Consider the following data:

- Statistics Canada has determined that those with less than a secondary education eat less fruit and vegetables and have higher rates of obesity.
- In terms of socio-economic status, obesity rates are higher among Canadian women in middle- and upper-middle-income households compared with highest-income households, while men in lower-middle-income households are less obese than those in highest-income households.
- Physical activity levels are higher among Canadians who have a positive social support network and are in more frequent contact with their friends and family.
- People who work in physically active jobs have a lower likelihood of being obese.
- People who are obese as children are more likely to be obese as young adults.
- Neighbourhoods that have better street lighting, sidewalks, recreational facilities, and playgrounds have more physically fit individuals living in them.
- In 2004, off-reserve Aboriginal adults had an obesity rate 1.6 times higher (38 percent) than the Canadian average of 23 percent.
- In 2004, 21 percent of Canadian children aged 2 to 5, 26 percent of those aged 6 to 11, and 29 percent of youth aged 12 to 17 were overweight or obese. Measured (as opposed to self-reported) obesity has increased 2.5 times in the last two decades.
- Mental health problems are associated with eating disorders such as anorexia, bulimia, and binge eating. Girls and women are affected more than boys and men.

SOURCES: King, Fitzhugh, Bassett, McLaughlin, Strath, et al., 2001; Health Canada, 2002; Addy, Wilson, Kirtland, Ainsworth, Sharpe, et al., 2004; Shields, 2005; Tjepkema, 2005; CIHI, 2006; Pan, Cameron, Des Meules, Morrison, Craig, et al., 2009.

dysmorphic disorder (excessive concern about a perceived defect in one's physical features) called *muscle dysmorphia*, which is a preoccupation that one's body is too small and inadequately muscular (Phillips & Castle, 2001). Muscle dysmorphia may lead to potentially dangerous abuse of anabolic steroids, and studies indicate that 6 to 7 percent of high school boys have used these drugs (Kanayama & Pope, 2012). While the cause of body dysmorphic disorder is unknown and is probably multifactorial, involving genetic, neurobiological, evolutionary, and psychological factors, social pressures for boys and men to be large and muscular almost certainly contribute to the development of muscle dysmorphia (Phillips & Castle, 2001; Kanayama & Pope, 2012). This disorder may be accompanied by an eating disorder.

Body Composition

body composition the proportion of lean tissue to fat in the body

Body composition refers to the proportion of lean tissue to fat in the body. Determining this proportion can provide an indicator of overall health and fitness in relation to weight and age. Many factors, including sex, age, heredity, activity, overall nutrition, and eating patterns, affect body composition.

Your body needs fat for fuel and other purposes, but if you consume too much fat and neglect physical activity, you end up with non-essential fat stored in various areas of your body. Adults over 30 tend to carry more fat on their frames than younger people do. Generally, women accumulate more fat than men do, and it tends to be distributed more evenly over the entire body (among men, the fat tends to accumulate more on the trunk and less on the extremities). Abdominal obesity is one of the six components of *metabolic syndrome*—a cluster of risk factors that increase an individual's likelihood of developing cardiovascular diseases, diabetes, and a number of other conditions (Grundy, Brewer, Cleeman, Smith, Lenfant, et al., 2004).

But being overweight is not the same as being obese, because many physically fit people are overweight from muscle gain (muscle is heavier than fat). Of course, people can be overweight because they carry excess fat, but it is important to distinguish between the concepts of overfat and overweight.

All fat in your body is classified as either essential or non-essential fat. Essential fat is required for normal functioning of your body. Deposits of this fat can be found in your muscles, heart, brain, spinal cord, nerves, lungs, and liver. Fat serves as an energy reserve, a regulator of body functions, an insulator against heat loss, and a protector against physical shock.

Non-essential or storage fat is stored below the surface of the skin and around major organs. Although some fat is vital for insulation and organ protection, too much can put you at risk for disease.

Recent research has suggested that obese individuals who are otherwise healthy—free of all obesity-related co-morbidities (category 0) or with subclinical levels of obesity-related co-morbidities such as pre-diabetes, pre-hypertension, occasional dyspnea (difficulty breathing), and mental illness (category 1)—could live just as long as their lean counterparts (Kuk, Ardern, Church, Sharma, Padwal, et al., 2011). Kuk and colleagues (2011) found that it is better to engage in a healthy lifestyle that includes physical activity rather than repeatedly trying to lose weight, because most people regain the weight they lose. It is believed that the cycling of weight loss and gain may be more detrimental than maintaining an elevated body weight and exercising if the person has no other health issues.

Somatotypes

Your body composition is affected by your **somatotype** (body type). Most people have a genetic predisposition toward a specific somatotype, although it is often mixed with some traits of a second somatotype. There are three somatotypes: ectomorphic, mesomorphic, and endomorphic.

- An *ectomorph* has a low percentage of fat in the body, small bones, a small amount of muscle, and a high metabolic rate. With this light build and slight muscular development, ectomorphs usually have a harder time gaining weight, and spend more time on strength training and less on cardiorespiratory training.
- A *mesomorph* has a low to medium percentage of fat in the body, medium to large bones, a large amount of muscle, and a medium to high metabolic rate. Many mesomorphs have a large chest and long torso, and are able to build muscle easily.
- An *endomorph* has a high percentage of fat in the body, large bones, a small amount of muscle, and a low metabolic rate. This body type tends to have a stocky build, wide hips, and a tendency to gain weight. Because this weight gain accumulates around the middle, endomorphs have difficulty losing weight. They need to pay close attention to their diet, and focus on cardiorespiratory training over strength training.

Although your somatotype is inherited and cannot be changed, diet and exercise can reduce the percentage of fat in your body.

somatotype
there are three somatotypes (body types): ectomorphic, mesomorphic, and endomorphic

Metabolism

Metabolism describes the chemical processes that occur within a living cell or organism that are necessary for maintaining life. Some substances are broken down to yield energy for vital processes (for example, carbohydrates are broken down into glucose), while other substances are synthesized (such as muscle tissue and cells).

DID YOU KNOW?

Each 5-unit increment in BMI above 25 kg/m^2 is associated with increases of 29 percent risk for overall mortality, 41 percent for vascular mortality, and 210 percent for diabetes-related mortality.

SOURCE: Yusuf, Hawken, Ounpuu, Bautise, Franzosi, et al., 2005.

Basal Metabolism

Body composition is also affected by **basal metabolism**, the amount of energy a body at rest needs to maintain essential functions. The **basal metabolic rate (BMR)** is the speed at which energy is used by the body. Factors affecting the BMR include age, sex, and level of physical activity.

Your metabolism affects your ability to lose or gain weight. A high metabolic rate makes it easier to burn fat and lose weight. If your metabolism is not working properly, you will find it more difficult to keep your weight stable or to lose weight.

Cutting calories lowers your metabolic rate. Your body senses the reduction in energy intake and slows down the burning of fat to protect the fat it has. After about three months your metabolic rate levels off and you no longer lose weight. If you return to your old eating habits, your body will store more fat than it used to because the metabolic rate remains depressed. Eventually you may gain back all the weight, and even put on more.

When you fast for at least six to eight hours, the body protects its fat reserves by starting to break down protein instead of fat for energy. Because protein is an im-

basal metabolism
the amount of energy a body at rest needs to maintain essential functions

basal metabolic rate (BMR)
the speed at which energy is used by the body

portant constituent of muscle and other tissues, fasting harms key parts of the body. (This is true to an even greater extent in the extreme cases of anorexia and bulimia.)

The key to maintaining a healthy weight is to combine proper eating (as described in Chapter 8) with a good exercise program. A program of cardiorespiratory exercise 30 minutes a day, every day of the week, will improve your cardiovascular system, increase your metabolic rate, and burn fat. Weight and strength training for 20–30 minutes a day, three to five days a week, will increase your muscular strength and endurance, make you leaner, and have a beneficial effect on bone density.

Measuring Overweight and Obesity

Health Canada (2003) has developed a weight classification system to identify weight-related health risks in populations and individuals over 18 years old. This system categorizes individuals' risks based on body weight, and is measured by body mass index (BMI) and the level of abdominal fat as determined by waist circumference (WC). For those 65 years and older, "the normal range may begin slightly above a BMI of 18.5 and extend into the overweight range" (Health Canada, 2000, p. 10). Under the current Canadian guidelines for body weight classification, the term *overweight* refers to anyone with a BMI of 25.0 to 29.9. The term *obese* refers to someone with a BMI of 30 or more (Health Canada, 2000). BMI is calculated by dividing your body weight in kilograms by the square of your height in metres (Health Canada, 2000). For example, someone who is 1.8 metres tall and weighs 71 kilograms would have a BMI of 21.9 (that is, $71/1.8^2 = 21.9$).

Go to **assignment 7.1** (in the appendix) and determine your BMI.

What Does the BMI Score Mean?

For adult males and females, a BMI greater than 30.0 indicates obesity. Underweight adult males and females have a BMI of less than 18.5. Being underweight increases the risk of undernutrition, osteoporosis, infertility, and impaired immunocompetence (Health Canada, 2003). A very low BMI also alerts health-care professionals to the possibility of anorexia or similar problems. In Canada almost one-half of Canadians are overweight or obese, while a similar proportion is in the normal weight range, and a very small proportion is underweight (Health Canada, 2010). Canadians rank in the middle of the G8 countries in terms of the proportion of the population that is obese. See Table 7.1 for an overview of body weight classifications.

It is important to note that a high BMI is not necessarily a problem for competitive athletes and bodybuilders (whose BMI may be high because their muscle mass is greater than average), pregnant or lactating women, children, and sedentary elderly people. Other tools are needed to assess the body composition of these groups. We do know that overweight status indicates some risks to health. Research suggests that regular physical activity can decrease the risk of several health problems. Equally, a nutritious diet has been shown to decrease some of the risks associated with being overweight.

TABLE 7.1

Canadian Guidelines for Body Weight Classification in Adults

Classification	BMI category (kg/m^2)	Risk of developing health problems
Underweight	< 18.5	Increased
Normal weight	18.5–24.9	Least
Overweight	25.0–29.9	Increased
Obese Class I	30.0–34.9	High
Obese Class II	35.0–39.9	Very high
Obese Class III	≥ 40.0	Extremely high

SOURCE: Health Canada, 2000; adapted from WHO, 2000.

Edmonton Obesity Staging System

Recent research has shifted the health focus from how big people are to how sick they are. Sharma and Kushner (2009) have developed a more holistic understanding of the potential impact of weight on an individual's health and functioning. The Edmonton Obesity Staging System (EOSS) categorizes obesity-related co-morbidities in five stages (0 to 4) to complement anthropometric indices (measurements of the percentage of fat a person has) and determine the best course of treatment for a specific individual. The co-morbidity variables include type 2 diabetes, hypertension, high blood cholesterol, osteoarthritis, liver disease, kidney disease, limitations of physical functioning, metabolic syndrome, and hypertriglyceridemic waist (large waist measurement combined with a high proportion of fatty acids in the blood). The EOSS goes beyond simply rating patients on a scale. Researchers consider not only the cardiometabolic risk or the consequences of excess weight, but also the mental and functional problems that obese patients may encounter. Future research will determine the validity of this index (Padwal, Pafewski, Allison, & Sharma, 2011).

Waist Circumference

Waist circumference (WC) is an indicator of health risks associated with excess abdominal fat. WC measurement can be used for individuals with a BMI in the 18.5–34.9 range. For BMIs equal to or exceeding 35.0, WC measurements do not provide additional information regarding the level of risk.

waist circumference (WC) an indicator of health risk associated with abdominal fat

Go to **assignment 7.2** (in the appendix) to determine your waist circumference.

Health Risk Classification

Excess fat around the waist and upper body (also described as an apple-shaped body) is associated with greater health risks than excess fat in the hip and thigh area (a pear-shaped body). A WC at or above 102 centimetres (40 inches) for men and 88 centimetres (35 inches) for women is associated with an increased risk of developing health problems such as type 2 diabetes, heart disease, and high blood pressure. The risk of developing health problems increases as WC increases beyond these cut-off points. Therefore, individuals who are overweight but not obese and who have a higher BMI are in a lower risk category. In other words, their muscle weighs more, and they are at less risk as long as they keep abdominal fat off. However, even if a person's BMI falls within the normal weight range, a high WC indicates some health risk. A marked weight change—either a gain or loss—may place someone at risk even if he or she remains within the same BMI category. Unhealthy weight-loss practices, such as restrictive eating habits, can also increase a person's risk of health problems, even for those of normal weight (Health Canada, 2003). See Table 7.2 for an overview of health risk classifications.

TABLE 7.2 Health Risk Classification Using Both BMI and WC

		BMI		
		Normal	Overweight	Obese Class 1
WC	< 102 cm (males) < 88 cm (females)	Least risk	Increased risk	High risk
	≥ 102 cm (males) ≥ 88 cm (females)	Increased risk	High risk	Very high risk

SOURCE: Adapted from National Institutes of Health, 1998.

Skinfold Measurements

skinfold measurement measurement of fat just below the skin surface at five points on the body to determine the percentage of body fat

The Canadian Society for Exercise Physiology (1996) recommends **skinfold measurement** for determining whether people whose BMI is greater than 27 are truly overweight or overfat. Unlike BMI measurement, skinfold measurement takes body type into account. The procedure involves using calipers to measure skinfolds at five points on the body. Fitness club staff or your college fitness instructor may be available to assess your body composition this way.

Waist-to-Hip Ratio Measurement

waist-to-hip ratio (WHR) measurement a method for assessing body composition, based on the relationship between the girth of the waist and the girth of the hips

Waist-to-hip ratio (WHR) measurement is based on the relationship between the girth of the waist and the girth of the hips. Most people store excess fat either around the middle (making the body apple-shaped) or on the hips (making the body pear-shaped). It is generally accepted that people who carry their extra weight around the middle face a greater health risk than those who carry it on the hips. Nevertheless, obese people are at greater risk than non-obese people, no matter where the excess fat is stored.

Turn to **assignment 7.3** (in the appendix) and determine your WHR.

For men, a WHR of 1.0 or greater indicates that excess fat is being carried around the middle, increasing the health risks associated with hypokinetic diseases (diseases related to lack of physical activity). For women, the crucial number is 0.8 or greater.

Eating Disorders

Overweight is not the only kind of body image problem that occurs in our society. Western society's obsession with thinness as the ideal—especially in women, as seen in magazines, movies, and advertisements—causes many people, both male and female, constant anxiety about their weight and body shape. Many assume that being thin equates with being attractive, successful, in control, and popular, while being overweight signifies being weak-willed, lazy, and out of control. (Of course, this assumption is untrue, as many thin people feel unhappy, unhealthy, and unpopular!) Poor self-image and underlying emotional problems may cause an individual to develop an eating disorder.

Eating disorders carry with them a high risk of other mental and physical illnesses that can even lead to death. Eating smaller or larger portions of food than usual is common, but for some people, portion size turns into a compulsion and their eating behaviours become extreme. If they succeed in losing weight, they gain a temporary sense of achievement. But because caloric deprivation lowers basal metabolic rate and increases the likelihood of binge eating, such people tend to regain the weight, causing them greater dissatisfaction and lower self-esteem. Losing and regaining weight then becomes a vicious cycle.

Extreme and repeated dieting can exact a physical toll, including anemia (low iron in the blood), delayed or absent menstruation, dehydration, high cholesterol, hair loss, nail destruction,

FACTS ABOUT . . .

Dieting and Weight Loss

- At any given time, 70 percent of women and 35 percent of men are dieting.
- One out of five women in Ontario between the ages of 20 and 34 is underweight.
- 40 percent of nine-year-old girls have dieted, despite being within healthy weight ranges.
- 80 percent of 18-year-old women have dieted.
- Approximately 3 percent of women will be affected by an eating disorder during their lifetime.

SOURCES: Health Canada, 2002; Bear, 2011.

and change of liver function. Muscle and lean tissue are lost first, because the body protects its fat, which is required for hormonal functions. The risk of dying from heart disease is 70 percent higher in those with fluctuating weight than in those whose weight remains stable, regardless of initial weight, blood pressure, smoking habits, cholesterol level, or level of physical activity (Bear, 2011).

Psychologically, dieting can cause depression, mood swings, reduced sexual interest, and impaired concentration and judgment. Some people develop alcohol dependency and anxiety disorders, particularly if bullying is a factor in their compulsion to lose weight. In extreme cases, bullying has led to suicide and even murder—all because of how people looked and felt.

Law enforcement officers may come to recognize a number of eating disorders as they deal with individuals in policing. These include anorexia nervosa, bulimia nervosa, binge eating disorder, and female athlete triad disorder. Treatment of eating disorders usually involves hospitalization and behavioural therapy to help the person regain control over his or her perception of body image, eating habits, and self-esteem in relation to friends and family (Bear, 2011).

FYI

Warning Signs of Eating Disorders

The following behaviours may indicate that someone you care about has an eating disorder:

1. a marked decrease or increase in weight that is not related to a medical condition
2. a preoccupation with food
3. unusual eating habits, such as cutting up food into tiny pieces, playing with food, or hiding/disguising uneaten food
4. hiding or hoarding of large amounts of food in unusual places (for example, bedroom, closet)
5. a preoccupation with weight
6. constant dissatisfaction with weight and body size/image despite weight loss, clothing size, etc.
7. negative and self-critical comments about body shape, size, and physical appearance
8. behavioural changes including isolation, depression, irritability, or loss of trust in friends
9. frequent trips to the washroom, especially after meals
10. smell of vomit in the washroom or on the breath
11. abuse of laxatives, diet pills, or diuretics
12. excessive exercising or multiple, daily trips to the gym
13. wearing of baggy clothes to mask weight gain or loss

Help is available

Help for eating disorders is available, for you and the person you care about. Contact:

- Healthy Eating: www.mhp.gov.on.ca/en/healthy-eating
- What's Eating You?: www.whatseatingyou.com
- National Eating Disorder Information Centre: www.nedic.ca
- Dieticians of Canada: www.dietitians.ca
- Nutrition—Centers for Disease Control: www.cdc.gov/nutrition

Anorexia Nervosa

anorexia nervosa
an eating disorder in which individuals do not eat enough to maintain a healthy body weight

Anorexia nervosa is a serious medical and psychiatric disorder. People who suffer from it do not get enough calories to maintain a healthy body weight. They usually begin at a normal or slightly above-average weight, and then starve themselves and exercise excessively to burn calories. These individuals refuse to maintain a normal body weight and have a distorted perception of the shape or size of their bodies (American Psychiatric Association, 1994). Anorexia often begins during adolescence, when many people have poor self-confidence and self-image.

Bulimia Nervosa

bulimia nervosa
an eating disorder in which individuals have an intense fear of overweight and overfat that causes binge eating followed by self-induced vomiting

People who suffer from **bulimia nervosa** may be able to maintain a normal weight but have an intense fear of being overweight and overfat. They have a distorted body image. Bulimia is characterized by uncontrollable binge eating followed by self-induced vomiting. Many bulimics rely on laxatives and diuretics to prevent food from being absorbed by their bodies. The majority of bulimics are women in their late teens or early 20s who have suffered a critical incident. They have difficulty handling emotions like depression, loneliness, and anger. They also have low self-esteem and tend to come from families with high expectations. The eating disorder may be an attempt to gain control over one part of their life.

Besides bingeing and purging, symptoms of bulimia include fluctuations in weight, dental decay, salivary gland enlargement, bowel problems or digestive complaints, and feelings of guilt and depression (American Psychiatric Association, 1994; Stice, 2002; Jacobi, Hayward, de Zwaan, Kraemer, & Agras, 2004).

DID YOU KNOW?

Although statistically more females than males are diagnosed with anorexia and bulimia, approximately 10 percent of those with eating disorders are male. Men who are runners, wrestlers, bodybuilders, and jockeys appear to be at higher risk than the general population.
SOURCE: Wolf, 1991.

Binge Eating Disorder

binge eating disorder (BED)
an eating disorder associated with obesity, where the person alternately eats obsessively and then diets and restricts eating; the disorder is diagnosed if the person does not follow the binge eating with compensatory behaviours such as vomiting, excessive exercise, or laxative abuse

Binge eating disorder (BED) is diagnosed if the binge eating is not followed by compensatory behaviours such as vomiting, excessive exercise, or laxative abuse. This disorder is associated with obesity. BED usually starts during adolescence or young adulthood. Men are more likely to be affected by BED than by other eating disorders. Individuals with BED who are obese must contend with negative societal attitudes toward obesity. As a result, many become isolated and lose self-esteem. They are hungry because they have been dieting or restricting their eating in response to that hunger. Many overeat to comfort themselves, to avoid uncomfortable situations, or to numb their feelings. They feel that they are out of control and unable to stop eating.

Female Athlete Triad

female athlete triad
an eating disorder among female athletes that is defined by three conditions: disordered eating, amenorrhea, and osteoporosis

The **female athlete triad** was first described in the early 1990s. This condition is defined by three signs: disordered eating, amenorrhea, and osteoporosis. Although researchers are still debating the prevalence of female athlete triad, many women who suffer from it may not be diagnosed (Yeager, Agostini, Nattiv, & Drinkwater, 1993). The concern is not only for the performance of these athletes but also for their future health.

Disordered Eating

The first sign in the female athlete triad is the precipitating event for the triad (Yeager et al., 1993). "Disordered eating" refers to a broad spectrum of abnormal eating behaviours (Sanborn, Horea, Siemers, & Dieringer, 2000). At the severe end of the spectrum are athletes who meet the diagnostic criteria for anorexia or bulimia. At the other end of the spectrum are athletes who consume fewer calories than their body requires. They may appear to be eating a healthy diet, but they are not consuming enough calories. Whichever end of the spectrum applies to a woman, this mismatch of energy needed versus what she is consuming creates an energy drain on the endocrine system, which in turn leads to the second and third signs of the triad.

Amenorrhea

Amenorrhea is the cessation of menstrual periods for three or more consecutive cycles. It is the result of insufficient estrogen production by the ovaries. Missing periods is a warning sign that something is not right in the female body. Confirmation by medical diagnosis is important and should not be ignored. Women who do not menstruate for more than three or four months can lose bone strength.

Amenorrhea is associated with a condition known as *anorexia athletica*, in which people exercise excessively because they believe this will help them master their bodies and give them a sense of power, control, and self-respect. These excessive behaviours may lead to amenorrhea. Some of the symptoms include over-exercise, being fanatical about weight and diet, taking time away from school, work, and relationships to exercise, a focus on the outcome of exercising rather than the fun of participating, a belief that self-worth is dependent on physical results, disappointment with training outcomes, and making statements such as, "It's okay to exercise this much because I'm an athlete" (National Eating Disorder Information Centre, 2005).

Osteoporosis

Osteoporosis is another consequence of inadequate estrogen. Yeager and colleagues (1993) describe osteoporosis in the female athlete triad as "premature bone loss or inadequate bone formation." They point out that the failure to build bone at a normal rate or losing bone density at a young age leads to short- and long-term problems, including stress fractures and early bone mineral density loss. After the age of 30, women can expect to lose an average of 0.5 percent of bone density per year, a rate that accelerates to 2 percent after menopause (Yeager et al., 1993). Without estrogen, these young athletes may never be able to maximize bone mineral density.

Treatment for female athlete triad disorder takes multiple approaches. In addition to medical diagnosis and supervision, the athlete requires nutritional education and some form of counselling to deal with the disorder.

It is important for athletes not to skip meals and snacks; they need to maintain enough energy for competition. Snacking on foods such as bagels, cheese, unsalted nuts and seeds, raw vegetables, fruit, and granola

FYI

Female Athlete Triad Update

In 2007, the American College of Sport Medicine (ACSM) redefined female athlete triad disorder as a continuous spectrum, as follows:

- Disordered eating has been replaced with a spectrum ranging from "optimal energy availability" to "low energy availability with or without an eating disorder."
- Amenorrhea has been replaced with a spectrum ranging from "eumenorrhea" (normal menstruation) to "functional hypothalamic amenorrhea" (cessation of menses due to a problem with the hypothalamus gland).
- Osteoporosis has been replaced with a spectrum ranging from "optimal bone health" to "osteoporosis."

ACSM emphasizes that energy availability is the cornerstone on which the other two components of the triad rest. Without correction, the impact of this syndrome is not fully realized until menopause, when bone loss is accelerated.

SOURCE: Nattiv, Loucks, Manore, Sanborn, Sundgot-Borgen, et al., 2007.

bars will aid in acquiring the required amount of iron, calcium, and protein. It is also important for female athletes to keep track of their menstrual periods and to discuss any irregularities with a physician.

If you recognize the symptoms of any eating disorder in yourself or a friend, do not hesitate to do something about it. There are excellent counselling services available that can help individuals get back on track and get proper medical attention. As a police officer, while you are not qualified to make diagnoses, you can watch for signs that should not be ignored. These may include physical or sexual abuse, emotional abuse (teasing, harassment, or bullying), perfectionism, behavioural rigidity, and substance abuse in elite-performance and competitive sports, in which body shape and size are factors.

KEY TERMS

anorexia nervosa, 154
basal metabolic rate (BMR), 149
basal metabolism, 149
binge eating disorder (BED), 154
body composition, 148
body mass index (BMI) , 146
bulimia nervosa, 154
female athlete triad, 154
skinfold measurement, 152
somatotype, 149
waist circumference (WC), 151
waist-to-hip ratio (WHR) measurement, 152

EXERCISES

Multiple Choice

1. The following signs all indicate an eating disorder except
   a. unusual eating behaviours such as cutting up food into very small pieces, playing with food, or hiding or disguising food that is uneaten
   b. disordered eating, amenorrhea, and osteoporosis
   c. an intense fear of being overweight and overfat
   d. satisfaction with body weight and body shape or size
   e. uncontrollable binge eating followed by self-induced vomiting
2. What is one health risk associated with obesity?
   a. type 2 diabetes
   b. glaucoma
   c. nerve disorder
   d. indigestion
   e. hernia
3. Which of the following is true about overweight?
   a. it is defined as "excessive abdominal fat"
   b. it is possible to be obese and not overweight
   c. overweight and obesity mean the same thing
   d. it is possible to be overweight but not obese
   e. overweight is the same as being underweight
4. Which of the following is a characteristic of anorexia nervosa?
   a. intense fear of fat
   b. denial of appetite
   c. avoidance of food
   d. excessive exercising
   e. all of the above
5. The female athlete triad is characterized by
   a. disordered eating, amenorrhea, and osteoporosis
   b. disordered eating, dysmenorrhea, and weight gain
   c. weight gain, amenorrhea, and excessive exercise
   d. weight gain, amenorrhea, and osteoporosis
   e. none of the above
6. Basal metabolic rate (BMR) is
   a. the sum of all the processes by which food energy is used by the body
   b. the body's total daily energy expenditure
   c. the energy required to digest a meal
   d. the speed at which energy is used by the body
   e. the energy required to start your day
7. The body mass index (BMI) is determined by
   a. skinfolds
   b. body weight
   c. body height
   d. body weight and body height
   e. body weight and skinfolds
8. The three somatotype bodies are
   a. ectomorphic, endomorphic, and mesomorphic
   b. ectomorphic, endomorphic, and mendomorphic
   c. ectomorphic, mesomorphic, and cytomorphic
   d. endomorphic, mesomorphic, and octomorphic
   e. endomorphic, mesomorphic, and mendomorphic

9. A high BMI may indicate
- **a.** a low immune system
- **b.** overweight
- **c.** anorexia
- **d.** a healthy body
- **e.** none of the above

10. The waist-to-hip ratio (WHR) provides an estimate of
- **a.** fatness
- **b.** location of regional fat deposition
- **c.** cholesterol
- **d.** athletic potential
- **e.** the percentage of fat in your body

11. Bulimia nervosa is associated with all the following except
- **a.** fear of becoming obese
- **b.** restricted eating patterns
- **c.** periods of bingeing and purging
- **d.** high levels of physical activity
- **e.** suffering from a critical incident

12. The body mass index measures
- **a.** the relationship between height and weight
- **b.** bioelectrical impedance
- **c.** girth (or circumference) at various body sites
- **d.** anorexia nervosa
- **e.** percentage of body fat

13. An eating disorder characterized by excessive preoccupation with food, self-starvation, and/or extreme exercising to achieve weight loss is known as
- **a.** bulimia nervosa
- **b.** anorexia nervosa
- **c.** binge eating disorder
- **d.** social physique anxiety
- **e.** satiety

14. Jadie is 1.65 metres tall and weighs 60 kilograms. Her BMI is approximately
- **a.** 20
- **b.** 21
- **c.** 22
- **d.** 23
- **e.** 24

15. Those who suffer from female athletic triad see the effects of osteoporosis
- **a.** when they are young
- **b.** both when they are young and when they reach menopause
- **c.** when they reach menopause
- **d.** after they are 80 years old
- **e.** only if they don't stop poor eating habits

Short Answer

1. What issues surround overweight and obesity in Canada?

2. Describe the three somatotypes.

3. Explain the terms *body mass index* and *waist-to-hip ratio.*

4. Determine the BMI for an adult female who is 1.70 metres tall and weighs 55.0 kilograms. Comment on the result.

5. What is the waist circumference a measure for? What is a healthy circumference for men? For women? Why?

6. Why is fasting a poor way to lose weight? What is a more appropriate way to modify body weight?

7. How are eating disorders not just physical problems? How might this affect your job as a police officer?

8. What methods are available to assess your body composition?

REFERENCES

Addy, C.L., Wilson, D.K., Kirtland, K.A., Ainsworth, B.E., Sharpe, P., et al. (2004). Associations of perceived social and physical environmental supports with physical activity and walking behavior. *American Journal of Public Health, 94*(3), 440–443.

American Psychiatric Association. (1994). *Diagnostic and statistical manual of mental disorders* (4th ed.). Washington, DC: Author.

Bear, M. (2011). Dieting and weight loss: Facts and fiction. Information sheet. Toronto: National Eating Disorder Information Centre. http://www.nedic.ca/knowthefacts/dietingfacts.shtml.

Canadian Institute for Health Information (CIHI). (2006). *Hospital morbidity database.* Ottawa: Author.

Canadian Society for Exercise Physiology (CSEP). (1996). *Canadian standardized test of fitness interpretation and counselling manual.* Ottawa: Author.

Community Foundation of Canada. (2011). *Health: Obesity. Canada's vital signs 2011.* http://www.vitalsignscanada.ca/2011_2health-e.html.

Grundy, S.M., Brewer, H.B. Jr, Cleeman, J.I., Smith, S.C. Jr., & Lenfant, C. (2004). Definition of metabolic syndrome: Report of the National Heart, Lung, and Blood Institute/American Heart Association Conference on Scientific Issues Related to Definition. *Circulation, 109*(3), 433–438.

Health Canada. (2000). *Canadian guidelines for weight classification in adults.* Ottawa: Author.

Health Canada. (2002). *A report on mental illnesses in Canada.* Catalogue no. 0-662-32817-5. Ottawa: Author.

Health Canada. (2003). *Canadian guidelines for body weight classification in adults.* Ottawa: Author.

Health Canada. (2010). *Healthy Canadians—A federal report on comparable health indicators 2010.* Ottawa: Author. http://www.hc-sc.gc.ca/hcs-sss/pubs/system-regime/index-eng.php.

Jacobi, C., Hayward, C., de Zwaan, M., Kraemer, H., & Agras, W.S. (2004). Coming to terms with risk factors for eating disorders: Application of risk terminology and suggestions for a general taxonomy. *Psychological Bulletin*, *130*(1), 19–65.

Kanayama, G., & Pope, H.G. Jr. (2012, June). Illicit use of androgens and other hormones: Recent advances. *Current Opinion in Endocrinology, Diabetes and Obesity*, *19*(3), 211–219.

Katzmarzyk, P.T., & Janssen, I. (2004). The economic costs associated with physical inactivity and obesity in Canada: An update. *Canadian Journal of Applied Physiology*, *29*(1), 90–115.

King, G.A, Fitzhugh, E.C., Bassett, D.R., McLaughlin, J.E., Strath, S.J., et al. (2001). Relationship of leisure-time physical activity and occupational activity to the prevalence of obesity. *International Journal of Obesity and Related Metabolic Disorders*, *25*, 606–612.

Kuk, J.L., Ardern, C.I., Church, T.S., Sharma, A.M., Padwal, R., et al. (2011). Edmonton Obesity Staging System: Association with weight history and mortality risk. *Applied Physiology, Nutrition and Metabolism*, *36*, 570–576.

National Eating Disorder Information Centre (NEDIC). (2005). Anorexia athletica. http://www.nedic.ca/knowthefacts/definitions.shtml.

National Institutes of Health (NIH). (1998). *Clinical guidelines on the identification, evaluation and treatment of overweight and obesity in adults: The evidence report.* Bethesda, MD: Author.

Nattiv, A., Loucks, A.B., Manore, M.M., Sanborn, C.F., Sundgot-Borgen, J., et al. (2007, October). American College of Sports Medicine position stand. The female athlete triad. *Medicine and Science in Sports and Exercise*, *39*(10), 1867–1882.

Padwal, R.S., Pafewski, N.M., Allison, D.B., & Sharma, A.M. (2011). Using the Edmonton Obesity Staging System to predict mortality in a population-representative cohort of people with overweight and obesity. *Canadian Medical Association Journal.* doi:10.1503/cmaj.110387.

Pan, S.Y., Cameron, C., DesMeules, M., Morrison, H., Craig, C.L., et al. (2009). Individual, social, environmental and physical environmental correlates with physical activity among Canadians: A cross-sectional study. *BMC Public Health*, *9*, 21. doi:10.1186/1471-2458-9-21.

Phillips, K.A., & Castle, D.J. (2001). Body dysmorphic disorder in men. *British Medical Journal*, *323*, 1015–1016.

Pope, H.G., Phillips, K.A., & Olivardia, R. (2000). *The Adonis complex: The secret crisis of male body obsession.* New York: Free Press.

Public Health Agency of Canada (PHAC). (2011). *Obesity in Canada. A joint report from the Public Health Agency of Canada and the Canadian Institute for Health Information.* Catalogue no. hps-107/2011 E-PDF. Ottawa: Authors.

Sanborn, C.F., Horea, M., Siemers, B.J., & Dieringer, K.I. (2000, April). Disordered eating and the female athlete triad. *Clinics in Sports Medicine*, *19*(2), 199–213.

Sharma, A.M., & Kushner, R.F. (2009). A proposed clinical staging system for obesity. *International Journal of Obesity*, *33*(3), 289–295.

Shields, M. (2005). Overweight Canadian children and adolescents. *Nutrition: Findings from the Canadian Community Health Survey.* Catalogue no. 82-620-MWE2005001. Ottawa: Statistics Canada.

Shields, M. (2010). Fitness of Canadian adults: Results from the 2007–2009 Canadian Health Measures Survey. *Health Reports*, *21*, 1–15.

Stice, E. (2002). Risk and maintenance factors for eating pathology: A meta-analytic review. *Psychological Bulletin*, *128*(5), 825–848.

Tjepkema, M. (2005). Measured obesity: Adult obesity in Canada. *Nutrition: Findings from the Canadian Community Health Survey.* Catalogue no. 82-620-MWE2005001. Ottawa: Statistics Canada.

Tjepkema, M. (2006). Adult obesity. *Health Reports*, *17*(3), 9–25.

Wolf, N. (1991). *The beauty myth: How images of beauty are used against women.* New York: William Morrow.

World Health Organization (WHO). (2000). *Obesity: Preventing and managing the global epidemic: Report of a WHO consultation on obesity.* Geneva: Author.

Yeager, K.K., Agostini, R., Nattiv, A., & Drinkwater, B. (1993). The female athlete triad: Disordered eating, amenorrhoea, osteoporosis. *Medicine and Science in Sports and Exercise*, *25*(7), 775–777.

Yusuf, S., Hawken, S., Ounpuu, S., Bautista, L., Franzosi, M.G., et al. (2005). Obesity and the risk of myocardial infarction in 27,000 participants from 52 countries: A case-control study. *Lancet*, *366*(9497),1640–1649.

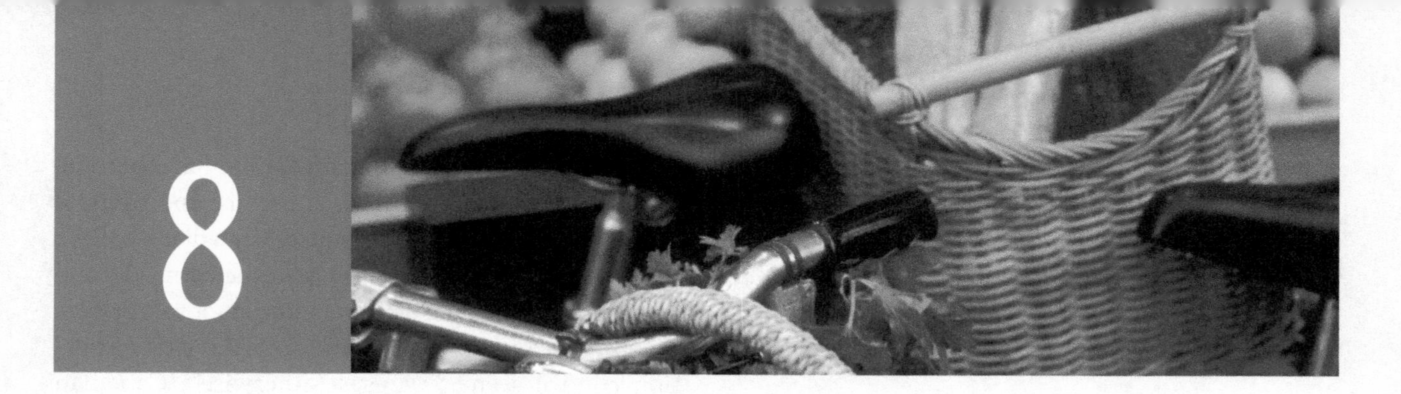

Nutrition

LEARNING OBJECTIVES

After completing this chapter, you should be able to:

- Describe nutritional trends in Canada.
- Understand the importance of maintaining a healthy weight, and the role of portion sizes and food labelling.
- Describe the role of the six basic nutrients: water, carbohydrates, protein, fats, vitamins, and minerals.
- Understand glycemic index and glycemic load.
- Describe the role of fibre in a healthy diet.
- Make better food choices using *Eating Well with Canada's Food Guide* and the DASH diet.
- Explain the importance of proper nutrition while working shifts.
- Determine which nutrition information, including websites, is valid and reliable.

OVERVIEW

Over the past 20 years, police officers—like other Canadians—have become better informed about nutrition. Yet, most Canadians' dietary and exercise habits remain poor. A 2011 survey reported that 78 percent of Canadians believe they eat nutritiously, yet "the preponderance of skipped meals, rushed meals, and meals without fresh fruits or vegetables; the expansive consumption of soft drinks; the excessive intake of caffeine, and the lack of portion control seen … suggest otherwise" (Canadian Council of Food and Nutrition, 2011).

Given the demands of shiftwork in particular, there is a tendency for police officers to consume fast-food meals, which are high in fat and sodium, between stressful calls. Compounded with the lack of regular exercise, these habits put them at risk for high cholesterol, elevated triglycerides, and overall body fat, potentially leading to diabetes and cardiovascular disease (see Chapters 11 and 12).

This chapter addresses the topic of nutrition with the view that good dietary choices are made over the course of a lifetime—not just over a police career.

FACTS ABOUT . . .

Nutrition in Canada

- According to recent data, overweight and obese adult Canadians—60.9 percent of men and 43.7 percent of women—are at increased health risk because of excess weight.
- In children, body weight and self-esteem are inversely related. For each BMI unit increase, self-esteem scores decrease by 4.8 percent. Children who watch more TV are particularly susceptible to weight gain, and those who take medications for mental health issues may experience increased appetite, making healthful dietary changes difficult to accomplish.
- Canadians now spend an average of 30 percent of their food budget on drive-through, take-out, and delivery food services. About half the participants of a recent survey reported eating such meals at least once a day.
- The highest consumers of fast food are men aged 19 to 30. The most popular items include pizza, hamburgers, hot dogs, chicken wings, french fries, coffee, and soft drinks.
- Women are more likely than men to consume fruit and vegetables. In 2010, 49.9 percent of females consumed fruit and vegetables five or more times daily, compared to 36.4 percent of males. Yet, although Canada's Food Guide recommends greater consumption of dark green and orange vegetables, the most common ones chosen by Canadians are potatoes, salad, and corn. Fruit choices tend to be seasonal and consumed as a snack or dessert.
- In choosing protein foods, Canadians are more likely to select high-fat, high-sodium processed meats (sausages, ham, bacon) rather than fish or legumes (lentils and beans).
- When people eat alone, they tend to eat things that are convenient yet less nutritious—more packaged and processed foods, including fewer basic food groups (grains, protein, fruits and vegetables, dairy products).

SOURCES: PHAC, 2010a, 2001b; Wang, Wild, Kipp, Kuhle, & Veugelers, 2009; Panagiotopoulos, Ronsley, Elbe, Davidson, & Smith, 2010; Dieticians of Canada, 2010a; Garriguet, 2004; Pérez, 2002.

Maintaining a Healthy Weight

A person's weight is the result of many factors, including height, genes, metabolism, behaviour, and environment. It is important that you learn how to balance the energy that you take in (calories) with the energy that you expend (exercise). For most people, maintaining this balance means consuming fewer calories and exercising more. In addition to making healthy food choices that are lower in fats (especially saturated and trans fatty acids), cholesterol, added sugars, and salt, Canadians need to pay attention to portion sizes. These topics will be covered later in this chapter.

The well-known risks of overweight and obesity include high blood pressure, high blood cholesterol, coronary heart disease, and stroke. But there is also a correlation between body weight and gallbladder disease, arthritis, sleep apnea, and some cancers (PHAC, 2009; Katzmarzyk & Janssen, 2004; Guh, Zhang, Bansback, Amarsi, Birmingham, & Anis, 2009).

If you are overweight or obese, simply losing as little as 10 percent of your current weight can lower your risks for these diseases. It is reasonable and safe to lose one-half to one kilogram per week. Losing more per week puts you at risk for gaining the weight back. Along with making healthier eating choices, you have to make a commitment to increase your level of physical activity (see Chapter 2 on goal setting and behavioural changes). Although weight-loss medication and weight-loss surgery may be optional for a small percentage of the population, for most people, changing eating habits and becoming more active are the keys to sustained weight loss.

Turn to **assignment 8.1** (in the appendix) to determine your understanding of portion size and how this affects the amount of physical activity you need to do if you consume certain foods.

Function of Food

Most Canadians have abundant choices with respect to food: grocery stores, cafeterias and restaurants, even vending machines. College and university students face particular obstacles in ensuring a nutritious diet (time constraints, lack of cooking facilities, money pressures), but education, motivation, and determination can make a difference.

Food provides nutrients that have physiological and biochemical functions in the body. There are **six basic nutrients**: water, carbohydrates, protein, fats, vitamins, and minerals. Their functions are:

six basic nutrients
the basic nutrients that the body requires to function efficiently: water, carbohydrates, protein, fats, vitamins, and minerals.

- *To promote growth and development of muscle, soft tissues, and organs.* Protein does most of the work for growth and repair, with the assistance of calcium and phosphorus in the skeletal building blocks.
- *To provide energy to the body.* Carbohydrates and fats contribute predominantly, although protein assists as a fuel source if needed.
- *To regulate metabolism.* Your body's enzymes are proteins that work with vitamins and minerals to regulate your metabolism.

Maintaining your energy balance and a nutrient-dense diet, a prudent training regime, proper timing of nutrient intake, and adequate rest and recovery are cornerstones to enhancing performance and seeing gains in your physique. It is important that you understand the basics of nutrition if you want to succeed in becoming and staying fit throughout your career.

Basic Nutrients

Our bodies require six basic nutrients to function efficiently: water (the most important), carbohydrates, protein, fats, vitamins, and minerals. In total, these substances provide 45 essential nutrients, which our bodies assimilate through digestion. Failing to consume the right nutrients in appropriate quantities inevitably leads to ill health.

Water

Water is the transportation medium in the body. Our bodies are about 60 percent water (the brain is composed of approximately 70 percent water, while our bones have about 22 percent water). Children have a higher percentage of water than adults. Women have less water than men, and people who have more fatty tissue have less water than those with less fatty tissue. Water cools and purifies the body's tissues, carries carbohydrates and protein through the bloodstream, participates in biochemical reactions, aids in digestion and absorption, and helps regulate body temperature. Water helps in getting rid of waste through urine, and drinking a lot of water correlates with a lower risk of developing kidney stones and colon and bladder cancer. Water also acts like a lubricant and a cushion for the joints. It protects sensitive tissue like the spine and is the fluid in the eye.

Police officers are often required to stand outdoors in hot weather for hours at a time. Dehydration (lack of body fluids) can quickly set in, so always carrying a source of water is important. Even a loss of 2 percent of your body weight through perspiration results in a decline in performance; a loss of 5 percent can result in fatigue, weakness, lethargy, dizziness, headache, and elevated heart rate. These symptoms can progress to cramps, confusion, inability to swallow or move, and failing kidney function. If you are thirsty, you are already dehydrated.

In general, a person should drink at least eight glasses (about 2 litres) of water a day. Those who are exercising, on a weight-loss program, or ill, need more water. It is advisable to drink at least 500 millilitres of water before any physical activity that lasts an hour or more, and to consume more fluids afterward, including those that restore electrolyte balance, such as sports drinks and juices. The most common electrolytes are sodium, potassium, magnesium, chloride, and calcium. Electrolytes assist in heart and nerve functions, muscle control, coordination, and the body's ability to absorb fluid.

hyperhydration water "intoxication," characterized by an abnormal increase in the body's water content

Besides dehydration, electrolyte imbalance can also be caused by **hyperhydration**, or water intoxication. Consuming too much water can result in a potentially fatal disturbance in brain function when electrolytes, specifically sodium, are diluted beyond safe limits. As your water level rises, the cells begin to swell, and the brain cannot handle the swelling. Symptoms of water intoxication include headache, nausea, vomiting, fatigue, restlessness, muscle weakness, spasms or cramps, and decreased consciousness or coma.

Deficiency of sodium is called hyponatremia; other electrolyte imbalances can happen with low calcium (hypocalcemia) and potassium (hypokalemia). Electrolyte imbalance rarely occurs through physical activity, but may result from other conditions such as severe burns, prolonged diarrhea or vomiting, or liver or kidney disease. Adequate consumption of properly formulated electrolyte-containing beverages as part of a fluid replacement regime may help prevent or reduce the risk of hyponatremia (Tipton, 2006).

Hydrating for an athletic event is slightly different from general hydration. Although it is recommended to avoid dehydration during exercise by continually consuming fluids, some athletes use glycerol-containing drinks to help them compete. Glycerol's osmotic properties reduce urine production, thus retaining water in the body longer for cardiovascular and thermo-regulatory functions to improve exercise capacity (Goulet, 2010). Concerns about this practice include delayed onset of sweating and reduced sweat rate, resulting in decreased ability to dissipate heat.

Instead of inducing hyperhydration with glycerol, a less expensive, safer, and more practical approach is to consume about 500 millilitres of water two hours before going to bed

FYI

Calculating Hydration

There are a number of ways to calculate how much water you should consume daily.

1. You should consume 6–12 glasses of water daily (a glass being 250 millilitres for women and 350 millilitres for men).
2. Another way to is to halve your weight in pounds to calculate the number of ounces of fluid you should be consuming daily. For example, if you weigh 160 pounds, then you should drink at least 80 ounces (2.37 litres) of water daily.
3. Another calculation based on body weight is:

   Body weight in pounds × 0.55 = ____ daily ounces of water; divide this figure by 8 to arrive at the number of glasses of water to drink per day. For example, if you weigh 160 pounds, then you should have approximately 88 ounces (2.6 litres) of water daily.

the night before an exercise or competition, and another 500 millilitres of fluid (juice, milk, or water) first thing the next morning. Then, one should drink (a) just enough water to maintain optimal hydration, (b) 300–500 millilitres of a diluted sports drink (3–4 percent) one hour before exercise, and then (c) an additional 300–500 millilitres (1–2.5 percent) 25 minutes before exercise.

Turn to **assignment 8.2** (in the appendix) and determine how much water you should consume daily.

Carbohydrates

The past few years have seen a lot of confusion over the consumption of carbohydrates. Because they are a staple of most people's diet, you need to learn about the differences among them in order to make better choices.

Eating carbohydrates often and in large quantities is known to increase the risk of diabetes and coronary heart disease. As a result, high-protein diets, such as Atkins and South Beach, have led people to believe that all carbohydrates are bad for you, but this is an oversimplification. Easily digested carbohydrates—such as white bread, white rice, pastries, sugared sodas, and other highly processed foods—may indeed contribute to weight gain and interfere with weight loss. But whole grains, beans, fruits, vegetables, and other intact carbohydrates do just the opposite; they promote good health.

Carbohydrates provide glucose (a sugar), which acts as fuel for the body. Excess glucose is stored as glycogen in the liver, and in muscles in small amounts, and when needed, is broken back down into glucose.

The muscular energy needed for high-intensity exercise is obtained mostly from carbohydrates. Ingestion rapidly replenishes carbohydrate stores, with the excess being converted into fat and stored in adipose (fat) tissue.

The digestive system handles all carbohydrates in a similar fashion. It tries to break them down into single sugar molecules so that they can cross into the bloodstream and be used for fuel for physical activity and proper organ function. This process converts most digestible carbohydrates into glucose.

Blood glucose is the only fuel used by the cells of the central nervous system (CNS) and red and white blood cells. When glucose is depleted, the liver breaks down fatty acids for energy, producing ketone bodies in the process. Ketones are acidic compounds derived from fat and certain amino acids. Normally rare in the blood, they help feed the brain when carbohydrates are not available, but disturb the body's acid–base balance and result in loss of minerals (Strychar, 2006). For the CNS to function optimally, blood glucose concentrations need to be above 4 millimoles per litre (mmol/L), the standard unit used to measure cholesterol in the blood. Normal levels are between 4 and 8 mmol/L. Below 3 mmol/L, hypoglycemia (low blood sugar) can produce symptoms of weakness, hunger, dizziness, and shivering; left too long, it may lead to unconsciousness and irreversible brain damage. A glucose level above 11 mmol/L is considered hyperglycemia. Symptoms include thirst, frequent urination, and fatigue (Diabetes Canada, 2012). For more information on blood glucose, refer to Chapter 11.

There are three types of carbohydrates: simple carbohydrates (sugars), complex carbohydrates (starches), and dietary fibre. Simple carbohydrates

DID YOU KNOW?

Fasting—the act of willingly refraining from some or all food, drink, or both for a period of time—may result in rapid weight loss but exacts a huge toll on the body. Deprived of glucose, the body begins to break down protein, reducing lean muscle mass rather than body fat. Paradoxically, fasting also slows the metabolism, making it harder to lose weight.

SOURCE: Strychar, 2006.

provide only quick spurts of energy. These sugars are linked to obesity, cardiovascular diseases, and reduced insulin sensitivity. Many of our processed foods contain simple sugars. Complex carbohydrates are the foundations of healthy eating. Consuming whole-grain products every day, for example, reduces the risk of heart disease and cancer (Aune, Chan, Lau, Vierira, Greenwood et al., 2011; Rautiainen, Larsson, Virtamo, & Wolk, 2012). Refined grains lack nutritional content, especially zinc, vitamin E, and magnesium. Whole-grain options include whole wheat, brown rice, 100 percent rye bread, spelt, buckwheat, and quinoa. Dietary fibre is indigestible material that aids in lowering blood cholesterol and facilitates digestion and elimination.

Carbohydrates come primarily from plant foods; milk is the only animal source. The best sources of carbohydrates—fruits, vegetables, and whole grains—deliver essential vitamins and minerals, fibre, and a host of important phytonutrients (plant-based nutrients, also called phytochemicals). Phytonutrients are compounds, found in vegetables and fruits, that are not used for normal functions of the body but have a beneficial effect on health or disease. An example is flavonoids, which are found in berries, herbs, and vegetables, and are associated with a decreased risk for cancer owing to their antioxidant and anti-inflammatory effects.

Understanding the Glycemic Index

DID YOU KNOW?

Your brain uses only glucose as a source of energy; without it, your ability to think is compromised. This is why many school boards have adopted breakfast programs.

The basic building block of a carbohydrate is a sugar molecule—a simple union of carbon, hydrogen, and oxygen. Starches and fibres are essentially chains of sugar molecules. Some contain hundreds of sugars. Some chains are straight; others branch wildly.

The digestive system breaks down all carbohydrates (or tries to break them down) into single-sugar molecules, as only these are small enough to cross into the bloodstream. It also converts most digestible carbohydrates into glucose—also known as blood sugar—because cells are designed to use this as a universal energy source.

glycemic index (GI) the amount of blood glucose (sugar) levels of certain foods within two hours of digestion

The **glycemic index (GI)** relates to how the body digests food—that is, how much the carbohydrate-rich foods raise blood glucose levels in the first two hours of digestion (Jenkins, Wolever, Taylor, Barker, Fielden, et al., 1981). Your body's response depends on several factors, including age, activity level, insulin levels, time of day, amount of fibre and fat in the food, how processed the food is, and what you have ingested with the food.

The following factors affect the glycemic index:

1. *Processing* Grains that are milled and refined (had the bran and germ removed) will have a higher glycemic index than whole grains.
2. *Type of starch* Some starches are easier to break down than others. For example, potatoes (GI=111) are digested and absorbed faster than sweet potato (GI=51).
3. *Fibre content* The more the fibre content, the less digestible the carbohydrate. Hence, less sugar is delivered.
4. *Ripeness* The riper the fruit or vegetable, the higher the glycemic index. For example, an underripe banana has a GI of 30, whereas an overripe banana has a GI of 48.

5. *Fat and acid content* The more fat or acid a food or meal has, the slower the carbohydrates are converted to sugar and absorbed.
6. *Physical form* Finely ground grain is more rapidly digested than a more coarsely ground grain, making it more glycemic.

The glycemic index ranges from 0 to100, with glucose being 100. High-glycemic foods—those that are starchy or sugary, such as simple carbohydrates—will increase the body's sugar levels rapidly. Within 30 minutes of ingestion, your body senses that energy levels are declining, which leaves you hungry again and running to the fridge (or fast-food outlet), even if you've just eaten loads of calories. Low-glycemic foods slowly increase sugar levels in the blood. These foods are generally lower in fat and higher in fibre, and are a rich source of vitamins, minerals, and antioxidants. A lower glycemic index suggests slower rates of digestion and absorption of the sugars and starches in the foods. This translates into a lower insulin demand, better long-term blood glucose control, and a reduction in blood lipids. Because insulin's other job is to tell your body to store fat, higher insulin levels in your blood make you more likely to convert your food to body fat rather than usable energy.

Understanding the glycemic index (Table 8.1) will help you if you are trying to lose weight or control diabetes. If your blood sugar rises too quickly, your brain

TABLE 8.1 Examples of Low-, Medium-, and High-Glycemic Index Foods

FOOD GROUP	LOW-GLYCEMIC INDEX FOODS (<60*)	MEDIUM-GLYCEMIC INDEX FOODS (60–85*)	HIGH-GLYCEMIC INDEX FOODS (>85*)
Sugars	• Fructose	• Sucrose	• Glucose
Breads and cereals	• Pumpernickel bread • All-Bran cereal • Barley • Oatmeal and oat bran	• Bagel • Bran muffins • Shredded Mini Wheats • Oatmeal (porridge) • Long-grain white rice (boiled 15–25 minutes)	• White bread • French baguette • Corn Flakes • Rice Krispies • Instant white rice
Dairy products	• Milk (skim and full-fat) • Yogurt	• Low-fat ice cream	
Fruits, vegetables, and legumes	• Unripe banana • Apple, berries, apple juice • Peach (fresh), pear • Yams • Black beans • Chickpeas (garbanzo beans) • Lentils (dhal), peas • Soybeans • Peanuts	• Overripe banana • Mango • Orange juice • Papaya • Peaches in heavy syrup • New potatoes (white or red)	• Carrots • Parsnips • Baked potato (russets) • Instant potatoes • Watermelon
Processed foods	• White spaghetti noodles • Vermicelli • Tomato soup	• Popcorn • Soft drinks • Most cookies	• Jelly beans • Rice cakes

* Glycemic index scores are based on a score out of 100.

SOURCE: Adapted from Foster-Powell, Holt, & Brand-Miller, 2002.

signals your pancreas to release more insulin, which opens the cells to glucose to be used as energy by the muscles, while any excess gets stored as fat. The more glucose your cells take in, the higher your blood sugar. Then, as the pancreas slows the release of insulin, your blood glucose dips. This is the reason that when you eat a chocolate bar, you first feel an energy rush, then lethargic and hungry. Excess secretion of insulin leads to fatigue, weight gain, and potentially, type 2 diabetes.

Besides overweight and diabetes, high-glycemic index foods have been linked to increased risk for coronary heart disease (Beulens, de Bruijne, Stolk, Peeters, Bots, et al., 2007), macular degeneration (Chiu, Milton, Klein, Gensler, & Taylor, 2009), colorectal cancer (Higginbotham, Zhang, Lee, Cook, Giovannucci, et al. 2004), and ovulatory infertility (Chavarro, Rich-Edwards, Rosner, & Willett, 2007).

One thing that the glycemic index can't tell us is how much digestible carbohydrate a food delivers. For example, some foods that contain a lot of water (such as watermelon) have a high glycemic index, but actually deliver only a small amount of carbohydrates. As a result, researchers developed the concept of **glycemic load (GL)**, which is a measurement that is determined by multiplying a food's glycemic index by the amount of carbohydrates it delivers. This gives a more accurate estimate of how much the food will affect blood glucose levels. In general, a glycemic load of 20 or more is high, 11 to 19 is medium, and 10 and under is low. As an example, a boiled carrot has a GI of 49 but a GL of 2. Dense white pasta has a high glycemic index and a high glycemic load—commercially prepackaged macaroni and cheese has a GI of 64 and a GL of 33 (University of Sydney, 2011).

Knowing glycemic levels can be a useful meal-planning tool once individuals determine their responses to different foods. In general, low-glycemic foods are helpful for those who want to lose weight. Low-glycemic foods gradually increase sugar levels in the bloodstream to sustain energy for longer periods of time. Because the sugars are slowly released, you will have more energy and also be less likely to want to eat more.

If you exercise and then consume high-glycemic foods soon after a workout, it will help you recover by raising low blood sugar after intense exercising. Low-glycemic foods are helpful in maintaining blood sugar levels for long periods of exercise. Many endurance athletes try to balance the consumption of high- and low-glycemic foods to maintain constant energy levels and avoid energy spikes and troughs.

TOP TIPS ...

For Low-Glycemic Choices

- Start the day with a whole grain such as steel-cut oats, whole wheat bread, or whole oats. Also use whole-grain breads for lunches and snacks.
- Try quinoa for breakfast or after a workout. It offers complete protein and low-glycemic carbohydrates.
- Try whole barley in place of refined white rice. In addition to being a low-glycemic food, barley has cholesterol-lowering fibre.
- Limit potatoes to only a few days a week. Instead, try brown rice, bulgur, wheat berries, millet, and hulled barley.
- Try whole wheat pasta. If it's too chewy, mix it with white pasta.
- Add more beans, peas, and lentils to your diet. They are a good source of slowly digestible carbohydrates and contain protein and minerals, as well.
- Nuts such as almonds, walnuts, and pistachios help lower cholesterol and reduce heart disease risk.
- A low-carbohydrate diet can and should include daily portions of low-glycemic foods such as fruits, vegetables, and whole grains for essential vitamins, minerals, and phytonutrients.

glycemic load (GL)
a measure of how quickly a food is converted into sugar in relation to how much sugar it contains

dietary fibre
food components that cannot be digested, found exclusively in plants; the two types of dietary fibre are insoluble and soluble

Dietary Fibre

Dietary fibre is the term for food components (such as cellulose) that cannot be digested. All fibre-containing foods contain a combination of insoluble and soluble fibre. Dietary fibre is a carbohydrate and is found exclusively in plants. When we consume refined grains, the fibre has been removed and what is left lacks a number of nutrients (including zinc, vitamin E, and magnesium). One indicator that you are consuming too many refined products is that as the day goes on, you experience abdominal bloating.

Insoluble fibre is found in wheat bran and wheat bran cereals, brown rice, whole-grain foods, fruits (such as raspberries and blackberries), and vegetables (such as broccoli and green peas). Insoluble fibre helps push food through the intestinal tract, promoting regularity and preventing constipation. This is important in chronic conditions such as irritable bowel syndrome, colitis, and diverticulitis.

Soluble fibre is found in oat bran, oatmeal, legumes (dried beans, peas, and lentils), pectin-rich fruit (apples, strawberries, and citrus fruits), and psyllium (a popular ingredient in breakfast cereals). When mixed with water, soluble fibre forms a gel. It binds to fatty substances in the intestine and carries them out as waste. Soluble fibre is important in lowering low-density lipoproteins (LDL, or "bad" cholesterol) in the prevention of cardiovascular disease. As well, it helps regulate the body's use of sugars, keeping hunger and blood sugar in check. This helps prevent and treat diabetes.

One way to tell if you are consuming enough fibre is your regularity. For proper bowel function you should be going one to three times daily. Less than that indicates constipation, which means sugars and fat have more time to sit in your intestine to be absorbed. Moving one's bowels more often, on the other hand, may indicate that the nutrients from food are not being absorbed. It is important to keep the fibre moving through your system by consuming enough water.

It is recommended that adult men and women consume 30 to 50 grams of fibre daily, depending on caloric needs (National Institutes of Health, 2006). This amount, however, will vary with age and health status (such as pregnancy).

Here are some ways to improve your fibre intake:

- Check food labels for fibre-filled whole grains like whole oats or whole wheat. Make sure that whole grains are the first ingredient listed and contain at least 3 grams of fibre per serving.
- To reach your daily fibre goal, you'll need to include fibre-rich foods at every meal. An average side salad of iceberg lettuce, tomatoes, cucumber, and onion yields only 2.6 grams of fibre for each 2-cup serving.
- Choose whole fruit instead of juice. Not only do fruits have more fibre, they have fewer calories than their liquid counterparts. Pressing fruit to obtain juice leaves much of the fibre behind. Five prunes contain 3 grams of fibre, while a half-cup of canned prune juice has only 1 gram.
- While whole wheat bread has three times the fibre of white bread, one slice of whole wheat bread still has only 1.6 grams of fibre.
- Fluids are important and water is the ideal choice, but you can also supply some of your fluid requirements with milk, juice, soup, and even tea. Drinking more fluids is especially important when increasing fibre intake.
- Try to eat more beans. They are a cheap source of fibre, complex carbohydrates, protein, and other important nutrients.
- Introduce flax seeds slowly into your diet. Flax is a soluble fibre that results in constipation in the beginning if you eat too much and don't consume enough water.

A word of caution: Consuming too much fibre can lead to certain risks, including dehydration (if the fibre absorbs too much water), reduced bodily absorption of important minerals, and nutritional and energy deficiencies if the fibre replaces other foods.

When starting a high-fibre diet it is important to go at it slowly and drink plenty of water. One of the side effects is increased gas and bloating until your body adjusts to the intake.

Protein

amino acids the fundamental constituents of proteins; amino acids can be divided into two types—complete (essential) and incomplete

Protein is found throughout your body in muscles, bones, skin, and hair. It makes up enzymes that power many biochemical reactions and builds hemoglobin, which carries oxygen in your blood. There are 22 building blocks called **amino acids** that provide the raw material to build over 10,000 proteins in your body. Amino acids are the main ingredient that goes into the production of antibodies, muscles, hormones, enzymes, and skin and hair cells.

Unlike carbohydrates or fats, which are stored in your body, you require a daily supply of protein. Children and infants need protein for growth, and adults need it to maintain health. Under certain extreme circumstances, such as starvation, the body may use amino acids as fuel.

Proteins that contain all the amino acids needed to build new proteins are called complete proteins and are found in animal sources—meat and fish, milk, and cheese products. Incomplete protein sources lack one or more of the essential amino acids and are found in fruits, vegetables, grains, and nuts.

Our bodies need to consume approximately 0.8–1 gram of protein per kilogram of body weight over the course of the day. Consuming less than this amount may result in the body's going into starvation mode and breaking down muscle instead of fat stores as a fuel source. (This is why it is very important to eat breakfast, as your body assumes starvation mode after six to eight hours of not eating.)

Too much protein in your diet may lead to high cholesterol, heart disease, and other diseases such as gout. A high-protein diet may put additional strain on the kidneys when extra waste matter (the end product of protein metabolism) is excreted in urine. This is why high-protein diets and over-consumption of protein supplements may not be healthy.

If not enough protein is consumed, growth failure, loss of muscle mass, decreased immunity, and weakening of the heart and respiratory systems can result, which can lead to death. Protein malnutrition can also lead to a condition known as kwashiorkor (a childhood malnutrition disease).

When choosing protein-rich foods, pay attention to what comes along with the protein. Vegetable sources of protein like beans, nuts, and whole grains also offer fibre, vitamins, and minerals. The best animal protein choices are fish and

FYI

Vegetarianism

People choose to be vegetarians for a number of reasons. Some do it to reduce the risks of obesity, heart disease, hypertension, type 2 diabetes, and certain cancers (particularly colorectal cancer). Others do not want to eat animals that have been slaughtered, while others find chewing meat difficult.

A well-planned vegetarian diet carries some nutritional benefits, such as a lower level of saturated fats, cholesterol, and animal protein, as well as higher levels of carbohydrates, fibre, magnesium, potassium, folate (a water-soluble B vitamin), antioxidants such as vitamins C and E, and phytochemicals (American Dietetic Association and Dietitians of Canada, 2003). There are a number of variations of vegetarianism, including pesco-vegetarianism (which allows some fish in the diet), lacto-ovo vegetarianism (includes dairy products and eggs), and veganism (eating only plant-based foods).

Vegetarians run the risk of deficiencies in some areas: protein, iron, calcium, zinc, and B vitamins. If you are contemplating a vegetarian diet, be sure to investigate alternative sources of these nutrients (such as soy products for protein and iron from spinach and other vegetables; see Tables 8.3 and 8.4).

poultry. Lean cuts of red meat, in moderate-sized portions, may be eaten occasionally. A 200-gram (6-ounce) steak has about 40 grams of protein but also about 38 grams of fat, 14 of them being saturated (which equates to about 60 percent of your recommended daily fat intake). The same amount of salmon has 34 grams of protein and 18 grams of fat, 4 of them saturated. Of concern is that moderate consumption of red meats is linked to colon cancer (World Cancer Research Fund, 2007), heart disease, and diabetes (Aune, Ursin, & Veierod, 2009).

It is important to get protein from a variety of sources. Vegetarians must be sure to consume the proper combination of plant proteins (dry beans, lentils, nuts, soy foods, sprouted seeds, grains, spirulina, and chlorella or blue-green algae) to achieve this balance. While most people who follow Canada's Food Guide will get enough protein in their diet, protein supplements may be useful for some individuals. The most efficient protein supplement is protein powder, which is more concentrated than pills.

In choosing a protein supplement, make sure it uses high-quality protein isolated from whey (extracted at low temperatures to prevent the breakdown of the amino acids themselves), as long as you do not have a dairy allergy. Protein supplements consist of whole protein (such as egg, milk, rice, hemp, or soy protein), individual amino acids, or combinations of individual amino acids. These do not have an advantage over food sources of protein, but they may offer convenience.

Protein Supplementation to Build Muscle Tissue

The timing of protein intake is important. Research shows that protein consumed with carbohydrates within an hour after exercise stimulates the release of insulin and growth hormone, and therefore, the growth of muscle mass (Poole, Wilborn, Taylor, & Kerksick, 2010).

Some research indicates that during the maintenance phase of body building, recommended protein intake is 1.2 grams per kilogram of body weight for maintenance of muscle mass. During the muscle-building phase, protein intake of 1.4–1.8 grams per kilogram of body weight is recommended. During the tapering or cutting phase, body builders significantly decrease their caloric intake. During this phase of calorie and carbohydrate restriction, protein needs increase to 1.8–2.0 grams of protein per kilogram of body weight to compensate for the use of protein for energy during this hypocaloric phase (Kleiner, 2000).

Research does not support protein intake in excess of 2.0 grams per kilogram of body weight. Excess protein intake is associated with dehydration and may be related to excessive urinary calcium losses and inadequate carbohydrate intake. Impairment of kidney function has also been associated with excessive protein intake (American Kidney Fund, 2002).

FYI

High-Protein, "Low-Carb" Diets for Weight Loss

High-protein, low-carbohydrate diets have become popular in recent years. They permit foods rich in fat as well as protein, but prohibit consumption of starchy foods, legumes, fruits, and sugar.

These diets may result in rapid and substantial weight loss, but the weight is likely to be regained quickly. A loss of 2–4 kilograms in the first week is common (mainly due to water loss), but weight loss is slow after that. Fatigue, constipation, and high blood cholesterol levels are some of the side effects.

Concerns about high-protein diets include the fact that they are high in saturated fats, very low in calcium (increasing the risk of osteoporosis), and low in fibre; fibre intake is usually less than 10 grams per day, while 30–50 grams is recommended.

When deprived of carbohydrates, your body responds in a fashion similar to fasting. The breakdown of protein and fats produces ketone bodies, which can lead to kidney damage. Thus, it is important to consume more water than the diet may recommend. Finally, high-protein diets lack many essential vitamins and minerals due to a lack of vegetables, fruits, and grains.

Some research suggests that this diet may be appropriate for diabetics, as the low-fat content found in some lower-carb diets may reduce risks of cardiovascular disease, type 2 diabetes, and obesity (Bradley, Spence, Hamish Courtney, McKinley, Ennis, et al., 2009).

Fats

fatty acids
the fundamental constituents of fats; fatty acids can be divided into two types—saturated and unsaturated

Fats are a source of essential **fatty acids** and other substances that, in small amounts, are used to synthesize hormones and cell membranes. Fatty acids are also a fuel source. Any excess is stored as body fat that may be used for future energy needs. Without physical activity, high-fat diets lead to weight gain and sometimes obesity, which can result in increased risk for heart disease and diabetes.

Knowing how much of which fats to include in your diet has become increasingly difficult. It's not just the amount that matters but the type that makes the difference—some fats are good at lowering the risk of certain diseases. Since Canadian legislation that compels the labelling of all prepackaged foods, manufacturers are now required to indicate unhealthy trans fatty acids on labels—in the past, we consumed them without knowing.

Fats break down into a myriad of fatty acids (chemically, long chains of carbon molecules with hydrogen atoms attached) that play an essential role in various bodily functions, including hormone production, cell growth and maintenance, and transportation and storage of fat-soluble vitamins (A, D, E, and K). Fatty acids also help the immune system to function and, when stored in triglyceride molecules as fat, they can become a vital source of energy.

Each gram of fat contains nine calories, no matter which fat it is. Some fats make food taste good, while other fats make us feel full (it takes longer for them to leave the stomach). Figure 8.1 outlines the percentage of saturated fat in common oils and fats.

FIGURE 8.1 Percentage of Saturated Fat in Common Oils and Fats

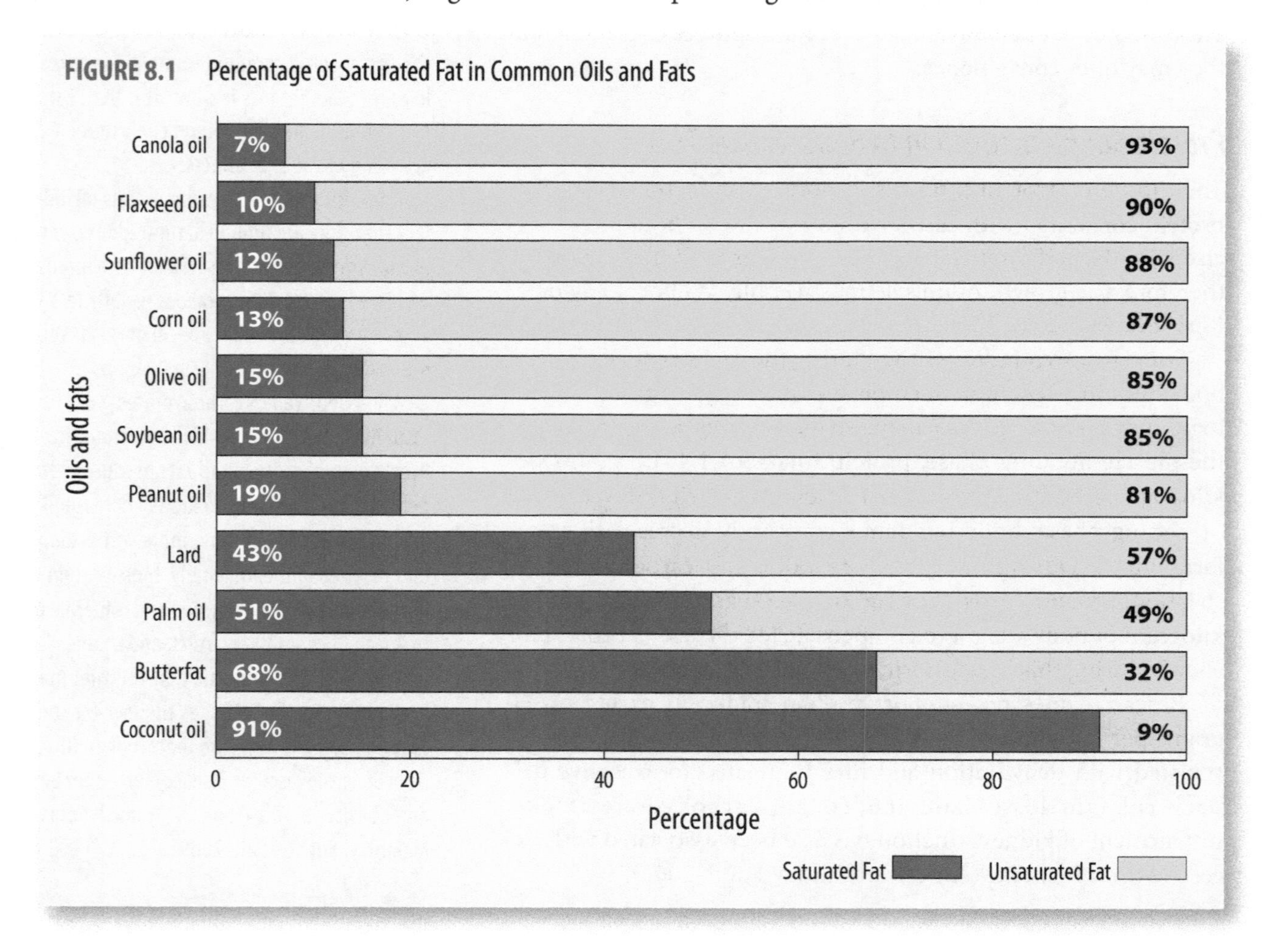

Understanding the Differences Among Fats

Fat is an important part of a healthy diet, providing energy (calories) as well as fatty acids. The body uses one fat—**cholesterol**—as a starting point to make estrogen, testosterone, vitamin D, and other vital compounds. Fat influences how our muscles will respond to insulin's signal to open up cells and allow sugar in.

cholesterol
a waxy, fat-like substance important for normal body function that travels through the blood and is linked to atherosclerosis

There are four main types of fatty acids: saturated fatty acids, monounsaturated fatty acids, polyunsaturated fatty acids, and trans fatty acids. Most fats and oils contain a mixture of all four types, but such mixtures usually have a higher proportion of one particular type of fatty acid.

Saturated Fats

Saturated fats (so called because the fatty acids are completely saturated with hydrogen atoms) are solid at room temperature. They raise the level of low-density lipoproteins (LDL, or "bad" cholesterol) and increase a person's risk for heart disease. LDLs carry cholesterol from the liver to the rest of the body. When there are too many in the bloodstream, they begin to deposit on the artery walls. Your diet should contain no more than 10 percent saturated fats. Foods that have saturated fats include animal products (for example, poultry, the marbled fat in steak, eggs, and full-fat dairy), as well as tropical oils such as coconut, palm, and palm kernel oils. If you consume 1,800 calories a day, you should be getting a maximum of 60 grams total of fat per day and only 20 grams of saturated fats.

Unsaturated Fats

Unsaturated fats are not completely saturated with hydrogen atoms. They are liquid at room temperature and are subcategorized as either monounsaturated or polyunsaturated, depending on which fatty acids are present in greater concentration. In general terms, monounsaturated and polyunsaturated fatty acids tend to lower the risk of heart disease.

Monounsaturated fats protect against heart disease by lowering LDL levels and also reduce the risk of certain cancers. These fats are a part of the so-called Mediterranean diet, which is rich in fruits, vegetables, legumes, olive oil, and nuts. Monounsaturated fats contribute to lowering risk for both heart disease and cancer. Canola and peanut oils, avocados, some margarines, and nuts such as almonds and hazelnuts are also excellent sources of these fats.

Polyunsaturated fats (PUFAs) are subdivided into three categories: omega-3 fatty acids, omega-6 fatty acids, and omega-9 fatty acids. Because the body can't make these, we need to consume them in our diet.

Omega-3 fatty acids are three fatty acids—eicosapentaenoic acid (EPA), docosahexaenoic acid (DHA), and alpha-linolenic acid (ALA). These fatty acids help prevent heart disease by lowering harmful triglycerides and blood pressure, reducing heart rhythm abnormalities, and preventing blood clots (thus reducing the risk of strokes and embolisms). They also have anti-inflammatory properties, thus reducing inflammation in rheumatoid arthritis and colitis. They are believed to help fight wrinkles and depression. Food sources include oily, cold-water fish such as salmon, mackerel, herring, and sardines for EPA and DHA. You can find ALA in flax seeds and flaxseed oils, canola oil, soybeans and soybean oil, and walnuts, and in smaller amounts in dark green, leafy vegetables.

Omega-6 fatty acids are found in linoleic acid, a second essential fatty acid. They help lower LDL cholesterol but need to be eaten in moderation, as in large quantities they can lower HDL ("good") cholesterol. They are important for reduction of inflammation in the body and are used to treat diabetic neuropathy, rheumatoid arthritis, allergies, eczema, and breast cancer. Sources include safflower, sunflower, corn, soybean, and sesame oils, as well as almonds, pecans, Brazil nuts, sunflower seeds, and sesame seeds. It is also found in evening primrose, borage, and blackcurrant seed oils. The recommended ratio of omega-6 to omega-3 fatty acids in a healthy diet is 4:1. The conservative estimate is that Canadians are getting 10:1; there is concern that we are consuming too much omega-6, so there is now a push to consume more omega-3s. For a good source of essential fatty acids, the ideal serving size of nuts is 60 millilitres, or one-quarter cup (Health Canada, 2012b).

Unlike omega-3 and omega-6, omega-9 fatty acids are a family of unsaturated fatty acids that are classified as non-essential. They are found in olive oil (oleic acid) and canola and refined sunflower oils (erucic acid), the latter two of which were developed for cooking at high temperatures.

Understanding Cholesterol

blood cholesterol the cholesterol produced by the liver

dietary cholesterol the cholesterol in food

Cholesterol is a waxy, fat-like substance that is important for normal body function. It aids cellular function and hormone production. Cholesterol travels through the blood packaged with other fats and proteins. When **blood cholesterol** is too high, it settles on the inside walls of blood vessels, clogging them (atherosclerosis; see Chapter 12). Twenty-five percent of our cholesterol is **dietary cholesterol** (from exogenous, or outside, sources), while 75 percent is blood cholesterol, manufactured by the body (endogenous source). Familial hypercholesterolemia (genetic high blood cholesterol) is believed to be due to a mutant gene, which releases cholesterol in the body and increases the risk of heart attacks. Most people make more cholesterol in their bodies than they consume in their diet. These cholesterols travel as lipoproteins (Durstine, 2005). There are two key kinds of lipoproteins:

low-density lipoprotein (LDL) cholesterol "bad" cholesterol; it can build up in the arteries and cause health problems

- **Low-density lipoprotein (LDL) cholesterol**, often referred to as "bad" cholesterol, is linked to heart disease and stroke. Although approximately one-half of LDL is removed by the liver within two to six hours after its formation, the rest can travel for approximately two days with the chance of binding to arteries and veins. This form of cholesterol is decreased through diet by decreasing fat intake, increasing dietary fibre, and maintaining good body composition through aerobic activity.

high-density lipoprotein (HDL) cholesterol "good" cholesterol; it helps clean out undesirable LDL deposits

- **High-density lipoprotein (HDL) cholesterol** is known as the "good" form of cholesterol. These particles scavenge cholesterol from the bloodstream and the arterial walls and take it back to the liver for disposal. It is increased through exercise, cessation of smoking, and weight reduction.

Total blood cholesterol levels should not exceed 6.2 mmol/L. LDL cholesterol should not be above 4.14 mmol/L, and HDL cholesterol should be greater than 0.9 mmol/L. Many people have their cholesterol levels checked by their doctor, but many are also not aware of what levels are acceptable. RCMP officers are required to have their levels checked for their annual physical. Although most men do not normally have this test done until they are 40 years old (and women not until 50 years old), you can ask your doctor what your levels are, and if they are high, what you can do about them. It is your right to know and make educated decisions about this aspect of your health and reduce your risk of cancer and cardiovascular diseases. The recommended intake for cholesterol consumption is less than 300 milligrams per day (Food and Nutrition Board, 2002).

Trans Fatty Acids

Trans fatty acids, often called **trans fats**, are created when a vegetable oil undergoes hydrogenation, a chemical process in which hydrogen is added at high temperature to make the oil solid. The process is commonly used in food processing to prolong the shelf life of packaged products and keep them more solid and resistant to chemical change. Fried foods and fast foods tend to be higher in trans fats. Trans fats are commonly used in baked goods and snack foods, including donuts.

trans fats
unsaturated fatty acids that have been hydrogenated to give them a longer shelf life; diets high in trans fats increase the risk of atherosclerosis and coronary heart disease

Trans fatty acids raise the risk of developing heart disease by raising the so-called bad LDL cholesterol and lowering good HDL cholesterol (Oomen, Ocké, Freskens, van Erp-Baart, Kok, et al., 2001; Health Canada, 2007a). Some questions have been raised about whether trans fatty acids increase the risk for type 2 diabetes. Trans fats have also been implicated in some cancers (Adams & Standridge, 2006).

In 2007, Health Canada made it mandatory for Canadian food companies to place the amount of trans fatty acids on their Nutrition Facts labels. Prior to 2007, it appeared as "hydrogenated" or "partially hydrogenated fats" or "vegetable shortening" on labels. Over one-quarter of Canadians aged 31 to 50 get more than 35 percent of their total calories from fat, the threshold beyond which health risks increase (Garriguet, 2004). While trans fat is considered somewhat more harmful than its cousin, saturated fat, too much of either greatly increases the risk of heart disease (Neergaard, 2007). Canada was the first country to introduce mandatory labelling of trans fat. The intent was to help Canadians make healthier choices and force food companies to reduce or eliminate trans fats from their products (Health Canada, 2007a).

Ways to Minimize Your Risks and Reduce Fat

Many people who have made an effort to lower their fat intake have still become obese. The so-called Western diet, low in fruits, vegetables, and whole grains, is high in red meat, processed meats, refined grains, potatoes, and sugary drinks—the opposite of the Mediterranean diet, which is high in unsaturated fats, vegetables, fruit, legumes, nuts, whole grains, yogurt, and some cheese. Western dietary habits increase the risk for metabolic syndrome, which can lead to heart disease and type 2 diabetes (Kastorini, Milionis, Esposito, Giugliano, Goudevenos et al., 2011).

To ensure that your diet has no more than 10 percent saturated fats and a maximum of 35 percent total dietary fat, here are some tips:

- Avoid full-fat dairy foods, fried foods, and high-fat bakery products.
- Follow Canada's Food Guide suggestions to choose lower-fat dairy products, less red meat, leaner meats, and foods prepared with little or no fat.
- Eat one or more good sources of omega-3 fats every day—such as fish, walnuts, canola or soybean oil, ground flax seeds, or flaxseed oil—to help prevent heart disease.

- Read the labels on packages before you buy. This practice is important for products such as cookies and crackers that advertise themselves as "low-fat." Many have replaced fat with added sugars, refined flour, salt, and trans fats. Avoid foods with labels that list "hydrogenated" or "partially hydrogenated" oils.
- Choose, but limit, soft margarines labelled as being free of trans fatty acids or made with non-hydrogenated fat. In cooking and at the table, use liquid vegetable oils rich in polyunsaturated and monounsaturated fats, such as olive, canola, sunflower, safflower, corn, and peanut oils.
- Fry foods less often. Try baking, broiling, and poaching instead.
- Do not replace high-fat foods with highly processed or refined carbohydrate foods like white bread, white rice, or potatoes. Just eat smaller portion sizes of products like skim milk and low-fat cheeses and low-fat meats.
- When you eat out, ask about the fat content of foods on the menu. Fast-food restaurants must now make their caloric content available for customers to read.
- Exercise at 70–85 percent of your MVO_2 for 40–90 minutes at least five times a week to reduce your risk factors associated with heart disease.

Table 8.2 categorizes food according to fat content to help you select lower-fat foods.

Vitamins

A vitamin is an essential, non-caloric, organic nutrient needed in small amounts in the diet. Vitamins act as facilitators for other nutrients, helping digestion, absorption, metabolism, and the building of structures in the body. Vitamins fall into two categories—fat soluble and water soluble. Fat-soluble vitamins (A, D, E, and K) are found in the fats and oils of food and are generally absorbed into the lymph system

TABLE 8.2 Learning to Choose Lower-Fat Foods

FOOD GROUP	HIGHER-FAT FOODS	LOWER-FAT FOODS
Dairy products	• Evaporated whole milk • Whole milk • Ice cream • Whipping cream • Sour cream • Cream cheese • Cheese (cheddar, Swiss, American) • Regular cottage cheese • Coffee creamers or non-dairy creamers • Mozzarella-filled pizza crusts	• Evaporated fat-free (skim) or reduced-fat (2 percent) milk • Low-fat (1 percent), reduced-fat (2 percent), or fat-free (skim) milk • Sorbet, sherbet; low-fat or fat-free frozen yogurt or ice cream • Imitation whipped cream made with fat-free milk • Plain low-fat yogurt • Fat-free or reduced-calorie cheeses • Low-fat (1 percent) or reduced-fat (2 percent) cottage cheese • Part-skim-milk ricotta cheese • Low-fat (1 percent) or reduced-fat (2 percent) milk powder
Cereals, grains, and pastas	• Pasta with cream sauces (Alfredo, rosé) • Pasta with cheese sauce • Granola	• Rice or noodles (spaghetti, macaroni, etc.) • Pasta with red sauce (marinara) • Pasta with vegetables (primavera) • Bran Flakes, Rice Krispies • Oatmeal • Reduced-fat granola

FOOD GROUP	HIGHER-FAT FOODS	LOWER-FAT FOODS
Meat, fish, and poultry	• Cold cuts or luncheon meats (bologna, salami, liverwurst, etc.) • Hot dogs • Bacon or sausage • Regular ground beef • Poultry with skin • Duck or goose • Oil-packed tuna • Beef (chuck, rib, brisket) • Pork (spareribs, untrimmed loin) • Frozen breaded fish or fried fish • Whole eggs • Frozen dinners (containing more than 13 grams of fat per serving)	• Low-fat cold cuts (95–97 percent fat-free luncheon meats) • Lower-fat hot dogs • Canadian bacon or lean ham • Extra-lean ground beef or turkey • Chicken or turkey without skin (white meat) • Water-packed tuna (rinse to reduce sodium content) • Beef (round, loin) with external fat trimmed • Pork tenderloin or trimmed, lean smoked ham • Fish or shellfish, unbreaded (fresh, frozen, or canned in water) • Egg whites or egg substitutes • Frozen TV dinners (with less than 13 grams of fat per serving and lower in sodium) • Turkey sausage, drained well • Vegetarian sausage (made with soy protein)
Baked goods	• Croissants • Donuts, muffins • Party crackers • Cake (pound, chocolate, yellow) • Cookies	• Hard French rolls • Soft, brown whole wheat rolls • English muffin • Reduced-fat or fat-free muffins or scones • Bagels • Low-fat crackers (choose lower in sodium) • Saltine or soda crackers (choose lower in sodium) • Cake (angel food, white, gingerbread) • Reduced-fat or fat-free cookies (graham crackers, ginger snaps, fig bars)
Snacks and sweets	• Nuts • Ice cream (including cones or bars) • Custards or puddings made with whole milk	• Popcorn (air-popped or light microwave) • Fruit or vegetables • Frozen yogurt, frozen fruit, or pudding bars • Pudding made with skim milk
Fats, oils, and salad dressings	• Regular margarine or butter • Regular mayonnaise • Regular salad dressings • Oils, shortening, or lard	• Light spread margarines • Calorie-reduced margarine such as Becel • Light mayonnaise or salad dressing • Reduced-calorie salad dressings • Herb-flavoured or wine vinegar • Non-stick cooking spray • Applesauce or fruit puree in baked goods to replace butter or oil
Miscellaneous	• Canned cream soups • Canned beans with bacon or franks • Gravy (homemade with fat) • Fudge sauce • Guacamole dip	• Canned broth-based soups • Canned baked beans in tomato sauce • Gravy mixes made with water or homemade with the fat skimmed off or removed (chilled and hardened) • Chocolate syrup • Cucumber slices or lettuce leaves • Salsa

SOURCE: National Institutes of Health, Department of Health and Human Services, n.d.

with the help of bile. They travel in the blood in association with protein carriers. Fat-soluble vitamins are stored in the liver or fatty tissue and can build up to toxic concentrations. Water-soluble vitamins are absorbed directly into the bloodstream and, instead of being stored to any great extent, are excreted in the urine. Water-soluble vitamins (B vitamins and vitamin C) can be easily leached out of food by cooking and washing with water. Although foods do not supply toxic levels of water-soluble vitamins, supplements may result in toxic levels.

Vitamins are important in many ways. B vitamins, found in legumes, oats, and leafy green vegetables, help convert food to energy and promote healthy skin, hair, muscles, and brain function. However, vitamin B12 is found only in animal sources (such as meat, fish, milk, and eggs) or fortified products, so a strict vegan needs to be aware of possible deficiencies in B12, which are linked to heart disease and stroke (Humphrey, Fu, Rogers, Freeman, & Helfand, 2008). Vitamin C, found in foods such as citrus fruits, tomatoes, leafy green vegetables, and sweet peppers, helps the body form collagen, a protein that is the primary component of the body's white fibrous connective tissue. Vitamin C also contributes to the formation of teeth, bones, cartilage, skin, and capillaries (the smallest blood vessels), and strengthens the immune system.

Table 8.3 summarizes key information about vitamins.

Minerals

Minerals, which are found in all body tissues and fluids, play a role in nerve function, muscle contraction, and metabolism. They are responsible for fluid and electrolyte imbalance (increased sodium concentration in response to water loss) and acid–base balance or pH (the kidneys control pH balance by excreting more or less acid). Minerals are the main components of bones and teeth. The major minerals include calcium, chloride, magnesium, phosphorus, potassium, sodium, and sulphur. Trace minerals include iodine, iron, zinc, selenium, fluoride, chromium, copper, manganese, and molybdenum. We require very small amounts of minerals—an excess of any mineral can create imbalances with other minerals and become toxic.

Table 8.4 summarizes key facts about minerals.

Understanding the Role of Sodium

Sodium is a mineral necessary for transmission of nerve impulses, muscle contraction, maintaining pH balance and, at the cellular level, pumping nutrients (like potassium) and fluid in and out. Yet, over-consumption of sodium can lead to high blood pressure—a major risk factor for stroke, heart disease, and kidney disease.

We consume sodium in the largest quantity in salts. While the recommended maximum daily intake is 1,500 milligrams per day, the average Canadian consumes about 3,400 milligrams of sodium (Health Canada, 2011). Over 75 percent of the sodium we consume is found in processed foods, such as deli meats, pizza, sauces, and soups. It is found in condiments and dressings, and occurs naturally in milk, fresh meats, fruits, and vegetables.

There is an initiative by the Canadian government to limit daily sodium intake to 2,300 milligrams by 2016 (Health Canada, 2011). As a result, nutrition labels on prepackaged foods now indicate the amount of sodium contained per serving.

Turn to **assignment 8.3** (in the appendix) to gain a greater awareness of your sodium intake.

TABLE 8.3 Major Vitamins

	VITAMIN	MAJOR FUNCTIONS	FOOD SOURCES	DEFICIENCY SIGNS AND SYMPTOMS	TOXICITY SIGNS AND SYMPTOMS
FAT-SOLUBLE	*A*	Vision, antioxidant, growth, reproduction, immune system	Fortified dairy products, liver, eggs, dark green leafy vegetables, yellow vegetables	Poor vision in dim light, blindness, anemia, diarrhea, poor growth, frequent infections	Blurred vision, growth retardation, abdominal cramping, pain in calves
	D	Bone and tooth development and growth	Fortified milk, eggs, liver, exposure to sun	Rickets (deformed bones)	Mental and physical retardation, excessive thirst, kidney stones
	E	Antioxidant, protects cell membranes	Vegetable oils, whole grains, green and leafy vegetables	Anemia, leg cramps, muscle degeneration	Discomfort, mimics the effects of anti-clotting medication
	K	Synthesis of blood-clotting proteins, assists in regulating blood calcium	Leafy green vegetables, liver, milk, cabbage-type vegetables	Hemorrhage	Jaundice, interference with anti-clotting medication
WATER-SOLUBLE	*Thiamine (B1)*	Energy metabolism, normal appetite function	Pork, liver, nuts, dried beans and peas, whole-grain cereals	Beriberi (paralysis), edema, chronic constipation, heart failure, confusion, depression	Sweating, nausea, restlessness, tightness of the throat
	Riboflavin (B2)	Energy metabolism, supports normal vision and healthy skin	Milk, yogurt, leafy green vegetables, meats, whole-grain and enriched breads and cereals	Enlarged purple tongue, hypersensitivity to light, skin rash	Bloodshot eyes, abnormal sensitivity to light, lesions of the skin
	Niacin (B3)	Increases levels of HDL in the blood and modestly decreases the risk of cardiovascular events	Dairy products, eggs, enriched breads and cereals, fish, lean meats, legumes, nuts, and poultry	Pellagra characterized by diarrhea, dermatitis, and dementia; mild deficiency slows metabolism, decreases tolerance to cold, and causes irritability, poor concentration, anxiety, apathy	Skin flushing, itching, dry skin and skin rashes including eczema; persistent toxicity may lead to dyspepsia (indigestion), nausea, and liver toxicity
	B6	Coenzyme for fat and protein metabolism, helps make red blood cells	Protein-rich foods, green and leafy vegetables, whole grains	Anemia, skin rash, irritability, muscle twitching	Depression, fatigue, nerve damage, headaches
	Folate (B9)	DNA production, anti-stress vitamin; prevents neural tube defects and assists in a healthy nervous system	Green leafy vegetables, oranges, nuts, liver	Anemia, depression, spina bifida in developing embryo	Itching, rashes, mental changes, shortness of breath, sleep disturbances
	B12	Coenzyme in new cell synthesis, maintains nerve cells	Animal products (meat, milk, cheese, eggs)	Anemia, fatigue, nerve degeneration	Diarrhea, blood clots, signs of allergic reactions
	C	Antioxidant, scar tissue formation, bone growth, strengthens immune system, aids in iron absorption	Citrus fruit, dark green vegetables, cabbage-type vegetables, strawberries, cantaloupe, tomatoes	Anemia, frequent infections, bleeding gums, failure of wounds to heal	Nausea, abdominal cramps, diarrhea, gout symptoms; deficiency symptoms may appear at first with withdrawal of high doses

SOURCE: Adapted from Sizer & Whitney, 1997; Dietitians of Canada, 2012.

TABLE 8.4 Major Minerals

MINERALS	MAJOR FUNCTIONS	FOOD SOURCES	DEFICIENCY SIGNS AND SYMPTOMS	TOXICITY SIGNS AND SYMPTOMS
Calcium	Builds and maintains bones and teeth, needed for muscle and nerve activity, regulates blood pressure and blood clotting	Milk products, fortified tofu and soy milk, salmon, broccoli, dried beans	Weak bone growth, rickets, stunted growth, muscle spasms, osteoporosis	Kidney stones, decreased zinc absorption
Sodium	Maintains acid–base balance in body fluids, needed for muscle and nerve activity	Salt, cured foods, bread, milk, cheese	Muscle cramps, headaches, weakness, swelling	Hypertension, kidney disease, heart problems
Potassium	Necessary for nerve function, maintains fluid balance	Whole grains, fruits (bananas), vegetables	Muscular weakness, confusion	Heart failure, death
Magnesium	Regulates enzyme activity, necessary for nerve function	Green leafy vegetables, whole grains, nuts	Muscular weakness, convulsions, confusion	Risk increases with kidney failure; nausea, diarrhea, appetite loss, muscle weakness, extremely low blood pressure and irregular heartbeat
Zinc	Component of several enzymes and the hormone insulin, maintains immune function, necessary for sexual maturation and reproduction	Meat, fish, poultry, whole grains, vegetables	Improper healing of wounds, poor growth, failure to mature sexually	Gastrointestinal problems, anemia, cardiovascular vessel diseases
Selenium	Component of an enzyme that functions as an antioxidant	Seafood, liver, vegetables and grains grown in selenium-rich soil	May protect against certain cancers and heart disease	Nerve damage
Iron	Component of hemoglobin, involved in the release of energy	Liver, red meats, and enriched breads and cereals	Anemia	Hemochromatosis (a rare iron metabolism disease)

SOURCE: Adapted from Sizer & Whitney, 1997; National Institutes of Health, Office of Dietary Supplements, n.d.

TOP TEN TIPS . . .

For Lowering Sodium Intake

1. Buy unsalted and low-sodium foods whenever possible. Look for words such as "sodium free," "low sodium," "reduced sodium," or "no added salt" on the package.
2. Compare food labels. Buy products with the lowest amounts of sodium. Look for foods that contain less than 360 milligrams of sodium per serving.
3. You can also use the "% Daily Value" (% DV) on the label to compare products to see whether the food has a little or a lot of sodium. Here is a good guide: 5 percent DV or less is a little and 15 percent DV or more is a lot, so look for products with a sodium content of less than 15 percent DV.
4. Check food labels often, because product ingredients may change.
5. Buy fresh or frozen vegetables over canned ones (choose low-sodium if you have to buy canned products) and look for low-sodium content if you buy canned or bottled vegetable juices.
6. Enjoy grains such as barley, quinoa, and rice, which are naturally sodium free.
7. Buy unseasoned meats, poultry, fish, seafood, and tofu; choose unsalted nuts.
8. Flavour your food with lemon or pepper instead of adding salt, sauces, or gravy.
9. At restaurants, ask for gravy, sauces, and salad dressing on the side. Ask for food to be cooked without salt or monosodium glutamate (MSG), a seasoning very high in sodium.
10. Check the restaurant's nutritional information for menu items with a low sodium content.

SOURCES: Healthy Canadians, 2011a, 2011b; Health Canada, 2012a.

For more information about sodium and ways to reduce it in your diet, go to the Healthy Canadians website at www.healthycanadians.gc.ca/init/sodium/index-eng.php.

Nutrition Facts and Labelling

In 2007, Canada made nutritional labelling on prepackaged foods mandatory. Each label bears the following information:

- a Nutrition Facts table
- the list of ingredients, by weight
- any nutritional claims, which are optional

These measures are intended to help build awareness and understanding of the key features of nutrition in the foods that Canadians are eating, a matter of particular concern to those with allergies or dietary issues. By being informed of packaged foods' content, people can make healthier choices.

Labels list calories and 13 core nutrients, and give the percentage of the recommended daily value of each nutrient. There are some exemptions to labelling requirements (such as fresh fruit, vegetables, raw meat and poultry, individual bakery items, alcoholic beverages, coffee beans, teas, herbs, and spices); however, if the food is altered in any way (such as with added sweeteners, vitamins, or minerals), each item must be labelled appropriately. Standard formats make information easier to find and use.

FYI

How to Read a Nutrition Label

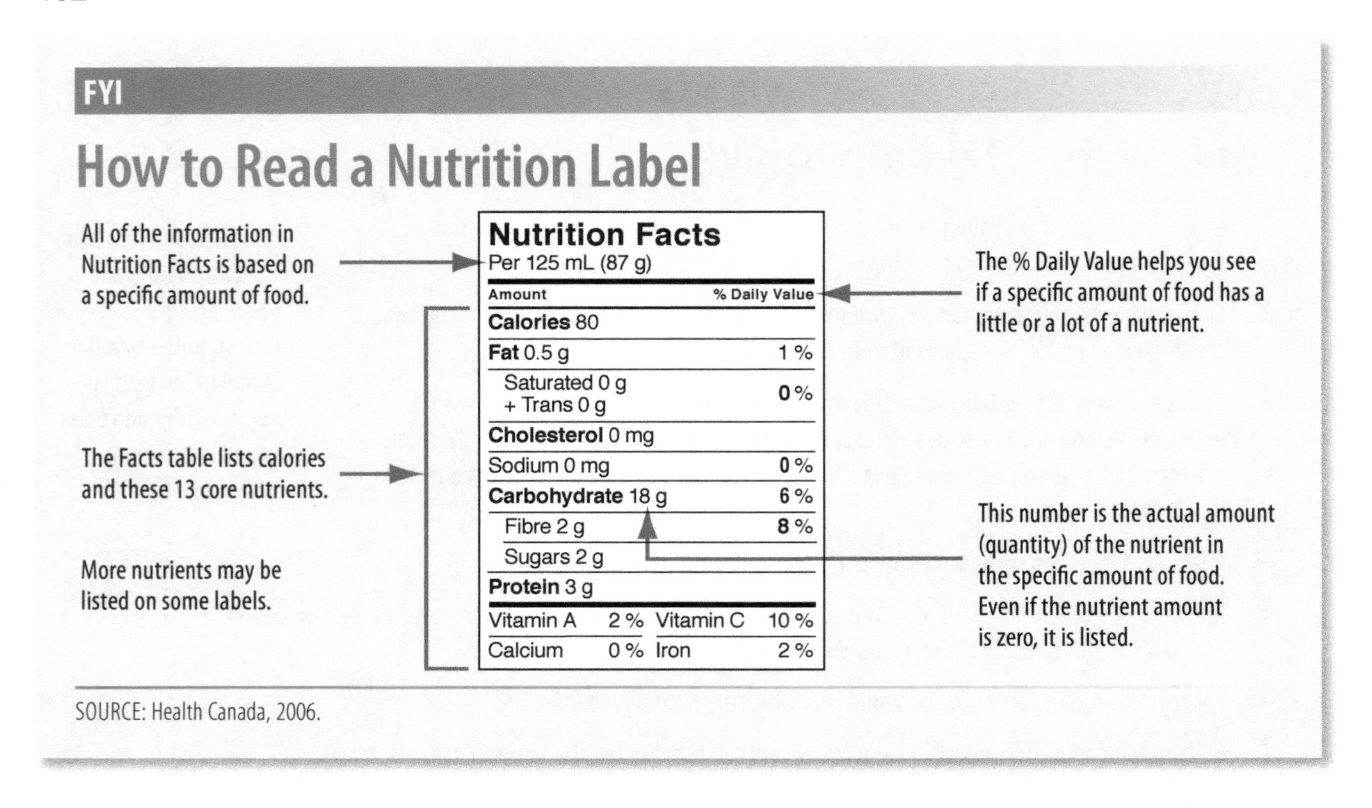

SOURCE: Health Canada, 2006.

Calories: Understanding the Caloric Value of Nutrients

kilocalorie (kcal) a measure of the amount of energy in food; also referred to as a calorie. An individual's energy needs are the number of calories he or she must consume to maintain health based on age, sex, weight, height, and activity level.

A calorie is a calorie is a calorie whether it comes from fat, protein, or carbohydrates. Also known as a **kilocalorie (kcal)**, a calorie is a measure of the amount of energy in food. An individual's energy needs are the number of calories he or she must consume to maintain health based on age, sex, weight, height, and activity level (Institute of Medicine, 2005). Just as gasoline powers your car, proper energy is required for your body. In terms of nutritional labelling, nutritional energy is recorded in kilocalories and kilojoules (kJ). Carbohydrates, fats, and proteins are the types of nutrients that contain calories and thus are the main energy sources for your body. In terms of energy density, food components have estimated energy values, while other substances found in food (water, non-digestible fibre, minerals, and vitamins) do not contribute to calculated energy density (Health Canada, 2007b). Caloric estimates are as follows:

- Fat has 9 kcal/g (37 kJ/g).
- Ethanol (alcohol) has 7 kcal/g (29 kJ/g).
- Protein has 4 kcal/g (17 kJ/g).
- Carbohydrate has 4 kcal/g (17 kJ/g).
- Polyols (sugar-free sweeteners) have 2.4 kcal/g (10 kJ/g).

The calories you eat are either converted to physical energy or stored within your body as fat after your limited carbohydrates are restored. Unless you lose those stored calories either by reducing caloric intake or by increasing physical activity so that you burn more calories, this fat remains in your body. Reducing the amount of fat and saturated fat in your diet is one way to limit your overall caloric intake. However, it is also important to reduce your overall food intake to reduce calories. Just because a product is fat free doesn't mean that it is calorie free.

Nutrient Content Claims

Nutritional claims on labels and packaging, such as "free," "low," or "reduced," can signal that a food has less of a certain component, such as calories, fat, saturated fat, or sodium. Such labels can help consumers moderate their intake of these components. Some labels also provide information on better options regarding fibre, vitamins, and minerals. Labelling can help people with diabetes choose foods lower in calories, carbohydrates, and fats.

Table 8.5 lists terms typically found on nutrition labels, with their meanings. Table 8.6 provides Health Canada's guidelines for any health claims related to a food product.

Turn to **assignment 8.4** to learn more about how to assess your foods.

TABLE 8.5 Common Nutrient Claims and What They Mean

TERM	MEANING
Free	An amount so small that it is considered nutritionally insignificant
Sodium-free	Less than 5 mg sodium (per serving)
Cholesterol-free	Less than 2 mg cholesterol and low in saturated fat (includes a restriction on trans fat) Not necessarily low in total fat
Low	Always associated with a very small amount
Low-fat	3 g or less of fat
Low in saturated fat	2 g or less of saturated and trans fat combined (per serving)
Reduced	At least 25 percent less of a nutrient compared with a similar product
Reduced in calories	At least 25 percent less energy than the food to which it is compared
Source	Always associated with a "significant" amount
Source of fibre	2 grams or more of fibre (per serving)
Good source of calcium	165 mg or more of calcium (per serving)
*Light**	When referring to a nutritional characteristic of a product, it is allowed only on foods that are either "reduced in fat" or "reduced in energy" (calories)

* Explanation on the label of what makes the food "light": this may refer to sensory characteristics, such as "light in colour." "Lightly salted" can be used when a food contains at least 50 percent less added sodium compared with a similar product.

SOURCE: Health Canada, 2002a.

TABLE 8.6 Guidelines for Making a Health Claim Related to a Food Product

TO MAKE A HEALTH CLAIM ABOUT ...	THE FOOD ...
Potassium, sodium, and reduced risk of high blood pressure	• must be low in (or free of) sodium • may also be high in potassium • must be low in saturated fatty acids • must be limited in alcohol • must have more than 40 calories if the food is not a vegetable or a fruit • must have a minimum amount of at least one vitamin or mineral
Calcium, vitamin D, regular physical activity, and reduced risk of osteoporosis	• must be high (or very high) in calcium • may also be very high in vitamin D • cannot have more phosphorus than calcium • must be limited in alcohol • must have more than 40 calories if the food is not a vegetable or a fruit
Saturated and trans fats and reduced risk of heart disease	• must be low in (or free of) saturated fat and trans fat • must be limited in cholesterol, sodium, and alcohol • must have more than 40 calories if the food is not a vegetable or a fruit • must have a minimum amount of at least one vitamin or mineral • must, if it is a fat or an oil, be a source of omega-3 or omega-6 polyunsaturated fatty acids
Vegetables and fruit and reduced risk of some types of cancers	• must be a fresh, frozen, dried, or canned fruit or vegetable; fruit or vegetable juice • must be limited in alcohol

SOURCE: Adapted from Health Canada, 2002b.

Eating Well for Life

Good nutrition, like regular physical activity, is something you practise over the course of a lifetime. The beneficial habits that will help carry you through your police career and into retirement can be formed now, during your student years.

Grocery Shopping 101

For the best nutritional content, look for fresh produce. Fresh produce just tastes better. However, many factors affect nutritional content, including crop variety, growing conditions, ripeness, how food is stored, and how it is processed and transported. For example, some vegetables—such as broccoli, green beans, kale, tomatoes, and soft fruits like peaches—lose nutrients more quickly when they travel long distances. So try to buy locally first if you can. Hardier foods—like apples, oranges, grapefruit, and carrots—can travel long distances and still keep their nutrients.

Canada's Food Guide

Canada's Food Guide first appeared during the Second World War, when food was rationed, as a way to ensure that Canadians did not become nutritionally deficient.

The current version, *Eating Well with Canada's Food Guide*, offers practical advice for healthy eating patterns. It also emphasizes physical activity to reduce the risk of obesity, type 2 diabetes, heart disease, certain cancers, and osteoporosis.

Based on scientific evidence to ensure that people are meeting their nutritional needs, Canada's Food Guide recommends the number of servings people should eat from each of the four food groups (vegetables and fruit, grain products, milk and alternatives, and meat and alternatives), plus a small amount of added oils and fats. Recommended servings differ for different ages, and there is a difference between males and females (see Table 8.7). People who are very active can choose extra servings from the four food groups, but must still ensure that their intake is low in fat, sugar, and salt.

FACTS ABOUT ...

Storing and Preparing Foods

- Store food properly to keep nutrients at their peak. Check whether fruits and vegetables should be stored in the fridge or at room temperature. For example, green beans should be refrigerated, as they can lose up to a quarter of their vitamin C when stored at room temperature for 24 hours.
- "Durable life" means the usual amount of time that an unopened food product, when stored under proper conditions, will retain its freshness, taste, nutritional value, and other qualities claimed by the manufacturer. The "best before" date, which must appear on prepackaged foods that will keep fresh for 90 days or less, tells you when the durable life period ends, although this does not guarantee product safety.
- Handwashing before handling food removes bacteria from your hands and reduces the possibility of contaminating the foods you touch.
- Wash raw fruits and vegetables with clean, running water before you prepare and eat them. Use a brush to scrub produce that has firm or rough surfaces, such as cantaloupes, carrots, oranges, and potatoes.
- To prevent the growth of harmful bacteria, make sure food is stored at or below 4 °C (40 °F). Refrigeration or even freezing doesn't kill bacteria; only proper cooking does.
- Because bacteria are carried in raw meat juices, meats should be stored and prepared separately from other foods.
- Meat should be defrosted and marinated in the refrigerator, as meat left out on a counter in temperatures above 4 °C (40 °F) can become contaminated. Fresh chicken and ground beef should be used within one to two days. After cooking, always put meat on a clean plate so that you don't contaminate it with the raw juices.
- Bacteria such as *E. coli*, *Salmonella*, and *Listeria* can be killed only by heat. Raw meat must be cooked to a safe internal temperature to avoid foodborne illness, as colour alone is not a reliable indicator.
- Cool food quickly using shallow containers. If it has been out for more than two hours, throw it out.

SOURCE: Canadian Food Inspection Agency, 2011.

To find out more about safe food handling, including an interactive guide, go to www.inspection.gc.ca, click on "Food" in the left-hand menu, then on "Food Safety Tips" and "Food Handling" in the subsequent menus that appear.

TABLE 8.7 Recommended Number of Food Guide Servings per Day*

		AGE GROUP (YEARS)								
		2–3	4–8	9–13	14–18		19–50		51+	
		Females and Males			Females	Males	Females	Males	Females	Males
FOOD GROUP SERVINGS PER DAY	*Vegetables and fruit*	4	5	6	7	8	7–8	8–10	7	7
	Grain products	3	4	6	6	7	6–7	8	6	7
	Milk and alternatives	2	2	3–4	3–4	3–4	2	2	3	3
	Meat and alternatives	1	1	12	2	3	2	3	2	3

* A healthy diet also includes a small amount (30–45 mL, or about 2–3 tablespoons) of unsaturated fat each day, including cooking oils, salad dressings, margarine, and mayonnaise.

SOURCE: Health Canada, 2012b.

For those trying to lose weight, it is very important to understand what a serving size entails. Table 8.8 gives suggested serving sizes, and Table 8.9 provides an easy way to gauge amounts of food.

TABLE 8.8 Canada's Food Guide Serving Examples

FOOD GROUP	EXAMPLES OF ONE SERVING
Vegetables and fruit	• 125 mL (1/2 cup) fresh, frozen, or canned vegetable or fruit or 100% juice • 250 mL (1 cup) leafy raw vegetables or salad • 1 piece of fruit
Grain products	• 1 slice (35 g) bread or 1/2 bagel (45 g) • 1/2 pita (35 g) or 1/2 tortilla (35 g) • 125 mL (1/2 cup) cooked rice, pasta, or couscous • 30 g cold cereal or 175 mL (3/4 cup) hot cereal
Milk and alternatives	• 250 mL (1 cup) milk or fortified soy beverage • 175 g (3/4 cup) yogurt • 50 g (1-1/2 oz) cheese
Meat and alternatives	• 75 g (2-1/2 oz)/125 mL (1/2 cup) cooked fish, shellfish, poultry, or lean meat • 175 mL (3/4 cup) cooked beans • 2 eggs • 30 mL (2 tbsp) peanut butter

SOURCE: Health Canada, 2012b.

TABLE 8.9 Estimating Amounts of Food (what the quantity looks like)

AMOUNT OF FOOD	SIZE ESTIMATE
3/4 cup of cereal	a small fist
1/2 cup of cooked rice, pasta, or potato	one-half baseball
1 baked potato	a fist or a bar of soap
1 muffin (equals two servings)	standard light bulb
1/2 bagel	small can of tuna
1 medium fruit	a baseball
1/2 cup (125 mL) of fresh fruit	one-half baseball
1/2 cup (125 mL) vegetables	small scoop of ice cream
1 oz (28 g) of low-fat or fat-free cheese	4 stacked dice or a pink eraser
2-1/2 oz (75 g) of lean red meat or poultry	computer mouse
2-1/2 oz (75 g) fish	eyeglass case
2 tbsp (30 mL) of peanut butter	1 ping-pong ball
1/2 cup (60 mL) nuts	2 egg cups
1 tsp (5 mL) of vegetable oil or mayonnaise	a quarter
1/2 cup of ice cream	one-half baseball
3/4 cup frozen yogurt	a baseball
1 oz (85 g) chocolate	package of dental floss

TABLE 8.10 Acceptable Macronutrient Ranges

AGE GROUP	PERCENTAGE OF TOTAL CALORIES FROM ...		
	CARBOHYDRATE	PROTEIN	FAT
1–3 years	45–65%	5–20%	30–40%
4–18 years	45–65%	10–30%	25–35%
19 years +	45–65%	10–35%	20–35%

SOURCE: Health Canada, 2012b.

Canada's Food Guide also calculates the acceptable ranges for macronutrients (carbohydrate, protein, and fat) in the diet, based on age group (Table 8.10). This approach offers flexibility for those who choose different diets to meet their physical needs. For example, the higher end of the range for protein may address athletes' needs.

The DASH Diet

The **Dietary Approaches to Stop Hypertension (DASH) diet** is a flexible and balanced eating plan that was developed to lower high blood pressure through reduction of sodium consumption. An excellent plan for weight loss, it emphasizes healthy foods and is heavy on fruit and vegetables, while balanced with the right amount of protein. It focuses on low-fat or non-fat dairy with whole grains, while emphasizing a high-fibre and low- to moderate-fat diet that is rich is potassium, calcium, and magnesium. The Heart and Stroke Foundation of Canada endorses the DASH diet (Heart and Stroke Foundation of Ontario, 2012), which reflects the principles of Canada's Food Guide. To see the publication *Your Guide to Lowering Your Blood Pressure with DASH*, go to the link listed under DASH Eating Plan listed in the appendix at the end of this chapter.

FYI

Making Wise Choices with the Four Food Groups

Whether you are at work, school, or home, you can make better choices to stay healthier using Canada's Food Guide.

FOOD GROUP	SHOULD INCLUDE ...
Vegetables and fruit	• eating dark green and orange vegetables daily • choosing vegetables and fruits prepared with little or no added fat, sugar, or salt • having vegetables and fruit more often than juice
Grain products	• making at least half your grain products whole grain each day • choosing grain products that are low in fat, sugar, and salt
Milk and alternatives	• drinking skim, 1 percent, or 2 percent milk at least twice daily • choosing low-fat alternatives to milk, including cheeses and yogurt
Meat and alternatives	• having meat alternatives such as beans, lentils, and tofu • eating at least two Food Guide servings of fish each week (see Guide for mercury warnings), such as Arctic char, herring, mackerel, salmon, sardines, and trout • selecting lean meats and alternatives prepared with little or no added fat or salt

Satisfy your thirst with water:

- Drink calorie-free water regularly to quench your thirst.
- Drink more water in hot weather and when you are active.

Shiftwork and Nutrition

Shiftwork has traditionally created barriers to access to healthy foods. But with the trend toward grocery stores that stay open 24 hours, people who work at night have more options. Some stores now provide pre-washed, ready-to-eat vegetables. And the broadening cultural demographics in Canada have increased the availability of more ethnically diverse food choices, which often provide healthier alternatives to the typical Western diet.

Chapter 15 deals with the specific stresses of shiftwork, including disturbed sleep. Sleep loss can lead to chronic fatigue, insulin resistance, excessive cortisol

DASH diet
a diet that follows Canada's Food Guide in order to reduce sodium, cholesterol, and fat in Canadians' diet

release (the "stress hormone"), anxiety/depression, obesity, and high cholesterol and blood pressure. Good nutrition can benefit your stress management and sleeping habits as well as your general health. Eating balanced meals and snacks at appropriate times and choosing healthy foods, such as fruits, vegetables, and whole grains, keeps your energy levels stable during your working hours and may also promote more restful sleep.

Particular nutrients and foods that may help you manage the stresses of shiftwork include the following:

- *Antioxidants* help repair, prevent, or limit oxidative damage—loss of electrons from atoms and molecules caused by free radicals (unstable molecules that may damage cells and lead to heart disease and cancer). Some of the best-known antioxidants include vitamins C and E, selenium (a trace mineral that helps reduce LDL cholesterol levels), and carotenoids (natural red, yellow, and orange pigments found in fruits and vegetables that help protect vitamin A and cells). The best sources of antioxidants include blueberries, cranberries, blackberries, raspberries, artichokes, raisins, and prunes.
- *B vitamins* promote wakefulness throughout the day or shift and encourage restful sleep. Vitamin B–rich foods include breads and beans, as well as various fruits, vegetables, and grains (see Table 8.3). If you take B vitamin supplements, it is important that you not consume them with coffee and take them with food during the day, not just before going to sleep.
- *Beta-carotene* is an antioxidant phytonutrient that can be converted into vitamin A when digested. Health benefits include enhancing sun protection, promoting heart health, and decreasing cancer mortality (Buijsse, Feskens, Schlettwein-Gsell, Ferry, Kok, et al. 2005). Top dietary sources include sweet potatoes, carrots, spinach, kale, and red bell peppers.
- *Calcium*, besides building strong, healthy bones and teeth, is involved in muscle contraction and relaxation, blood clotting, and blood pressure. Of special note: Caffeinated drinks increase the excretion of calcium that is stored in the body, specifically the bones. As you get older, calcium supplements only help you keep what bone you have left; they can no longer add to it. This is a concern with the physical demands of policing. You can add calcium in your diet by choosing calcium-rich snacks like cheese and yogurt, desserts such as puddings and custards, and by using skim milk powder or evaporated milk in baking, sauces, and shakes (see Table 8.4).
- *Iron* deficiency can lead to decreased immune function, loss of energy, and reduced capacity to learn. Iron-deficiency anemia is more prevalent in females and is characterized by a pale complexion, listlessness, irritability, and mental and physical fatigue. Iron can be found in meat, fish, and poultry, all of which contain heme iron, which is more easily absorbed by the body. It is also found in vegetables and grains (see Table 8.4).
- *Magnesium* is one of the most abundant minerals in the body. If you lack magnesium you may feel anxious, fatigued, and moody, and experience muscle and joint pain and restless legs syndrome. Foods rich in magnesium include Brazil nuts, soybeans, wheat bran, millet, seafood, legumes, and

dark green vegetables like kale or Swiss chard (see Table 8.4). If you take a magnesium supplement, be sure to take it with calcium, and later in the day rather than earlier.

- *Tyrosine* is one of the amino acids used to synthesize proteins. It is important for lucid and swift thinking. It releases dopamine, a neurotransmitter that increases heart rate and blood pressure, and stimulates metabolism and many of the body's energy reserves. Dopamine releases chemicals (for example, endorphins) that allow us to feel pleasure. A massive disturbance of dopamine regulation in the brain can result in the inability to respond emotionally or express feelings appropriately. Lack of dopamine is associated with conditions such as Parkinson's disease, schizophrenia, autism, and attention disorders. Tyrosine is found in eggs, soy products, fish, turkey, almonds, and avocados.
- *Tryptophan* is an amino acid that aids in releasing serotonin, a hormone that helps produce a stable mood and healthy sleep. It also helps in making niacin (vitamin B3), which facilitates the function of the digestive system, skin, and nerves. It helps with mental alertness and in converting food to energy. Serotonin triggers the release of melatonin, a natural chemical that helps you sleep. Tryptophan-rich foods include turkey, cheese, sesame and pumpkin seeds, yogurt, peanuts, and warm milk. If you take melatonin supplements, you should take them only for short periods when your shifts are changing, 30 minutes to one hour prior to going to sleep.

Snacking

For people who work shifts, snacking is a double-edged sword. Taking small amounts of healthy food at appropriate intervals can keep your energy levels stable during working hours. But snacking too much, or snacking on the wrong foods, can lead to consumption of empty and extra calories that results in weight gain, especially when you are not as physically active as you might be.

Without a healthy snack, our bodies experience a drop in blood sugar that saps energy and zaps concentration. Reach this level of hunger, and you're apt to gobble up the first edible thing within reach. Here are some points to consider when reaching for a snack (Dietitians of Canada, 2010b):

- Eat no more than three snacks per day, and keep each under 200 calories. Include foods from at least two of the four food groups.
- Eating empty calories from sweet, sugary foods will leave you unsatisfied. Boost your satisfaction and your satiety by choosing delicious and nutritionally dense snacks. Nuts, full of healthy unsaturated fats and protein, will fill you up. So will whole-grain breads or cereals and fruits and veggies, since they're packed with fibre that your body digests slowly.
- Think of snacks as mini-meals. Rather than pumping a bunch of empty extra calories into your daily tally, think of snacks as fuel to fill you up and to serve a nutritional purpose.
- Drink water often. Water has no calories. It quenches your thirst and helps you feel full.

- Make snacks as convenient to eat as possible. Put snacks into baggies at the beginning of the week. Select finger foods, like freshly popped popcorn with minimal salt; nuts and seeds; low-fat cheese sticks; and whole-grain crackers, pita, or English muffins. Or, pack a travel-sized spoon for scooping from a yogurt cup.
- Before the start of your work week, cut up vegetables so that they are ready to go whenever you are, whether to take to work or for eating right out of the fridge.
- Give your body a break between snacks. Eat a small serving, and then stow any remaining food out of sight. We tend to eat more when food is right in front of us.
- Skip individually prepackaged foods. For example, buy a large box of low-fat, low-sodium whole-grain crackers and place them in small baggies. Include a jar of natural peanut butter to stash at work.

Caffeinated Drinks

Caffeine, although not a nutritional food or supplement, is ubiquitous in our culture. Not only do we consume it in coffee and tea; it is also added to some carbonated drinks and certain drug products, such as cold and headache remedies. Caffeine is found naturally in the leaves, seeds, and fruit of a number of plants, including cocoa, kola, guarana, and yerba mate (the last two being herbs that are not always listed as caffeinated ingredients).

Caffeine is adrenaline (or stress) in a mug. It stimulates us and, theoretically at least, makes us more alert and wakeful with clearer thinking and better general body coordination. However, too much caffeine can result in restlessness, headaches, and dizziness, as well as insomnia, loss of fine motor control, and rapid breathing. Not only do caffeinated drinks dehydrate us; they also raise our cortisol (stress hormone) levels and decrease our metabolic rate. Caffeine can have a laxative effect on the digestive system, making it "lazy" and preventing the absorption of important nutrients. It can also interfere with the absorption of medication and iron. It fits the definition of an addictive substance because habituated individuals experience withdrawal symptoms, an increased tolerance over time, and physical cravings. As a result, two small cups of coffee should be your daily limit—that is, 400 milligrams of caffeine per day. Recent recommendations for children and adolescents suggest a daily intake of no more than 2.5 milligrams per kilogram of body weight (Health Canada, 2010).

One major concern for fitness professionals today is the popularity of "energy drinks." Not only do they contain caffeine, which must by law be labelled; they often include caffeine-containing herbs that do not have to be listed among the ingredients. This means that some drinks can have two or three times the caffeine content that is listed on the container. Some people ingest these as sports drinks to enhance their performance, mistakenly thinking that they provide energy and replenish electrolytes. Worse, some consume them when they are out drinking alcohol with friends in an attempt to delay alcohol's depressant effect and stay alert and awake.

In reality, these drinks cause irregular heartbeat, high blood pressure, and jitteriness. They can interfere with insulin sensitivity and cause headaches and fatigue. In extreme circumstances, energy drinks have caused death (Seifert,

FYI

Finding the Most Trustworthy Health Information on the Internet

Finding trustworthy health information on the Internet can be overwhelming. Here are some guidelines to help you determine the reliability and quality of the information you are reading.

1. Is the resource credible?
   - Are the author's name and professional credentials clearly stated? Is there contact information for the author or organization? Is the organization reputable?
   - Is medical information provided by a medical professional? Is evidence (scientific studies, research) provided to support the information?
2. Is the content relevant to you?
   - Does the content discuss the issue with enough detail?
   - Does the site contain original content, or does it only link to other sites?
   - Is the information presented in a Canadian context?
3. Does the site reflect a broad view of health?
   - Does the cited research recognize that health has many different facets, is dynamic and changing, is unique to different demographics, and is determined by many diverse factors?
4. Is the resource timely?
   - Is the information continually reviewed and updated? Is the date of the last revision clearly marked?
5. Is there clear and adequate disclosure?
   - Is the mandate of the information clearly stated? For example, is it a non-profit organization trying to promote nutrition, exercise, and active living, or is it a product company trying to sell you its goods?
   - Is the article biased or based on a conflict of interest? Are both sides of the issue presented? (For example, promotion of a vegetarian diet should indicate that there are other dietary options or clearly state that the viewpoint is just one side of a multifaceted issue.)
   - Are there commercial links or sponsorships tied to the site, or links you must access before entering the intended site?
   - If a site is collecting or requesting information about you, does it tell you exactly why it wants the information? Are the site's privacy guidelines stated? If you have to register to use the site, is the reason clear and is your privacy ensured?
6. Are there clear caution statements?
   - Does the site state that health information should not be a substitute for visiting a health professional?
   - If there are fees associated with use of the resources on the site, are they clearly explained?
7. Is the site user-friendly?
   - Is information presented in a clear manner? Can you contact the author/organization for additional information?
8. Does the site support a variety of activities?
   - Does it provide links to more information or resources on the topic? Does it offer screening tools, surveys, games, and activities to promote understanding? Does it give an opportunity for feedback?

SOURCE: Adapted from Canadian Health Network, n.d.

Schaechter, Hershorin, & Lipshultz, 2011). Given the physical demands and training required of police officers, and the concern about the negative effects of consuming these drinks prior to participation in physical activity, waivers now include a clause stipulating that the participant must not have consumed an energy drink for at least two hours prior to participation in fitness class, testing, or competition.

Staying awake on night shifts and then trying to sleep during the day is a challenge for officers who work shifts. Here are some caffeine-related tips that can apply to your career as a student, as well:

- Don't consume caffeinated products within six hours of going to sleep. If you want to have a caffeinated beverage, stick to green tea, which has less caffeine than some other beverages.
- For every cup of caffeinated drink consumed, drink two cups of water.
- Manage your diet to gain more energy. Eat smaller meals, eat healthier, and drink more water. Rather than have a cup of coffee, eat fruit on an empty stomach to boost your glucose levels and raise your energy.
- When you feel drowsy, take a short exercise break. This means getting out of the cruiser every hour or so to walk around.
- Whether or not they are caffeinated, stay away from soft drinks (carbonated or non-carbonated). They provide empty calories and have been linked to fatty liver disease (Nseir, Nassar, & Assy, 2010).

Some Final Thoughts

The bottom line comes down to making educated and healthy choices for yourself. Shiftwork does affect the availability of health-promoting foods; however, if you plan appropriately and prepare meals and snacks ahead of time, you can avoid the pitfalls of poor nutrition. If you want to stay healthy, follow the guidelines set out by Canada's Food Guide and ensure that you exercise. Make sure you read widely about nutrition and ask questions. If you need assistance to get on track with better eating habits, contact your doctor or a dietitian for advice.

How Food Companies Help Canadians with Healthy Eating

Food and Consumer Products of Canada (FCPC) speaks for companies while working with Canadian government agencies and industry to provide support to the government's commitment to nutrition, healthy lifestyles, and workplace wellness. These companies provide products, choices, and consumer information, using marketing and advertising strategies that meet the standards set by Agriculture and Agri-Food Canada. Here are some of the results of the FCPC's efforts:

- reducing hydrogenated oils in the food supply to help consumers limit consumption of trans fatty acids
- increasing the range of products with reduced levels of calories, sugar, fat, and salt, in line with current guidelines on healthy eating

- providing portion-sized options, such as single-serve packages and child-sized portions, in line with the varied needs of consumers
- attempting to add foods that supply vitamins and minerals to create nutritionally beneficial product choices
- providing nutritional information and education so that consumers can make informed choices, including labelling on packaged foods

Many companies provide websites that offer educational nutritional information about their products and healthy recipes. Some provide fun planners for physical activities, answer health questions, and offer promotional challenges or sponsored events, games, and contests to promote healthy living. Many have specialized areas for children, and some provide links to external health- or activity-based organizations. These include Active Healthy Kids Canada, Healthy Buddies, and the Long Live Kids Program. See the appendix at the end of this chapter for details.

Employee Wellness Initiatives

Many private sector companies are beginning to encourage their employees to make healthy food choices and engage in physical activity. Some companies provide flexible time schedules so that employees can participate in physical fitness programs throughout the day; nutritional counselling as a benefit option; and on-site fitness centres, weight-loss programs, and cafeteria facilities with healthy food selections. Some police services in Ontario have followed suit. There are a few services (Peel Regional Police Service, Toronto Police Service, Waterloo Police Service, York Regional Police Service, and the RCMP) that have fitness and lifestyle consultants who work directly to promote these activities.

APPENDIX: FURTHER INFORMATION ON NUTRITION

Here are some Canadian websites that can provide you with more health and nutrition information.

5 to 10 a Day

www.5to10aday.com

A campaign aimed at helping Canadians of all ages eat more fruits and vegetables as part of a healthy diet and active lifestyle.

Active Healthy Kids Canada

www.activehealthykids.ca

"Powering the movement to get kids moving." The 2012 Active Healthy Kids Canada Report Card looks at how physical activity affects such outcomes as mental health and body weight, which in turn affect levels of physical activity.

Anaphylaxis Canada

www.anaphylaxis.ca

Dedicated to helping people with severe allergies.

Canadian Cancer Society

www.cancer.ca

Provides cancer patients, their friends and family, and the general public with up-to-date information about cancer and cancer prevention.

Canadian Centre for Ethics in Sport

www.cces.ca/en/nutrition

Clear and consistent guidance on fuelling the body for athletic performance.

Canadian Diabetes Association

www.diabetes.ca

Information on nutrition and physical activity for the prevention and management of diabetes.

Canadian Food Inspection Agency

www.inspection.gc.ca

Dedicated to safeguarding food, animals, and plants to enhance the health and well-being of Canada's people, environment, and economy.

Canadian Foundation for Dietetic Research

www.cfdr.ca/sharing/CCFNLibrary.aspx

Information and advocacy on policy matters and critical food and nutrition issues in Canada.

DASH Eating Plan

www.nhlbi.nih.gov/health/public/heart/hbp/dash/new_dash.pdf

A guide to lowering blood pressure and reducing the amount of sodium you consume.

Dietitians of Canada

www.dietitians.ca

Interactive tools, tips, and fact sheets for healthy eating. Check out the Eating & Activity Tracker (eaTracker; see below) to get personalized advice about your current food choices. The website can also help you find a nutrition professional in your area.

eaTracker

www.eatracker.ca

An initiative of Dietitians of Canada to help Canadians track their daily food and activity choices, and track their progress. The eaTracker tool provides personalized feedback on calories, essential nutrients, activity levels, and body mass index (BMI).

Eat Right Ontario

www.eatrightontario.ca

Information on popular nutrition and healthy eating. Its monthly email newsletter provides timely updates. The site offers access to a dietitian via email or phone for specific information.

Food and Consumer Products of Canada

www.fcpc.ca

Works with government agencies and industry to provide support to the government's commitment to nutrition, healthy lifestyles, and workplace wellness.

Health Canada

www.hc-sc.gc.ca

Federal department responsible for helping Canadians maintain and improve their health while respecting individual choices and circumstances. Provides high-quality research on long-term health care and disease prevention, and encourages physical activity and healthy eating.

Healthy Buddies

www.healthybuddies.ca

Empowers elementary school children to live healthier lives by informing them about the three components of health: physical activity, nutrition, and mental health.

Heart & Stroke Health Check

www.heartandstroke.com

A not-for-profit food information program that provides information on choosing foods in grocery stores and restaurants that can be part of a healthy diet. On the home page, scroll down under "Manage Your Health" and click on "Health Information" and choose "Health Check."

Leslie Beck

www.lesliebeck.com

Leslie Beck, a Canadian registered dietitian and nutrionist, provides information about nutrition and exercise.

Long Live Kids Program

http://longlivekids.ca

A national child-focused initiative developed by Health Canada in partnership with Food and Consumer Products of Canada to support public awareness and an educational program that encourages children to eat smart, move more, and become media wise. Its program "The Science of Food" provides scientific information and activities to educate children about the importance of a balanced and nutritious diet.

Meal Planning Resource—Canadian Diabetes Association

www.diabetes.ca/diabetes-and-you/nutrition/meal-planning

Created to help diabetics eat tasty and healthy meals for good health and diabetes management. The manual contains information on a wide variety of topics, from eating out to recipe makeovers and physical activity.

Nutrition Resource Centre (NRC)

www.nutritionrc.ca/index.html

An initiative of the Ontario Public Health Association, funded by the Ontario Ministry of Health and Long-Term Care, NRC was established to increase the level of coordinated provincial support of nutritional promotion programming, resource development, dissemination, and support services for nutrition professionals.

Nutritional Labelling

www.hc-sc.gc.ca/fn-an/label-etiquet/nutrition/index-eng.php

Information regarding the regulation of and compliance with nutritional labelling for most prepackaged foods.

Osteoporosis Canada

www.osteoporosis.ca

Information on nutrition and physical activity for the prevention of osteoporosis.

Sodium 101

www.sodium101.ca

Information for consumers on sodium, including label reading, health effects, and tips for reducing sodium intake.

Trans Fats

www.hc-sc.gc.ca/fn-an/nutrition/gras-trans-fats/index-eng.php

Health Canada's information on trans fats, including frequently asked questions and information on the trans fat task force.

KEY TERMS

amino acids, 170
blood cholesterol, 174
cholesterol, 173
DASH diet, 187
dietary cholesterol, 174
dietary fibre, 168
fatty acids, 172
glycemic index (GI), 166
glycemic load (GL), 168
high-density lipoprotein (HDL) cholesterol, 174
hyperhydration, 164
kilocalorie (kcal), 182
low-density lipoprotein (LDL) cholesterol, 174
six basic nutrients, 163
trans fats, 175

EXERCISES

Multiple Choice

1. According to Canada's Food Guide, over half of your daily calories may come from
   - a. vitamins
   - b. minerals
   - c. fats
   - d. carbohydrates
   - e. proteins
2. What is the best advice for someone participating in a regular fitness program?
   - a. eat as much as you can
   - b. eat more protein
   - c. eat a balanced diet
   - d. eat fewer carbohydrates
   - e. reduce all fats
3. The guidelines in Canada's Food Guide do not include
   - a. enjoying a variety of foods from each of the four food groups daily
   - b. choosing higher-fat foods more often
   - c. emphasizing grain products, vegetables, and fruit
   - d. consuming a small amount of oils and fats
   - e. limiting salt, alcohol, and caffeine
4. Carbohydrates are stored in the liver and muscles in the form of
   - a. fatty acids
   - b. amino acids
   - c. glycogen
   - d. LDL
   - e. HDL
5. A good source of protein is ______________.
   - a. oranges
   - b. peanuts
   - c. meat
   - d. strawberries
   - e. squash
6. The body cannot survive without which nutrient for a prolonged period of time?
   - a. carbohydrates
   - b. proteins
   - c. fats
   - d. water
   - e. minerals
7. According to Canada's Food Guide, one serving of grain products would consist of
   - a. one large hamburger bun
   - b. one cup of hot cereal
   - c. three saltine crackers
   - d. one-half cup of cooked rice
   - e. one toasted bagel
8. Which is least likely to be true of complex carbohydrates?
   - a. they are high in fibre
   - b. they are low in calories
   - c. they are low in nutrients
   - d. they are low in saturated fats
   - e. they are low in amino acids
9. Which of the following is good advice for weight control?
   - a. eat as fast as you can so you don't think about food
   - b. space meals out equally throughout the day
   - c. skip lunch or breakfast if you don't feel hungry
   - d. eat a large dinner and a small lunch and breakfast
   - e. read a book while eating to take your mind off of food
10. "Empty calories" refers to
    - a. food that does not make you fat
    - b. calories with a low caloric content
    - c. regurgitation of food to prevent weight gain
    - d. food that is low in nutrients and high in calories
    - e. the apparent inability of thin people to gain weight

11. Which of the following is true of dietary fat?
    a. it is an essential part of the diet
    b. it should never be consumed by an athlete
    c. it should make up 40 percent of your total caloric intake
    d. it should be primarily saturated
    e. it has fewer calories per gram than carbohydrates

12. How many calories are found in a 4-gram serving of fat?
    a. 12 kcal
    b. 15 kcal
    c. 27 kcal
    d. 36 kcal
    e. 40 kcal

13. Complete proteins, containing all the essential amino acids, are found in
    a. legumes
    b. nuts
    c. animal products
    d. wild rice
    e. leafy green vegetables

14. Most experts agree that there is a link between excessive sodium intake and
    a. cancer
    b. hypotension
    c. blood clotting
    d. diabetes
    e. hypertension

15. Which is worst for you?
    a. butter
    b. tub margarine
    c. stick margarine
    d. low-sodium whipped butter
    e. light tub margarine

16. Four of these strategies have been clearly shown to keep blood pressure from rising. Which hasn't?
    a. cutting salt
    b. losing excess weight
    c. eating potassium-rich foods
    d. getting adequate calcium
    e. exercising regularly

17. ______________ are high in saturated fats.
    a. Corn oil and soybean oil
    b. Broccoli and cauliflower
    c. Whole milk and cheeses
    d. Bread and potatoes
    e. White and whole-grain rice

18. Which of the following is the best source for omega-3 fatty acids?
    a. wheat products
    b. berries
    c. corn oil
    d. pork
    e. sardines

Short Answers

1. What are the six basic nutrients?

2. What constitutes a balanced and healthy diet?

3. What percentages of total energy intake should come from proteins, fats, and carbohydrates? Fill in the chart.

AGE GROUP	PERCENTAGE OF TOTAL CALORIES FROM ...		
	CARBOHYDRATE	PROTEIN	FAT
1–3 years	__–__ %	__–__ %	__–__ %
4–18 years	__–__ %	__–__ %	__–__ %
19 years +	__–__ %	__–__ %	__–__ %

4. Why is fibre important to your diet?

5. What is the distinction between blood cholesterol and dietary cholesterol?

6. What are some ways to reduce fat in your diet?

7. What are vitamins and minerals, and why are they important in your diet?

8. What are the benefits and risks of consuming caffeine?

9. What is the basis of the DASH diet?

10. What are some ways to keep food safe and prevent you from getting sick?

REFERENCES

Adams, S.M., & Standridge, J.B. (2006). What should we eat? Evidence from observational studies. *Southern Medical Journal*, 99(7), 744–748.

American Dietetic Association and Dietitians of Canada. (2003). Position of the American Dietetic Association and Dietitians of Canada: Vegetarian diets. Public policy statement. *Canadian Journal of Dietetic Practice and Research, 64*(2).

American Kidney Fund. (2002). AKF warns about impact of high-protein diets on kidney health. http://www.atkinsexposed.org/atkins/79/American_Kidney_Fund.htm.

Aune, D., Chan, D.S., Lau, R., Vierira, R., Greenwood, D.C., et al. (2011). Dietary fibre, whole grains, and risk of colorectal cancer: Systematic review and dose-response meta-analysis of prospective studies. *British Medical Journal, 343,* d6617. http://www.ncbi.nlm.nih.gov/pubmed/22074852 .

Aune, D., Ursin, G., & Veierod, M.B. (2009). Meat consumption and the risk of type 2 diabetes: A systematic review and meta-analysis of cohort studies. *Diabetologia, 52,* 2277–2287.

Beulens, J.W., de Bruijne, L.M., Stolk, R.P., Peeters, P.H., Bots, M.L., et al. (2007). High dietary glycemic load and glycemic index increase risk of cardiovascular disease among middle-aged women: A population-based follow-up study. *Journal of the American College of Cardiology, 50,* 14–21.

Bradley, U., Spence, M., Hamish Courtney, C., McKinley, M.C., Ennis, C.N., et al. (2009). Low-fat versus low-carbohydrate weight reduction diets. *Diabetes, 58*(12), 2741–2748.

Buijsse, B., Feskens, E.J., Schlettwein-Gsell, D., Ferry, M., Kok, F.J., et al. (2005). Plasma carotene and alpha-tocopherol in relation to 10-y all-cause and cause-specific mortality in European elderly: The Survey in Europe on Nutrition and the Elderly, a Concerted Action (SENECA). *American Journal of Clinical Nutrition, 82*(4), 879–886.

Canadian Council of Food and Nutrition. (2011). Home plate. What consumers are eating behind closed doors. An initiative of the Canadian Council of Food and Nutrition. http://www.ccfn.ca/pdfs/Home_Plate_Jan28_FINAL_Report.pdf.

Canadian Food Inspection Agency. (2011). http://www.inspection.gc.ca.

Canadian Health Network. (n.d.). How to find the most trustworthy health information on the Internet. http://www.canadian-health-network.ca.

Chavarro, J.E., Rich-Edwards, J.W., Rosner, B.A., & Willett, W.C. (2007). Diet and lifestyle in the prevention of ovulatory disorder infertility. *Obstetrics and Gynecology, 110,* 1050–1058.

Chiu, C.J., Milton, R.C., Klein, R., Gensler, G., & Taylor, A. (2009). Dietary compound score and risk of age-related macular degeneration in the Age-Related Eye Disease Study. *Ophthalmology, 116*(5), 939–946.

Diabetes Canada. (2012). Signs and symptoms of hypoglycemia. http://www.diabetes.ca/Files/kwd_signs.pdf.

Dietitians of Canada. (2010a). Advertising of food and beverages to children. Position of Dietitians of Canada. http://www.dietitians.ca/Downloadable-Content/Public/Advertising-to-Children-position-paper.aspx.

Dietitians of Canada. (2010b). Healthy snacks for adults. http://www.dietitians.ca/Nutrition-Resources-A-Z/Factsheets/Healthy-Eating---General/Healthy-Snacks-for-Adults.aspx.

Dietitians of Canada. (2012). Functions and food sources of some common vitamins. http://www.dietitians.ca/Nutrition-Resources-A-Z/Factsheets/Vitamins/Functions-and-Food-Sources-of-Common-Vitamins.aspx.

Durstine, L. (2005). Understanding blood cholesterol. In *Action plan for high cholesterol* (pp. 1–12). American College of Sports Medicine. Champaign, IL: Human Kinetics.

Food and Nutrition Board, Institute of Medicine. (2002). Energy. In *Dietary reference intakes for energy, carbohydrate, fiber, fat, fatty acids, cholesterol, protein, and amino acids (macronutrients).* Washington, DC: National Academies Press.

Foster-Powell, K., Holt, S.H., & Brand-Miller, J.C. (2002). International table of glycemic index and glycemic load values: 2002. *American Journal of Clinical Nutrition, 76,* 5–56.

Garriguet, D. (2004). Overview of Canadians' eating habits. In *Nutrition: Findings from the Canadian Community Healthy Survey.* Ottawa: Statistics Canada Cat. no. 82-620-MIE-No. 2. http://publications.gc.ca/Collection/Statcan/82-620-M/82-620-MIE2006002.pdf.

Goulet, E.D.B. (2010). Glycerol-induced hyperhydration. A method for estimating the optimal load of fluid to be ingested before exercise to maximize endurance performance. *Journal of Strength and Conditioning Research, 24*(1), 74–78.

Guh, D.P., Zhang, W., Bansback, N., Amarsi, Z., Birmingham, C.L., & Anis, A.H. (2009). The incidence of co-morbidities related to obesity and overweight: A systemic review and meta-analysis. *BMC Public Health, 9,* 88. doi:10.1186/1471-2458-9-88.

Health Canada. (2002a). Nutritional labelling. Get the facts! http://www.hc-sc.gc.ca:fn-an:label-etiquet:nutrition:index_e.html.

Health Canada. (2002b). Table of diet-related health claims. Nutrition labelling toolkit for educators. Food and nutrition. http://www.hc-sc.gc.ca/fn-an/label-etiquet/nutrition/educat/te_background-le_point-08-table2-eng.php.

Health Canada. (2006). Nutritional labelling. http://www.hc-sc.gc.ca/fn-an/label-etiquet/nutrition/index-eng.php.

Health Canada. (2007a). Trans fat. It's your health. Cat. no. H50-3/196-2005E. ISBN #0-662-41771-2. http://www.hc-sc.gc.ca/hl-vs/alt_formats/pacrb-dgapcr/pdf/iyh-vsv/food-aliment/trans-eng.pdf.

Health Canada. (2007b). Guide to developing accurate nutrient values. http://www.hc-sc.gc.ca/fn-an/label-etiquet/nutrition/reg/guide-nutri_val_tc-tm-eng.php.

Health Canada. (2010). Caffeine. http://www.hc-sc.gc.ca/hl-vs/iyh-vsv/food-aliment/caffeine-eng.php.

Health Canada. (2011). Sodium in Canada. http://www.hc-sc.gc.ca/fn-an/nutrition/sodium/index-eng.php.

Health Canada. (2012a). Sodium. http://www.hc-sc.gc.ca/hl-vs/iyh-vsv/food-aliment/sodium-eng.php.

Health Canada. (2012b). Eating well with Canada's Food Guide. http://www.hc-sc.gc.ca/fn-an/alt_formats/hpfb-dgpsa/pdf/food-guide-aliment/view_eatwell_vue_bienmang-eng.pdf.

Healthy Canadians. (2011a). Choosing foods with less sodium: At the grocery store. http://www.healthycanadians.gc.ca/init/sodium/index-eng.php.

Healthy Canadians. (2011b). Choosing foods with less sodium: When eating out. http://www.healthycanadians.gc.ca/init/sodium/index-eng.php.

Heart and Stroke Foundation of Ontario. (2012). The DASH diet to lower high blood pressure. http://www.heartandstroke.on.ca/site/c.pvI3IeNWJwE/b.4119695/k.9ECB/The_DASH_Diet_to_lower_blood_pressure.htm.

Higginbotham, S., Zhang, Z.F., Lee, I.M., Cook, N.R., Giovannucci, E., et al. (2004). Dietary glycemic load and risk of colorectal cancer in the Women's Health Study. *Journal of the National Cancer Institute, 96*(3), 229–233.

Humphrey, L.L., Fu, R., Rogers, K., Freeman, M., & Helfand, M. (2008). Homocysteine level and coronary heart disease incidence: A systematic review and meta-analysis. *Mayo Clinical Proceedings, 83*(11), 1203–1212.

Institute of Medicine. (2005). *Dietary reference intakes for energy, carbohydrate, fiber, fat, fatty acids, cholesterol, protein and amino acids.* Washington, DC: National Academies Press.

Jenkins, D.A., Wolever, T.M., Taylor, R.H., Barker, H., Fielden, H., et al. (1981). Glycemic index of foods: A physiological basis for carbohydrate exchange. *American Journal of Clinical Nutrition, 34,* 362–366.

Kastorini, C.M., Milionis, H.J., Esposito, K., Giugliano, D., Goudevenos, J.A., et al. (2011). The effect of Mediterranean diet on metabolic syndrome and its components: A meta-analysis of 50 studies and 534,906 individuals. *Journal of the American College of Cardiology, 57,* 1299–1313.

Katzmarzyk, P., & I. Janssen. (2004). The economic costs associated with physical inactivity and obesity in Canada: An update. *Canadian Journal of Applied Physiology, 29,* 90–115.

Kleiner, S. (2000). Bodybuilding. In Rosenbloom, C. (Ed.), *Sports nutrition: A guide for the professional working with active people* (3rd ed.). Chicago: American Dietetic Association.

National Institutes of Health. (n.d.). Low-calorie, lower-fat alternative foods. Department of Health and Human Services, National Heart, Lung, and Blood Institute. Obesity Education. http://www.nhlbi.nih.gov/health/public/heart/obesity/lose_wt/lcal_fat.htm.

National Institutes of Health. (2006). DASH eating plan: Your guide to lowering your blood pressure with DASH. US Department of Health and Human Services. NIH Publications no. 06-4082. http://www.nhlbi.hih.gov/health/public/heart/hbp/dash/new_dash.pdf.

National Institutes of Health, Office of Dietary Supplements. (n.d.). Nutrient recommendations: Dietary reference intakes (DRI). http://ods.od.nih.gov/Health_Information/Dietary_Reference_Intakes.aspx.

Neergaard, L. (2007). As foods dump trans fat, are they really getting healthier? *Medbroadcast Health News.* Canadian Press. http://www.medbroadcast.com.

Nseir, W., Nassar, F., & Assy, N. (2010). Soft drinks consumption and non-alcoholic fatty liver disease. *World Journal of Gastroenterology, 16*(21), 2579–2588.

Oomen, C.M., Ocké, M.C., Freskens, E.J.M., van Erp-Baart, M.J., Kok, F.J., et al. (2001). Association between trans fatty acid intake and 10-year risk of coronary heart disease in the Zutphen Elderly Study: A prospective population-based study. *Lancet, 357,* 746–751.

Panagiotopoulos, C., Ronsley, R., Elbe, D., Davidson, J., & Smith, D.H. (2010). First do no harm: Promoting an evidence-based approach to atypical antipsychotic use in children and adolescents. *Journal of the Canadian Academy of Child and Adolescent Psychiatry, 19,* 124–137.

Pérez, C.E. (2002). Fruit and vegetable consumption. *Health Reports, 13*(3). Statistics Canada Cat. no. 82-003 (pp. 23–31). http://www.statcan.gc.ca/pub/82-003-x/2001003/article/6103-eng.pdf.

Poole, C., Wilborn, C., Taylor, L., & Kerksick, C. (2010). The role of post-exercise nutrient administration of protein and glycogen synthesis. *Journal of Sports Science and Medicine, 9,* 354–363. http://www.jssm.org/vol9/n3/1/v9n3-1pdf.pdf.

Public Health Agency of Canada (PHAC). (2009). Sleep apnea rapid response. Canadian Community Health Survey (2009). http://www.phac-aspc.gc.ca/cd-mc/sleepapnea-apneesommeil/ff-rr-2009-eng.php.

Public Health Agency of Canada (PHAC). (2010a). Overweight and obese adults (self-reported). Canadian Community Health Survey, 2010 Health Fact sheets. Cat no. 82-625-X. http://www.statcan.gc.ca/pub/82-625-x/2011001/article/11461-eng.htm#ft1.

Public Health Agency of Canada (PHAC). (2010b). Fruit and vegetable consumption. Canadian Community Health Survey, 2010 Health Fact sheets. Cat. no. 82-625-X. http://www.statcan.gc.ca/pub/82-625-x/2011001/article/11461-eng.htm#ft1.

Rautiainen, S., Larsson, S., Virtamo, J., & Wolk, A. (2012). Total antioxidant capacity of diet and risk of stroke: A population-based prospective cohort of women. *Stroke, 43*(2), 335–340. http://www.ncbi.nlm.nih.gov/pubmed/22135074.

Seifert, S.M., Schaechter, J.L., Hershorin, E.R., & Lipshultz, S.E. (2011). Health effects of energy drinks on children, adolescents and young adults. *Pediatrics, 127*(3), 511–528. doi:10.1542/peds.2009-3592.

Sizer, F., & Whitney, E. (1997). *Nutrition: Concepts and controversies* (7th ed.). Belmont, CA: Wadsworth.

Strychar, I. (2006). Diet in the management of weight loss. *Canadian Medical Association Journal, 174*(1). doi:10.1503/cmaj.045037.

University of Sydney. (2011). International GI Database. http://www.glycemicindex.com.

Tipton, C.M. (Ed.). (2006). Physiological systems and their responses to conditions of heat and cold. In *ACSM's Advanced Exercise Physiology* (pp. 550–551). Baltimore, MD: Lippincott, Williams & Williams.

Wang, F., Wild, T.C., Kipp, W., Kuhle, S., & Veugelers, P.J. (2009). The influence of childhood obesity on the development of self-esteem. Statistics Canada Cat. no. 82-003-XPE. *Health Reports, 20*(2). http://www.statcan.gc.ca/pub/82-003-x/2009002/article/10871-eng.pdf.

World Cancer Research Fund. American Institute for Cancer Research. (2007). *Food, nutrition, physical activity, and the prevention of cancer: A global perspective.* Washington, DC: Author. http://www.dietandcancerreport.org.

PART 4

Understanding and Managing Potential Health Problems

9

Diabetes

LEARNING OBJECTIVES

After completing this chapter, you should be able to:

- Understand the facts about diabetes as a disease.
- Describe the four types of diabetes, including prediabetes.
- Describe signs and symptoms associated with diabetes.
- Describe the complications associated with diabetes.
- Explain the risk factors associated with diabetes.
- Describe lifestyle modifications that officers who have diabetes must make in order to perform shiftwork.

OVERVIEW

diabetes
a chronic disease in which the body cannot properly use glucose for energy

glucose
a simple form of sugar that acts as fuel for the body

Diabetes is a chronic disease in which the body cannot properly use glucose for energy. **Glucose**, a component of carbohydrates and the main source of energy for the brain, comes from foods such as breads, cereals, pasta, rice, potatoes, fruits, and some vegetables. To use glucose for energy, your body needs insulin, a hormone secreted by beta cells in the pancreas. When your body has little or no insulin, the glucose builds up in your blood instead of being used for energy. This causes high blood glucose levels, also known as hyperglycemia.

High blood sugar is associated with diabetes. Normal glucose levels are between 4.0 and 7.0 mmol/L when fasting and between 5.0 and 10.0 mmol/L, two hours after eating (Canadian Diabetes Association, 2003). When blood glucose levels are consistently above 10 mmol/L, a person is hyperglycemic, which can lead to serious medical conditions (discussed below). These can have an impact on a law officer's career—for example, the ability to drive a cruiser or deal with an emergency.

Your liver stores glucose and releases it during the night. This means that in the morning, your blood glucose level is higher even if you didn't eat before going to bed. High blood glucose is a concern for those with type 2 (formerly known as "adult-onset") diabetes, because their liver releases too much glucose. Illnesses such as a cold, flu, or infection can raise your blood glucose as a stress response. Emotional stress (excitement, anger, worry) can also increase blood glucose. These circumstances can affect your ability to do your job.

Low blood sugar—hypoglycemia—is also associated with diabetes. When blood glucose levels are between 2.5 and 4.0 mmol/L, a person is hypoglycemic (discussed below). Individuals who skip meals, eat poorly (not enough carbohydrates), are more active than usual, or take more diabetes medication than normal will experience a drop in blood glucose. People whose blood glucose is this low should not drive or operate machinery, as their responses are impaired. Below 2.5 mmol/L, individuals are severely hypoglycemic and may experience loss of consciousness or seizures.

DID YOU KNOW?

Diabetics who cannot control their blood glucose levels may have their driver's licence revoked. For more information, contact the Canadian Diabetes Association.

SOURCE: Canadian Diabetes Association, 2012a.

The Changing Face of Diabetes in Canada

Diabetes is the sixth leading cause of death in Canada (Statistics Canada, 2011). By 1999–2000, about 5.1 percent of the Canadian population aged 20 and over (approximately 1.2 million people) had been diagnosed with diabetes (Murphy, Gorber, & O'Dwyer, 2005). By 2006–2007, diabetes had increased by over 21 percent, with approximately 2 million Canadians aged one year and older, or about one in 16, diagnosed with diabetes (5.9 percent of girls/women and 6.6 percent of boys/men) (PHAC, 2009). These figures equate to more than 9 million Canadians living with diabetes or prediabetes (Canadian Diabetes Association, 2011a).

As age increases, so does prevalence of the disease, with more men being affected than women (Health Canada, 2003b; PHAC, 2009).

Rates among Aboriginal peoples are almost triple the rate of the general population. A 2006–2007 survey (PHAC, 2009) noted that prevalence of diabetes is higher in First Nations youth and seniors. The Canadian Diabetes Association (2011a) estimates that Aboriginal people are five times more likely than the general population to develop type 2 diabetes.

Notably, one in three people with diabetes don't know they have it. On average, people have diabetes for seven years before diagnosis.

FACTS ABOUT . . .

Diabetes and Mortality

- Diabetes is a contributing factor in the deaths of approximately 41,500 Canadians each year. The gap between the death rates of diabetics and non-diabetics is greater in younger age groups.
- In 2001–2002, Canadian adults with diabetes were twice as likely as those without the disease to die prematurely. By 2006, mortality rates were four to six times higher than those without diabetes for adults aged 20 to 44.
- Mortality rates for adults aged 45–79 are two to three times higher for individuals with diabetes. Children in the 1-to-19-year age group have about a 10-year reduction in life expectancy.
- Approximately 80 percent of people with diabetes will die as a result of heart disease or stroke.
- More than 9 million Canadians live with diabetes or prediabetes. With more than 20 people being newly diagnosed with the disease every hour of every day, chances are that diabetes affects you or someone you know.

SOURCES: Canadian Diabetes Association, 2011a; Health Canada, 2003b; PHAC, 2009.

What Does the Future Hold?

In 2004, academic research estimated that there would be a 76.5 percent increase in the number of people living with diabetes by 2016 (Canadian Diabetes Association, 2004). However, the prevalence of diabetes in Ontario increased so much between 1995 and 2005 that today it has already exceeded the predicted global rate set for 2030, while the mortality rate fell by 25 percent from 1995 to 2005 (Lipscombe & Hux, 2007). The Canadian Diabetes Association now estimates that 285 million people worldwide are affected with diabetes. With a further 7 million people developing diabetes each year, this number is expected to reach 438 million by 2030 (Canadian Diabetes Association, 2011a).

Of great concern is the proportion of children and adolescents who are overweight, a significant risk factor for developing diabetes. The proportion of overweight children in Ontario has tripled over the past 30 years, and the evidence clearly indicates that overweight children tend to become overweight adults, thus increasing their risk of developing type 2 diabetes in their lifetime.

The financial burden of diabetes and its complications is enormous. Diabetics have two to three times higher medical costs over their lifetime. The cost of medication and supplies can reach $15,000 a year. Of greater concern is the cost to the Canadian health-care system, predicted to reach $16.9 billion a year by 2020 (Canadian Diabetes Association, 2011a).

Types of Diabetes

There are four types of diabetes (Canadian Diabetes Association, 2011b): type 1 diabetes, type 2 diabetes, gestational diabetes, and prediabetes (the newest type identified).

Type 1 diabetes occurs when the pancreas either no longer produces insulin or produces very little. About 10 percent of people with diabetes have this type. Type 1 diabetes usually begins in the first two decades of life. In this form of diabetes, the

type 1 diabetes
diabetes that occurs when the pancreas no longer produces insulin or produces very little

immune system destroys the insulin-producing cells of the pancreas. A combination of genetic factors and environmental stressors such as viruses are believed to trigger this form of diabetes. Treatment requires a strict diet, planned physical activity, home blood glucose testing several times a day, and multiple daily insulin injections. Type 1 diabetes has huge implications for an individual's health. The pain and discomfort of blood glucose monitoring and needle injections often lead to anxiety and fear. In fact, between 33 percent and 45 percent of insulin users avoid injections because of anxiety (Travis, 2008; Zambanini, Newson, Maisey, & Feher, 1999). Fatigue is also a symptom. Type 1 diabetes can result in a drastic reduction in one's quality of life, and shortens the average lifespan by 15 years (Health Canada, 2002; PHAC, 2009).

type 2 diabetes
diabetes that occurs when the pancreas cannot produce enough insulin or the body is unable to use the insulin effectively

FYI

Symptoms of Diabetes

Some of the symptoms of diabetes that individuals experience include the following:

- unusual thirst
- frequent urination
- unusual weight loss or weight gain
- extreme fatigue or lack of energy
- blurred vision
- frequent or recurring infections
- cuts and bruises that are slow to heal
- tingling or numbness in hands or feet

Note, however, that many people who have type 2 diabetes display no symptoms.

SOURCE: Canadian Diabetes Association, 2007b.

Type 2 diabetes (formerly known as adult-onset diabetes mellitus) occurs when the pancreas cannot produce enough insulin or the body is unable to use the insulin effectively. About 90 percent of diabetics have this type. Type 2 diabetes usually develops in obese individuals over the age of 40. This form of diabetes is now widely considered to be one of the components of a group of disorders called *metabolic syndrome*, which includes central obesity (extra weight around the middle of the body), insulin resistance, high cholesterol, lipid disorders, high blood pressure, a high risk of blood clotting, and disturbed blood flow to many organs (Health Canada, 2000). Obesity, physical inactivity, poor diet, aging, hormonal changes, and stress significantly increase the risk of type 2 diabetes. The disease may be controlled by diet, exercise, and oral medication. In addition, some people require insulin injections. Weight loss can also help to bring blood sugar into the normal range, as approximately 80 percent of people who develop type 2 diabetes are overweight (US Department of Health and Human Services, 2001). Life expectancy is also reduced in people with type 2 diabetes.

The mechanisms of type 2 diabetes are not fully understood. However, some experts believe it happens in three stages (American Diabetes Association, 2007):

- The first stage is called *insulin resistance*. Although insulin can attach to the liver and muscle receptors, this stage prevents insulin from moving glucose from the blood into the cells.
- The second stage is called *postprandial hyperglycemia*, which occurs when the pancreas cannot produce enough insulin and there is an abnormal rise in blood sugar after a meal.
- The third stage is termed *fasting hyperglycemia*, a state of elevated glucose levels most of the time. Elevated glucose impairs and possibly destroys beta cells, thereby stopping insulin production and causing full-blown diabetes.

gestational diabetes
a temporary condition in which hormonal changes associated with pregnancy and the growth demands of the fetus increase insulin needs to two to three times the normal level; generally occurs after the 24th week of pregnancy and resolves after delivery

Gestational diabetes is a temporary condition that occurs during pregnancy (generally after the 24th week) and resolves after delivery. Hormonal changes associated with pregnancy and the growth demands of the fetus increase insulin needs to two to three times the normal level. Gestational diabetes occurs in 2–10 percent of all pregnancies (Centers for Disease Control and Prevention, 2011). If gestational diabetes is diagnosed in a pregnant woman but not addressed, her baby is likely to be larger than normal (over 4 kilograms or 9 pounds), born with low glucose levels, and born prematurely. It increases the risk to both mother and child of developing type 2 diabetes. Women who gain over 14 kilograms (30 pounds) during pregnancy have an increased risk. Gestational diabetes may result in respiratory distress syndrome, low blood calcium, neonatal hypoglycemia (low blood sugar in the newborn infant), and pre-eclampsia (toxemia of pregnancy, a life-threatening condition). Most neonates born with diabetes die within their first year of life despite receiving medical care (Canadian Diabetes Association, 2008).

Prediabetes is a term for impaired fasting glucose or impaired glucose tolerance. It refers to blood glucose levels that are consistently higher than normal but not over 7.0 mmol/L. Although not everyone with higher glucose levels will develop type 2 diabetes, many will, especially when combined with other metabolic syndrome risk factors such as high blood pressure, high levels of low-density lipoprotein cholesterol (LDL, or "bad" cholesterol) and triglycerides, low levels of high-density lipoproteins (HDL, or "good" cholesterol), and a tendency toward abdominal obesity. Usually, those who have prediabetes have no symptoms but if glucose levels are not lowered, they are at increased risk for developing diabetes within 10 years. There is good news, though: you can reduce the risk of getting diabetes, and even return to normal blood glucose levels, with modest weight loss and moderate physical activity.

prediabetes
impaired fasting glucose or impaired glucose tolerance; refers to blood glucose levels that are consistently higher than normal but not over 7.0 mmol/L

Diabetes may also be caused by pancreatic disease or damage to the pancreas if the insulin-producing beta cells are destroyed.

Children and Diabetes

Although type 1 diabetes can develop in children only a few months old, it is somewhat rare for children under five years to develop this disease. The incidence increases with age through childhood and adolescence, and then decreases during adulthood. Usually, people are diagnosed with type 1 diabetes before the age of 30, most often during childhood or their teens.

Type 2 diabetes in children is on the rise. In the next 15 years, it is anticipated that the global incidence will increase by up to 50 percent (Canadian Diabetes Association, 2009). One of the biggest risk factors is being overweight. Over 26 percent of children between 2 and 17 are either overweight or obese, with 8 percent being obese (Tjepkema & Shields, 2004). More than 63 percent of children and youth in Canada are insufficiently active to obtain the health benefits associated with exercise (Canadian Diabetes Association, 2009).

One of the most significant issues is unrecognized hypoglycemia, which may be disruptive to children's performance and participation in physical activity (Pacaud, 2002). This may lead to metabolic control problems. Education, regular monitoring, and lifestyle choices can help regulate metabolism.

Complications Associated with Diabetes

Diabetes results in a reduction of functional health and premature death. These outcomes are attributed to the complications associated with consistently high blood glucose levels over a prolonged period of time. Many aspects of quality of life

FACTS ABOUT . . .

Diabetes Complications

Hospitalization data indicate that adults diagnosed with diabetes were also diagnosed with the following:

- three times the rate of hypertension
- three times the rate of ischemic heart disease and heart attack
- three times the rate of stroke
- four times the rate of heart failure
- six times the rate of chronic kidney disease
- 20 times the rate of lower-limb amputation
- 12 times the rate of hospitalization for end-stage kidney disease

SOURCE: PHAC, 2009, 2011.

FYI

Diabetic Dermopathy

Diabetic dermopathy, also known as shin spots or pigmented pretibial patches, is a skin condition usually found on the lower legs of people with diabetes. It is thought to result from changes in the small blood vessels that supply the skin and from minor leakage of blood products from these vessels into the skin. Many diabetics have problems with their feet, must keep them clean and dry, and must keep their toenails in good condition.

may be affected by diabetes. Chronically high levels of blood glucose may lead to heart disease and stroke, retinopathy, kidney disease, gangrene and amputation, nerve disease (including erectile dysfunction), and other complications.

Because of the chronic nature of diabetes and the number of associated complications, it is an expensive disease to treat, both in terms of health-care costs and the toll it takes on quality of life. Diabetes plays a pivotal role in end-stage organ (especially kidney) failure. Complications of diabetes are caused by persistently high blood glucose levels, high blood pressure, and high LDL cholesterol. Months and years of elevated levels can damage the blood vessels and nerves, increasing the risk for heart disease, blindness, nerve and kidney damage, and skin complications such as bacterial and fungal infections and diabetic dermopathy. Over time, all these complications due to diabetes may lead to diabetic retinopathy, neuropathy, kidney failure, and diabetic foot (described below).

Complications affect all types of diabetes (Canadian Diabetes Association, 2006a). They include:

- *Depression* This condition is twice as common in people with diabetes as in the general population. About 25 percent of patients with diabetes have symptoms of depression, and major depression is present in at least 15 percent of those afflicted.
- *Heart disease and stroke* Compared to the general population, diabetics have cardiovascular problems at a younger age and die from these events at rates much higher than people without diabetes (three times higher for men and five times higher for women). In fact, up to 80 percent of people with diabetes will die as a result of a heart attack or stroke. On average, people with diabetes at age 40 have the same level of risk as non-diabetics who are 55 years of age (Canadian Diabetes Association, 2008).
- *Digestive problems* These are relatively common among people with diabetes. Constipation affects 60 percent of diabetics. Diabetes is also linked to diarrhea, and is one of the most common causes of gastroparesis (delayed emptying of the stomach), which affects up to 75 percent of people with diabetes. Gastroparesis can cause bloating, loss of appetite, vomiting, dehydration, heartburn, nausea, an early feeling of fullness when eating, weight loss, erratic blood glucose levels, reflux, and spasms of the stomach wall.
- *Dental problems* Diabetes can contribute to dry mouth and a burning sensation on the tongue, which can lead to irritation of the lining of the mouth. If blood glucose levels are poorly managed, toothaches, bleeding of the gums, infection of the gum and bone tissues, and delayed healing responses may result.

- *Compromised men's sexual health* Diabetes causes damage to the walls of the blood vessels, which affects circulation and blood flow. Fifty percent of men will experience erectile dysfunction (ED) within 10 years of a diagnosis of diabetes. In fact, in up to 12 percent of men with diabetes, ED is the first sign that leads to the diagnosis of diabetes.
- *Thyroid disorders* Approximately one-third of people with type 1 diabetes have thyroid disease. The thyroid is a butterfly-shaped gland in the lower neck (just beneath the skin in the front of the windpipe) that regulates the body's metabolism. An overactive thyroid (hyperthyroidism) may increase insulin requirements, while an underactive thyroid (hypothyroidism) may decrease insulin requirements.
- *Diabetic retinopathy and other eye conditions* Diabetic retinopathy is the most common cause of blindness in people under age 65. About one in four people with diabetes experience this problem. Those who develop diabetes are also more likely to develop cataracts at a younger age and are twice as likely to develop glaucoma (increased intra-ocular pressure causing irreversible optic nerve damage). Nearly all people with type 1 diabetes and 60 percent of those with type 2 develop some form of diabetic retinopathy during the first 20 years they have the disease (PHAC, 2008). It is the leading cause of vision loss in Canadians under 50 (PHAC, 2008) and of adult blindness in Canada (Health Canada, 2003b). Diabetes causes the arteries in the retina to weaken and begin to leak, forming dot-like hemorrhages. Vision may begin to blur, floaters (caused by blood leaking into the retina) may drift in front of the visual field, and eyesight may decrease. With abnormal vessel growth and scar tissue, some people develop retinal detachment (separation of the sensory and pigment layers) and glaucoma.
- *Neuropathy* Damage to sensory nerves of the extremities can affect the transmission of nerve impulses and lead to loss of sensation, making people more prone to injury. Numbness and tingling in the feet is often the first sign, though symptoms vary depending on the nerve(s) and the part of the body affected. Because of poor circulation, wounds heal slowly or ineffectively. Some people suffer from pressure sores. Gangrene and amputation are more common in people with this complication.
- *Skin infections* These include bacterial infections (styes, boils, folliculitis, carbuncles, and nail infections) caused by *Staphylococcus*, as well as yeast-like fungal infections between the fingers and toes, corners of the mouth, armpits, groin, and so on.
- *Diabetic foot* This complication manifests as infection in the skin, muscles, or bones of the foot, resulting in poor circulation and neuropathy. The diabetic's compromised immune system can lead to the loss of sensation in the foot, reduced blood circulation, poor wound healing, death of the tissue, severe infection, gangrene, and potential amputation. Approximately 15 percent of individuals with diabetes will develop foot ulceration at some point in their life (American Podiatric Medical Association, 2007), and half of all leg amputations occur in people with diabetes (Foster & Edmonds, 2001).

- *Diabetic nephropathy* This is the most common cause of chronic kidney failure, which accounted for 35 percent of all new kidney failure cases in 2006 (PHAC, 2008). The kidneys lose the ability to filter out waste products, leading to a buildup of waste in the blood and, ultimately, end-stage kidney disease. Early intervention can prevent or delay the advance of diabetic kidney disease.

Risk Factors Associated with Diabetes

Some of the risk factors for developing diabetes include the following (Canadian Diabetes Association, 2007b):

- *Age* Incidence increases with age—throughout childhood and adolescence for type 1, and after 40 years of age in adults for type 2.
- *Being overweight* A BMI greater than 27 indicates a risk for developing type 2 diabetes and other health problems, including cardiovascular disease and premature death (Centers for Disease Control and Prevention, 2003; Health Canada, 2003a).
- *Having an apple-shaped figure* Individuals who carry most of their weight in the trunk of their bodies tend to have a higher risk of diabetes than those of similar weight with pear-shaped bodies (excess fat carried mainly in the hips and thighs). A waist measurement of more than 100 centimetres (39.5 inches) in men and 95 centimetres (37.5 inches) in women suggests an increased risk (Centers for Disease Control and Prevention, 2003).
- *Having a sedentary lifestyle* Lack of exercise and sitting for long periods of time can lead to being overweight, which increases the risk of diabetes and impedes glucose uptake.
- *Belonging to a high-risk group* People of Aboriginal, Hispanic, Asian, or African descent are three to five times more likely than the general population to develop diabetes. Aboriginal people, in particular, suffer a greater risk and burden of poor health compared to other Canadians. Of special note, diabetes also develops at an earlier age among First Nations people, and in recent years, type 2 diabetes has been diagnosed in First Nations children (First Nations and Inuit Regional Health Survey National Steering Committee, 1999). Almost one-third of First Nations women with diabetes report getting the diagnosis during pregnancy (Dean, 1998).

  Factors that pose a risk to Aboriginal populations are lifestyle and heredity. The relatively recent shift from traditional diets high in animal protein to "modern urban diets" high in carbohydrates, combined with decreased physical activity, has resulted in high levels of obesity that compound pre-existing risks for diabetes. Type 2 diabetes, in particular, is increasingly prevalent, as is its main risk factor—excess body weight. Rates of diabetes in First Nations escalated from 9.3 percent in 1995 to 15 percent in 2006–2007 (PHAC, 2009) and are higher in women than men, affecting this population at a younger age.
- *Family history* The genetic link for type 2 diabetes is stronger than the genetic link for type 1. Having a parent or sibling with the disease particularly increases risk (Centers for Disease Control and Prevention, 2003).

- *History of diabetes during pregnancy* Nearly 40 percent of women who have diabetes during their pregnancy go on to develop type 2 diabetes later, usually within 5 to 10 years of giving birth. Giving birth to a baby that weighs more than 4 kilograms (9 pounds) is a symptom of gestational diabetes (Centers for Disease Control and Prevention, 2003).
- *Dyslipidemia (high cholesterol) or other fats in the blood* More than 40 percent of people with diabetes have abnormal levels of cholesterol and similar fatty substances that circulate in the blood. These abnormalities appear to be associated with an increased risk for cardiovascular disease.
- *Impaired glucose tolerance* If blood sugar control and reaction to sugar loads are abnormal, there is a higher risk of developing type 2 diabetes within five years and developing cardiovascular disease (Centers for Disease Control and Prevention, 2003).
- *High blood pressure* Up to 60 percent of people with undiagnosed diabetes have high blood pressure (Centers for Disease Control and Prevention, 2003).
- *Prediabetes* In this condition, blood sugar levels are higher than normal but not high enough to be classified as type 2 diabetes. Left untreated, prediabetics often progress to type 2 diabetes.

Turn to **assignment 9.1** (in the appendix) and assess your risk for diabetes.

What Happens When You Are Hypoglycemic or Hyperglycemic?

Insulin shock is another term used for the condition of hypoglycemia or low blood sugar. Symptoms include shakes, sweating, trembling, dizziness, irritability, confusion, blurred vision, and hunger. In severe cases, low blood sugar may cause you to pass out. It is common in diabetics who take too much insulin, skip meals, drink too much alcohol, and exercise too vigorously. Treatment includes providing the individual with something to ingest that contains a high amount of glucose; this will increase blood sugar levels adequately in order to improve mental status. Such treatment can include tablets made of glucose or dextrose (these can be obtained at health food stores), fruit juices such as orange juice or apple juice, milk, 100 millilitres of regular soda pop, or table sugar (10–15 grams or 2–3 teaspoons) with water. Bystanders should not try to administer fluids by mouth to someone who is unconscious, because this may cause the person to aspirate (inhale the fluid into the lungs, which can cause serious complications).

Hyperglycemia is a condition caused by greater than normal glucose in the blood. Symptoms include increased thirst, frequent urination, dry mouth, nausea, vomiting, shortness of breath, and fatigue. Prolonged high levels can lead to ketoacidosis, which results when fat is used as the energy source rather than glucose, resulting in ketones (a chemical byproduct of the breakdown of fat) in the urine. This is more common in type 1 diabetes, and can lead to serious dehydration and coma. Symptoms of ketoacidosis include a slightly sweet breath odour (which smells like nail-polish remover), extreme dryness of the mucous membranes, weight loss, increased thirst and urination, weakness, abdominal pains, generalized aches, nausea and vomiting, and breathlessness (Canadian Diabetes Association, 2007a).

Living with Diabetes and Shiftwork

The province of Ontario designates certain medical conditions as possible grounds for disqualification to be hired as a police constable, for example, dialysis dependence or insulin dependence. In the latter case, the applicant will be referred to a specialist to determine whether he or she meets the medical standards for driving (in accordance with the driving fitness guidelines of the CMA and the Canadian Diabetes Association). Those candidates who are non-insulin-treated diabetics and do not have an understanding of how to control insulin levels through diet, medication, and exercise may be considered ineligible as well. (To learn more about medical requirements, refer to Ontario Association of Chiefs of Police, 2009, in the References.)

Shiftwork can be hard on everyone, but it can be especially challenging for those with diabetes. One of the biggest changes in recent years regarding diabetes management is taking responsibility for your own care. Shiftwork will increase your risk of a hypoglycemic incident. This pattern of work influences the body's circadian (daily) rhythms, which regulate processes such as hunger and fatigue, thus disrupting your body's internal clock and affecting blood glucose control from physical and mental stress.

Putting a plan in place will help you deal effectively with diabetes (Canadian Diabetes Association, 2006b; Diabetes UK, 2006):

- Prepare a written plan that you can share with your supervisor, including a medical plan and personal health identification.
- Wear personal health identification (such as a medical alert bracelet).
- Carry quick, easy-to-eat food that you can consume following a check of your blood glucose level.
- Have regularly planned meals. Snacking and strict adherence to certain mealtimes may not be as critical for people on regular, intermediate-acting, or premixed insulins; however, this approach is very important for somebody taking oral medications in place of injections.
- Carry your blood glucose meter with you in your cruiser. When you are driving for work or operating machinery (such as on snowmobile or water patrol), it is best that you check your levels every couple of hours to know how much insulin you need rather than risk a hypoglycemic reaction.
- Take regular rest breaks.
- Engage in regular physical activity. This is very important, especially if you are working the night shift.
- Manage your stress. Stress can increase your body's production of hormones that block the effects of insulin, causing your blood sugar to rise. As well, prolonged stress may lead to depression.

A great resource for more information on managing your weight, alcohol intake, blood pressure, cholesterol, and nutritional concerns such as eating out, glycemic index, and basic carbohydrates is the Canadian Diabetes Association at www.diabetes.ca.

Despite all the latest advancements in the treatment of diabetes, there are still complications that may preclude you from policing. Those who have foot problems may find it difficult to wear steel-toed boots on cold concrete for 12-hour shifts. Retinopathy may impair your vision, making it difficult to work as a patrol officer. Finally, shift rotation can be stressful. It is best to have shifts that rotate every two to three days and move "forward" (from morning to afternoon to night). The stress of shiftwork can be further compounded by adding court days to regular shifts.

Remember that *you* have to take care of you. Research suggests that lifestyle and type 2 diabetes are closely linked. This means that you can help prevent or delay the onset of the disease. A healthy diet, weight control, exercise, and stress management are important preventive steps.

DID YOU KNOW?

Studies have shown that through lifestyle changes, including moderate weight loss and regular exercise, the onset of type 2 diabetes can be delayed by up to 58 percent.

SOURCE: Knowler, Barrett-Connor, Fowler, Hamman, Lachin, et al., 2002.

A Final Word

With early diagnosis, you can manage diabetes fairly well. It is important that you learn as much about the disease as you can in order to make healthier life choices, and be sure to get tested every three years after you reach age 40.

You need to know what, when, and how much to eat in order to manage your blood sugar levels. You may need to add pills, insulin, or both to your lifestyle changes to achieve your blood glucose targets. You must also maintain a healthy weight, especially if you have type 2 diabetes. Exercise is known to lower blood sugar and enhance overall fitness. This will also help to keep your blood pressure at or below 130/80 and your cholesterol levels down.

Here are some additional suggestions to help prevent, delay, or manage diabetes:

- If you smoke, make a serious effort to quit.
- See an eye specialist on a regular basis to check for signs of eye disease.
- Exercise proper foot care, have your feet checked regularly by your physician, and keep your vaccinations up to date.
- Be nutritionally conscious when you are at work and home. You can find diabetes-friendly recipes on the website of the Canadian Diabetes Association (2012b), or research the DASH (Dietary Approaches to Stop Hypertension) diet at the National Heart, Lung, and Blood Institute (n.d.) (see References).
- Speak to a specialist if you are feeling overwhelmed or depressed about how diabetes is negatively affecting you.
- If your extremities feel numb or if you experience "pins and needles," advise your physician.
- Have your urine tested regularly for early signs of kidney disease.
- Have your teeth cleaned twice a year.

Stay healthy by asking your doctor the right questions. Be a proactive patient who is informed.

KEY TERMS

diabetes, 206
gestational diabetes, 208
glucose, 206
prediabetes, 209
type 1 diabetes, 207
type 2 diabetes, 208

EXERCISES

True or False?

1. You can help prevent or delay type 2 diabetes.
2. By far the most common form of diabetes is type 2 diabetes mellitus.
3. Risk factors for type 1 diabetes mellitus include family history, obesity, inactivity, and being a member of a high-risk population.
4. Type 1 diabetes mellitus is caused by an autoimmune reaction that destroys the beta cells of the pancreas.
5. Type 2 diabetes mellitus was previously called juvenile-onset or insulin-dependent diabetes.
6. When a pregnant woman develops diabetes mellitus it is called gestational diabetes.
7. Babies born to mothers with gestational diabetes often exhibit excessive birth weight.
8. In type 2 diabetes mellitus the body tissues become less sensitive to the effects of insulin.
9. Blurred vision is a symptom of low blood sugar.
10. Type 1 diabetes can be prevented or delayed through weight loss and exercise.

Multiple Choice

1. What symptom(s) may indicate that you should get checked for diabetes?
   - **a.** your feet swell up
   - **b.** you feel more energized than usual
   - **c.** you may be extra thirsty and lose weight quickly
   - **d.** you gain weight and are hungry
   - **e.** you experience heart palpitations
2. How often should you test your blood glucose?
   - **a.** it depends on the individual
   - **b.** every 24 hours
   - **c.** every couple of hours
   - **d.** before you eat
   - **e.** when you first get up and when you go to bed
3. What does diabetes have to do with your nerves?
   - **a.** it makes them more aware of your surroundings
   - **b.** it affects the transmission of nerve impulses
   - **c.** it interferes with blood flow to the tissues
   - **d.** it has nothing to do with your nerves
   - **e.** it sends feedback to the brain
4. What is the greatest risk factor for diabetes?
   - **a.** poor lifestyle choices
   - **b.** ethnic background and genetic susceptibility
   - **c.** eating too much sugar
   - **d.** smoking and drinking
   - **e.** exercising too much
5. What does diabetes have to do with erectile dysfunction?
   - **a.** it is not involved in sexual dysfunction
   - **b.** no one really understands the link
   - **c.** nerve damage affects the blood flow to the penis
   - **d.** it prevents the dysfunction
   - **e.** blood flow to the groin is decreased
6. What does diabetes have to do with dental care?
   - **a.** diabetes is unrelated to dental care
   - **b.** diabetes can cause gum disease and teeth problems
   - **c.** dentists want to be involved in your health care
   - **d.** diabetes affects the alignment of your teeth
   - **e.** diabetes medication promotes good dental health

7. What is diabetic ketoacidosis?
   a. the name of a diabetic research project
   b. a life-saving condition
   c. a form of indigestion caused by too much acid
   d. the breakdown of protein to use as an energy source in place of glucose
   e. the breakdown of fat to use as an energy source in place of glucose
8. What do diabetes pills do?
   a. they treat pancreas problems
   b. they help keep blood glucose in the target range
   c. they help to keep you regular
   d. they reduce pain
   e. they help digestive enzymes
9. How does diabetes affect your eyes?
   a. lack of insulin interferes with brain signals to the eyes
   b. lack of insulin reduces energy levels to the brain
   c. high blood glucose levels can damage blood vessels in the retina
   d. low blood glucose levels can cause cornea damage
   e. low blood glucose causes headaches behind the eyes
10. Who should check your blood glucose levels?
    a. only your doctor
    b. your doctor and a diabetic educator
    c. you
    d. you, your doctor, and a diabetic educator
    e. you don't have to check your levels outside of a medical checkup
11. How does diabetes affect your feet?
    a. it causes athlete's foot
    b. it causes feet to become very sweaty
    c. it causes blisters on the feet
    d. it affects the arch in your foot
    e. it causes nerve damage to the feet
12. Can children and young people develop type 2 diabetes?
    a. yes, but mostly adults develop type 2 diabetes
    b. yes, but they grow out of it
    c. no, only adults get type 2 diabetes
    d. no, because they exercise too much
    e. yes; children first develop type 1, which then becomes type 2
13. How does diabetes affect your kidneys?
    a. it affects the liver rather than the kidneys
    b. high blood glucose levels can affect the kidneys' filter system
    c. insulin gets blocked in the kidneys
    d. fat cells get blocked by the kidneys
    e. protein cells get blocked by the kidneys
14. Why is it important to check blood glucose levels with diabetes?
    a. regular checks don't change the condition of the disease
    b. regular checks ensure that blood glucose remains at a normal level
    c. regular checks ensure that you don't need to take insulin
    d. regular checks take your blood glucose levels down
    e. regular checks ensure you have enough fluids in your body
15. How is type 2 diabetes controlled?
    a. through insulin injections
    b. you don't need to do anything
    c. exercise and diet alone
    d. insulin, exercise, diet, and healthy lifestyle choices
    e. through a high carbohydrate diet
16. Which statement regarding prediabetes is incorrect?
    a. Prediabetes is a term for impaired fasting glucose or impaired glucose tolerance.
    b. More than 9 million Canadians live with diabetes or prediabetes.
    c. Symptoms show up quickly for those who develop prediabetes.
    d. Abdominal fat increases your risk of becoming prediabetic.
    e. Blood sugar levels are higher than normal but not high enough to be classified as type 2 diabetes.

17. If you have diabetes in your family, are you at risk?
   a. you definitely will get diabetes
   b. you aren't at any risk for diabetes
   c. if one person has diabetes, everyone will have diabetes
   d. you are at low risk for developing the disease
   e. you are at higher risk for developing the disease

18. What is neuropathy?
   a. sensory nerve damage
   b. the study of the brain
   c. nervous system surgery
   d. the study of kidney nerves
   e. the pathway of nerve transmissions

19. What signs might you see if someone is experiencing low blood glucose?
   a. the person is out of breath after a 1.5-mile run
   b. the person becomes emotional
   c. the person gets confused and may lose consciousness
   d. the person is not hungry
   e. the person can't do more than 10 curl-ups

20. How do you know if you have type 2 diabetes?
   a. you are more thirsty than normal and have blurry vision
   b. you feel really energetic but not very hungry
   c. a friend tells you that you have diabetes
   d. you are energetic and able to work out vigorously
   e. you are not thirsty after working out

Short Answer

1. What is the prevalence of diabetes in Canada?

2. Describe the difference between type 1 and type 2 diabetes.

3. Explain what prediabetes is and the impact it could have on your career.

4. What are five risk factors associated with type 2 diabetes?

5. What are five of the signs or symptoms of diabetes?

6. How does shiftwork affect diabetes?

7. Describe five ways to regulate your blood sugar levels.

8. What are three severe complications of diabetes?

9. How can you moderate diabetes risks?

REFERENCES

American Diabetes Association. (2007). Diagnosis and classification of diabetes mellitus. *Diabetes Care, 30,* 42–47.

American Podiatric Medical Association. (2007). Facts on diabetes and the foot. http://www.apma.org/faqsdiab.html.

Canadian Diabetes Association. (2003). Insulin: Things you should know. http://www.diabetes.ca/section_about/insulin3.asp.

Canadian Diabetes Association. (2004). Projection of prevalence and cost of diabetes in Canada: 2000–2016. *Canadian Journal of Diabetes, 28*(2), 1–8.

Canadian Diabetes Association. (2006a). About diabetes: Complications. http://www.diabetes.ca/diabetes-and-you/living/complications.

Canadian Diabetes Association. (2006b). About diabetes: Diabetes and shiftwork. http://www.diabetes.ca.

Canadian Diabetes Association. (2007a). About diabetic ketoacidosis. http://www.diabetes.ca.

Canadian Diabetes Association. (2007b). Are you at risk? http://www.diabetes.ca/diabetes-and-you/what/at-risk.

Canadian Diabetes Association. (2008). Diabetes + heart disease. http://www.diabetes.ca/getserious/heart-disease.

Canadian Diabetes Association. (2009). Researching the way to better diabetes care. Research report 2009. http://www.diabetes.ca/documents/about-us/Research_Report_-_2009.pdf.

Canadian Diabetes Association. (2011a). The prevalence and costs of diabetes. http://www.diabetes.ca/diabetes-and-you/what/prevalence.

Canadian Diabetes Association. (2011b). Diabetes and you. What is diabetes? http://www.diabetes.ca/diabetes-and-you.

Canadian Diabetes Association. (2012a). FAQs—Diabetes and driving. http://www.diabetes.ca/get-involved/helping-you/advocacy/faq/driving.

Canadian Diabetes Association. (2012b). Recipes. http://www.diabetes.ca/diabetes-and-you/recipes.

Centers for Disease Control and Prevention. (2003). National diabetes fact sheet: National estimates and general information on diabetes and prediabetes in the United States, 2003. Atlanta: US Department of Health and Human Services.

Centers for Disease Control and Prevention. (2011). National diabetes fact sheet: National estimates and general information on diabetes and prediabetes in the United States, 2011. Atlanta: US Department of Health and Human Services. http://diabetes.niddk.nih.gov/dm/pubs/statistics.

Dean, H. (1998). NIDDM among youth in First Nation children in Canada. *Clinical Pediatrics, 37*, 89–96.

Diabetes UK. (2006). Diabetes and the police officer: Guidance for the recruitment and employment of police officers with diabetes. http://www.diabetes.org.uk/Documents/Reports/police_Guidance_FINAL.pdf.

First Nations and Inuit Regional Health Survey National Steering Committee. (1999). *First Nations and Inuit Regional Health Survey: National report.* Ottawa: Health Canada.

Foster, A., & Edmonds, M. (2001). An overview of foot disease in patients with diabetes. *Nursing Standard, 16*(12), 45–52.

Health Canada. (2000). *Diabetes among Aboriginal (First Nations, Inuit and Métis) people in Canada: The evidence.* Ottawa: Author.

Health Canada. (2002). *Diabetes in Canada* (2nd ed.). Centre for Chronic Disease Prevention and Control Population and Public Health Branch. http://www.phac-aspc.gc.ca/publicat/dic-dac2/pdf/dic-dac2_en.pdf.

Health Canada. (2003a). Canadian guidelines for healthy weight classification in adults. Office of Nutrition Policy and Promotion. http://www.hc-sc.gc.ca/fn-an/alt_formats/hpfb-dgpsa/pdf/nutrition/weight_book-livres_des_poids-eng.pdf.

Health Canada. (2003b). *Responding to the challenge of diabetes in Canada.* Catalogue no. H39-4/21-2003E. Ottawa: Author.

Knowler, W.C., Barrett-Connor, E., Fowler, S.E., Hamman, R.F., Lachin, J.M., et al. (2002). Reduction in the incidence of type 2 diabetes with lifestyle intervention or metformin. *New England Journal of Medicine, 346*(6), 393–403.

Lipscombe, L., & Hux, J. (2007). Trends in diabetes prevalence, incidence and mortality in Ontario, Canada 1995–2005: A population-based study. *Lancet, 369*(9563), 750–756.

Murphy, K., Gorber, S.C., & O'Dwyer, A. (2005). *Population health impact of disease in Canada (PHI). Health state descriptions for Canadians: Diabetes.* Catalogue no. 82-619-MIE2005002. Ottawa: Statistics Canada.

National Heart, Lung, and Blood Institute. (n.d.). Healthy eating. [The DASH diet.] http://www.nhlbi.nih.gov/hbp/prevent/h_eating/h_eating.htm.

Ontario Association of Chiefs of Police (OACP). (2009, September). Constable selection system: Self assess! Medical requirements for candidates. http://www.mcscs.jus.gov.on.ca/stellent/groups/public/@mcscs/@www/@com/documents/webasset/ec075034.pdf.

Pacaud, D. (2002). Hypoglycemia: The Achilles heel of the treatment of children with type 1 diabetes. *Canadian Journal of Diabetes, 26*(3), 215–222.

Public Health Agency of Canada (PHAC). (2006, August). Diabetes in Canada. http://www.phac-aspc.gc.ca/publicat/dic-dac99/d07_e.html.

Public Health Agency of Canada (PHAC). (2008). National diabetes fact sheets, Canada 2008. Common complications of diabetes. http://www.phac-aspc.gc.ca/publicat/2008/ndfs-fnrd-08/ndfs_lwd-fnrd_vad-eng.php.

Public Health Agency of Canada (PHAC). (2009). *Report from the National Diabetes Surveillance System: Diabetes in Canada, 2009.* Catalogue no. HP32-2/1-2009E-PDF. Ottawa: Centre for Chronic Disease Prevention and Control.

Public Health Agency of Canada (PHAC). (2011). *Diabetes in Canada: Facts and figures from a public health perspective, 2011.* Catalogue no. HP35-25/2011E-PDF. Ottawa: Author.

Statistics Canada. (2011, November 1). Table 102-0561—Leading causes of death, total population, by age group and sex, Canada, annual, 2000 to 2008. CANSIM database. Catalogue no. 84-215-XWE. http://www5.statcan.gc.ca/cansim/a26;jsessionid=C29808782DB6E07BCF9CEE61DBE7CF51?lang=eng&retrLang=eng&id=1020561&pattern=102-0561..102-0563&tabMode=dataTable&srchLan=-1&p1=-1&p2=-1#F15.

Tjepkema, M., & Shields, M. (2004). *Nutrition: Findings from the Canadian Community Health Survey. Issue no. 1. Measured obesity: Adult obesity in Canada.* Ottawa: Statistics Canada.

Travis, L. (2008, September 10). One-third of patients with diabetes fear and dread insulin injections. *Endocrine Today*, *6*(16). http://www.i-port.com/downloads/Endocrine_Today.pdf.

US Department of Health and Human Services. (2001). Diet and exercise dramatically delay type 2 diabetes. http://www.hhs.gov/news/press/2001pres/20010808a.html.

Zambanini, A., Newson, R.B., Maisey, M., & Feher, M.D. (1999). Injection-related anxiety in insulin treated diabetes. *Diabetes Research in Clinical Practice*, *46*(3), 239–246.

10

Cardiovascular Disease

LEARNING OBJECTIVES

After completing this chapter, you should be able to:

- Comment on the impact of cardiovascular disease on Canadian society.
- Understand the basic anatomy of the heart and the etiology of various cardiovascular diseases.
- Describe six types of cardiovascular disease: ischemic heart disease, cerebrovascular disease, peripheral vascular disease, heart failure, rheumatic heart disease, and congenital heart disease.
- Describe four common cardiovascular diseases: arteriosclerosis, coronary heart disease, stroke, and hypertension.
- Describe the controllable and uncontrollable risk factors associated with cardiovascular diseases.
- List some of the symptoms of heart attacks and strokes.
- Make appropriate health decisions regarding your heart.

OVERVIEW

The term *cardiovascular disease* applies to any disease that affects the heart or blood vessels. Although much research—and media attention—has focused on diseases such as cancer, HIV/AIDS, and hepatitis B and C, cardiovascular disease was the leading cause of death until 2005 (Statistics Canada, 2011, p. 6). While mortality rates have declined in recent years, in 2008, 29 percent of all deaths in Canada were due to cardiovascular disease (Heart and Stroke Foundation of Canada [HSFC], 2012). Figure 10.1 shows the proportion of deaths attributable to the leading risk factors worldwide. The highest risk factor, by far, is high blood pressure (WHO, 2008, 2009).

Cardiovascular Disease: A Canadian Concern

Canadian statistics reveal that women have caught up to men when it comes to deaths from cardiovascular disease (HSFC, 2007c; Statistics Canada, 2011). In 1973, there were 23 percent fewer female than male deaths from heart disease and stroke (34,924 female deaths versus 45,404 male deaths). By 2003, the number of male deaths had decreased by 19 percent, to 37,004, while the number of female deaths *increased* by 5 percent to 36,823. By 2008, more women (34,909) than men (34,739) died of cardiovascular disease.

Of all cardiovascular deaths in 2008, 54 percent were due to ischemic heart disease, 20 percent to stroke, 23 percent to heart attack, and 3 percent due to other forms of heart disease (malfunctioning of the electrical system of the heart, viral heart infections, and heart muscle diseases) and vascular problems, including arteriosclerosis (hardening of the arteries), atherosclerosis (buildup of plaque in the arteries), and high blood pressure (Statistics Canada, 2011).

FIGURE 10.1 Distribution of Deaths Worldwide for Women and Men, 2004

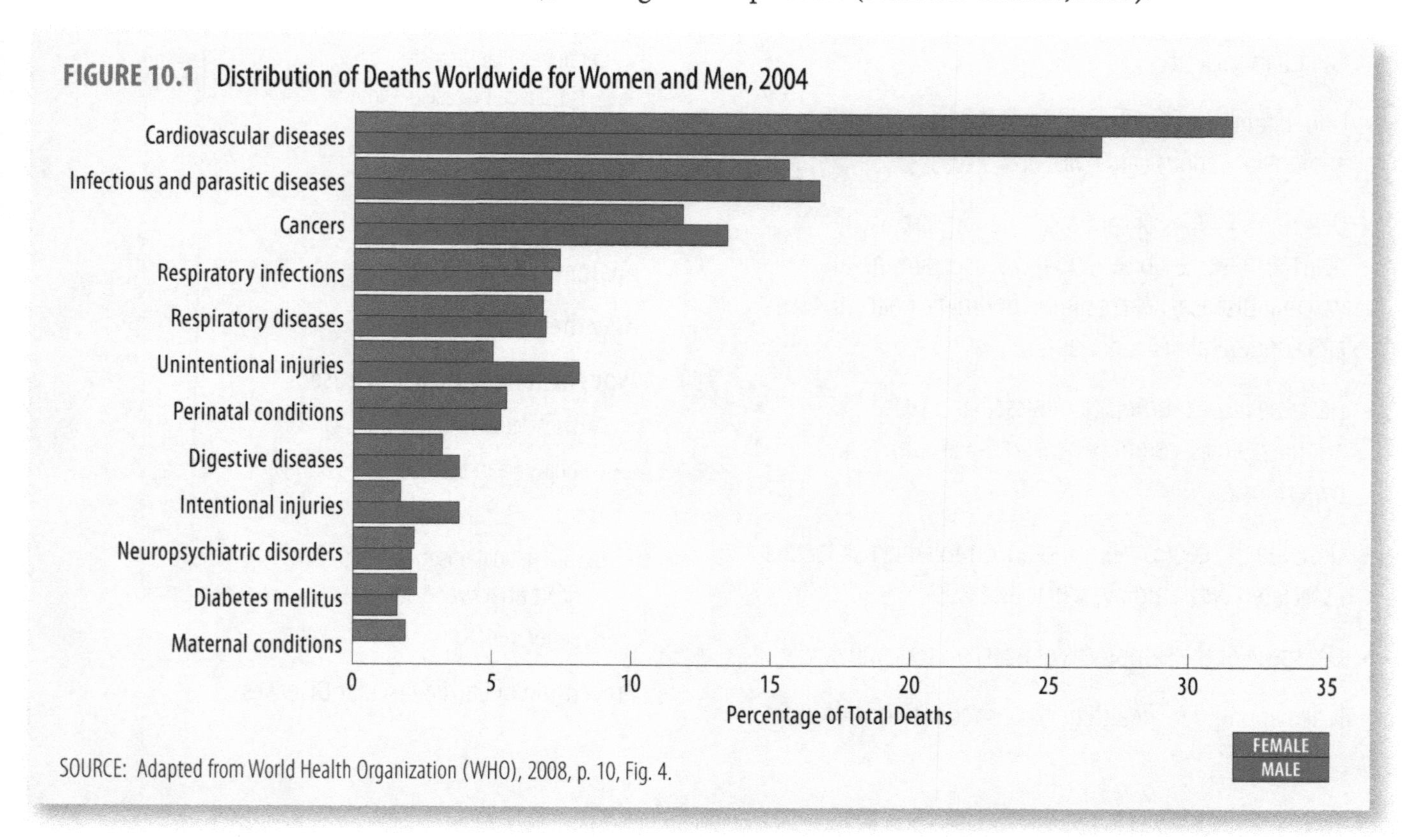

SOURCE: Adapted from World Health Organization (WHO), 2008, p. 10, Fig. 4.

Considerable research has identified the major risk factors for heart disease. It is important to manage the risks that you can influence, especially if you have other risk factors that are beyond your control.

Risk factors that you *cannot* control include age and gender (55 and over for women, 45 and over for men), ethnic descent (African, South Asian, and First Nations populations are at higher risk), and family history, which includes heart attacks or strokes before age 65, and angina.

Risk factors that you *can* control or manage include high blood cholesterol, high blood pressure (hypertension), lack of exercise, being overweight, smoking, drinking too much alcohol, stress, lack of fruit and vegetables in your diet, and diabetes (HSFC, 2001).

FYI

On the Job

In the spring of 2002, the RCMP's "O" Division had its officers' blood cholesterol levels tested. Almost 50 percent of those tested had high cholesterol readings (R. Seguin, RCMP "O" Division Fitness and Lifestyle Coordinator, personal communication, 2007). This finding has serious implications: combined with any other risk factors, high cholesterol can be life threatening. The stresses of shiftwork, the lack of available nutritious foods on night shifts, and, for some officers, limited involvement in exercise programs—especially for those who live and work in isolated locations—can be a deadly combination. As an officer, you need to be aware of the risks associated with the career that you have chosen.

Cardiovascular Disease: Not Just a Disease of Old Age

Canadians run a high risk of developing cardiovascular diseases. We know that 9 out of 10 Canadians have at least one risk factor associated with cardiovascular disease (smoking, alcohol, physical inactivity, overweight or obesity, high blood pressure, high blood cholesterol, less than recommended daily consumption of vegetables and fruit, diabetes, stress) (Public Health Agency of Canada [PHAC], 2009), and we've gone from 1 in 10 having three or more risk factors (HSFC, 2003) to 2 in 5 in 2009 (PHAC, 2009).

Cardiovascular disease is not restricted to elderly people. It is the number two killer for ages 25–64 years, the number three killer for ages 0–14 years, and the number five killer for ages 15–24 years (HSFC, 2007a).

Young people carry a high level of risk factors. Nearly 40 percent of teenaged girls are physically inactive. Nearly 25 percent of adults in their 20s are overweight. Twenty percent of young women in their later teens (18–19 years) and 25 percent of young men smoke cigarettes daily.

We know that women tend to be more physically inactive and have higher blood pressure after menopause. More men smoke, consume less than the recommended amounts of fruits and vegetables, and are overweight. All these risks can lead to cardiovascular disease. Many cardiac rehabilitative exercise therapists are seeing increasing numbers of patients who are between 25 and 50 years of age (J. Pepe, CSEP Certified Exercise Physiologist, personal communication, 2007).

Income and education also affect the prevalence of cardiovascular diseases. Those with higher levels of education tend to have increased knowledge and skills to undertake healthier behaviours. Individuals who live in poverty, however, must cope with meeting basic needs, and their lack of income may limit their ability to purchase healthy foods, engage in physical activity, and acquire medications that can improve health problems such as high blood pressure and diabetes.

Cardiovascular diseases (CVDs) have become the most costly contributors to health costs in Canada. In 2000, CVDs were the second most costly contributor to total Canadian health costs ($22.2 billion). In the same year, hospital care was the largest contributor to CVD health-care costs ($4.0 billion), while drugs cost $2.1 billion and physician care cost $1.5 billion. Premature death from CVDs results in an estimated $9.3 billion in lost productivity annually, while long-term disability costs us $4.2 billion, and short-term disability $1.2 billion (PHAC, 2009). A study by the Conference Board of Canada has projected that by 2020, total costs for CVDs could reach $28.3 billion (Browarski, Stonebridge, & Theriault, 2010, p. 15).

Cardiovascular Disease: Not Just a Man's Disease

The gap between men and women in the number of deaths from heart disease and stroke has reversed, with more women than men dying after a cardiovascular event such as a heart attack or stroke. In 2004, more women (8,667) died from stroke than did men (5,959) (HSFC, 2007c). The Heart and Stroke Foundation of Canada (2007c) has reported that women are 16 percent more likely than men to die within 30 days of a heart attack and 11 percent more likely than men to die within 30 days of a stroke. Issues that need to be addressed include education (including the role of the mass media) about risks and symptoms, poverty, geography, women's roles and control over their lives, and equality of access to services.

Older women face the greatest danger, because the risk of cardiovascular disease quadruples after menopause (Terry, Pencina, Vasan, Murabito, Wolf, et al., 2005). At menopause, the ovaries gradually stop producing the heart-protective hormone estrogen. There may be an increase in LDL or "bad" cholesterol and triglyceride levels, and a decrease in HDL or "good" cholesterol. Blood pressure also starts creeping up. Reduced estrogen may lead to an increase in body fat above the waist, which affects the way blood clots and the way the body handles sugars (prediabetes).

In 2008, 16 percent of women and 20 percent of men in Canada aged 15 years and older were smokers. The good news regarding this statistic is that it is the lowest level in more than four decades of monitoring smoking rates (Health Canada, 2007; Canadian Cancer Society, 2010). However, with smoking and the use of oral contraceptives combined, there is increased risk for blood clots and stroke in women (Stampfer, Hu, Manson, Rimm, & Willett, 2003).

Another frightening statistic is that almost 60 percent of adults aged 18 and older, or 14.1 million Canadians, are overweight or obese, with 53 percent of Canadian women aged 18 and older overweight or obese (Tjepkema, 2005). Obesity increases the risk of high blood pressure, diabetes, high blood cholesterol, heart disease, and stroke. With over 49 percent of women aged 12 and older inactive, women are doubling their risk of developing heart disease, doubling the risk of dying from cardiovascular disease, and increasing the risk of hypertension. If a woman becomes hypertensive, it increases the risk of cardiovascular disease by 3.5 times over that of a woman with normal blood pressure (Corrao, Becker, Ockene, & Hamilton, 1990). Women and men with high blood pressure at age 50 develop heart disease seven years earlier and die on average five years earlier than people with normal blood pressure at this age (Women's Heart Foundation, 2007). Combine any of these factors with diabetes, and the risk of developing cardiovascular disease becomes two to four times greater than that for women without diabetes (Centers for Disease Control and Prevention, 2011).

Cardiovascular Disease and Children

In Canada, rates of obesity among children and youth aged 2–17 years are increasing. In 1978–1979, just 3 percent of children and youth were obese; by 2009, 8.6 percent of children and youth aged 6–17 were obese (PHAC, 2011). An additional 18 percent of Canadian children and youth are overweight. This means more than one-quarter (26 percent) of children are carrying too much weight. Aboriginal groups tend to have a higher prevalence still of childhood obesity, with 16.9 percent of Métis, 20.0 percent of off-reserve First Nations, and 25.6 percent of Inuit young people self-reporting as overweight or obese (PHAC, 2011).

Excessive weight gain during adolescence and young adulthood may be one of the most important determinants of future development of heart disease and stroke (Connelly, 2005). Dr. Douglas Lee and colleagues (2009), of the Institute for Clinical Evaluative Sciences, say projections suggest that the rising prevalence of obesity in the current generation of adolescents will increase the prevalence of coronary heart disease by 5–16 percent by 2035.

PERSONAL PERSPECTIVE

Strokes and Smoking

A few years ago, a female graduate at our college suffered a mild stroke. She was 21 years old. The doctors determined that smoking, social drinking, and taking birth control pills contributed to her stroke. With a strong will, she has struggled with regaining her speech and the use of her arm and foot.

We all need to understand that what we consume can directly affect our bodies. Statistics indicate that women smokers who use birth control pills are 10–20 times more likely to have heart attacks or strokes than non-smoking women (HSFC, 2006c).

Here are some self-help resources to assist you if you are a smoker and are interested in quitting:

- One Step at a Time: Canadian Cancer Society .... www.cancer.ca
- How to Quit Smoking: Ontario Lung Association .... www.lung.ca
- Canadian Health Network ... www.canadian-health-network.ca
- Physicians for a Smoke-Free Canada .... www.smoke-free.ca
- QuitNet .... www.quitnet.org
- Quit Smoking Support ...... www.quitsmokingsupport.com
- Quit 4 Life: Health Canada ... www.quit4life.com
- Women's Health Matters .... www.womenshealthmatters.ca

Anatomy of the Heart

Located between your lungs, slightly to the left and behind your sternum, is your heart. It weighs between 200 and 425 grams and is about the size of your fist.

Your heart is designed to circulate blood. It pumps oxygen-rich blood to the rest of your body through a complex network of arteries, arterioles, and capillaries; deoxygenated (oxygen-poor) blood is carried back to the heart through the veins to send to the lungs to pick up oxygen and remove carbon dioxide.

DID YOU KNOW?

The average heart beats approximately 100,000 times a day, distributing about 7,200 litres (1,900 gallons) of blood. In your lifetime, it will beat approximately 2.5 billion times.

How the Heart Functions

Your heart is a pump with four chambers. The two upper chambers are referred to as the left and right atria, and the lower ones are the left and right ventricles. Separating the left and right sides of the heart is a wall of muscle called the septum. There are four valves that separate each chamber and prevent the blood from coming back when the heart is at rest (see Figure 10.2).

The right two chambers of your heart (right atrium and ventricle) pump the deoxygenated blood to the lungs and exchange the waste (carbon dioxide) for oxygen. The blood then returns to the left chambers of the heart (left atrium and ventricle). The left ventricle is the largest and strongest chamber. Its job is to push

FIGURE 10.2 Diagram of the Heart

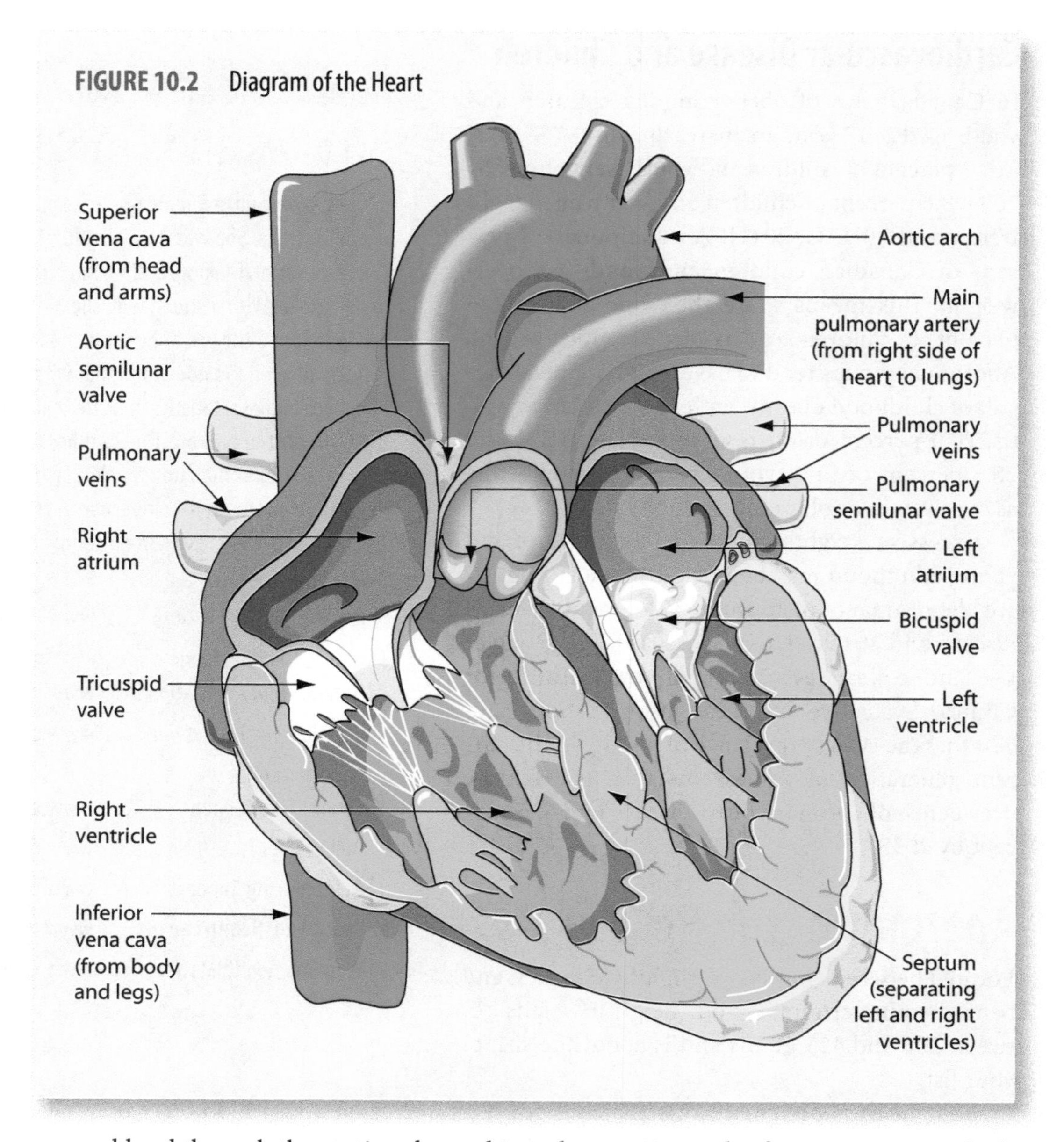

blood through the aortic valve and into the superior and inferior vena cava, which distribute the blood to the rest of the body.

An electrical impulse starts each heartbeat and causes the atria to contract. The impulse begins in a group of cells called the sinoatrial node (SA node). This node is the pacemaker of the heart. The electrical impulse spreads across into the lower part of the heart, stimulating the atrioventricular node (AV node), which causes the ventricles to contract and send blood pumping out with great force.

Types of Cardiovascular Disease

Cardiovascular disease refers to diseases of the heart and blood vessels throughout the body. There are six types of cardiovascular disease: ischemic heart disease, cerebrovascular disease, peripheral vascular disease, heart failure, rheumatic heart disease, and congenital heart disease (PHAC, 2010b).

Ischemic heart disease is the most prevalent type of cardiovascular disease. It refers to blockages of the coronary arteries that result in lack of oxygen (ischemia), chest pain (angina), and shortness of breath (dyspnea). Complete blockage results in a myocardial infarction, or heart attack.

ischemic heart disease
blockage of the coronary arteries resulting in lack of oxygen, angina, and dyspnea

Cerebrovascular disease (stroke) refers to diseases that involve problems with the circulation of blood to blood vessels in the brain. A complete blockage resulting in long-term effects is known as a *thrombotic* stroke (caused by a clot). Sometimes a blood vessel bursts in the brain, resulting in a *hemorrhagic* stroke. A blockage lasting less than 24 hours is referred to as a transient ischemic attack, or TIA.

cerebrovascular disease
interruption of circulation to the brain due either to clotting or hemorrhage

Peripheral vascular disease affects the circulation in the extremities, primarily in the legs, due to hardening of the arteries (arteriosclerosis). Patients complain about pain in their legs (especially when walking), cramping at night, and tingling or pain when legs are elevated or dangling. This condition can be associated with leg ulcers, foot cyanosis (blue tinge from poor circulation), and impotence (Creager & Libby, 2007).

peripheral vascular disease
reduced circulation to the extremities due to hardening of the arteries

Heart failure, also called *congestive heart failure*, occurs when the pumping action of the heart cannot provide enough blood to the rest of the body as it is needed. This happens as a result of damage to the heart muscle in the case of coronary heart disease, resulting in a myocardial infarction (heart attack). Heart failure may also be caused by infections (myocarditis) or by toxins (for example, excessive consumption of alcohol or use of some chemotherapy agents). The most common cause of heart failure is long-standing high blood pressure, which results in thickening of the heart and a reduced ability to pump blood effectively to the body. Complications include diminished kidney function, lung congestion (pulmonary edema), liver impairment (inability to get rid of toxins), poor absorption of nutrients and medicines by the intestines, and swelling (edema) in the ankles and feet. Other symptoms include shortness of breath, fatigue, chronic cough or wheezing, rapid or irregular heartbeat, lack of appetite, and fluid retention (National Heart, Lung, and Blood Institute, 2012).

heart failure
inability of the heart to pump enough blood to the body

Rheumatic heart disease begins with a bacterial infection in childhood that affects joints and heart valves. Untreated strep throat, or other infections with *Streptococcus* bacteria, can progress into rheumatic fever. While the body tries to fight the infection, the bacteria attacks one or more heart valves, although symptoms do not appear until years later. Rheumatic fever is more common in developing countries or where there is little access to health care.

rheumatic heart disease
defects in heart valve function resulting from an infection by *Streptococcus* bacteria

Other infections can attack the inner tissues of the heart, including valves (endocarditis) and the outer tissue overlying the heart (pericarditis).

Of special note is a condition called bacterial endocarditis. This is an infection of the heart's inner lining (endocardium) or the heart valves. Endocarditis can damage or destroy heart valves as bacteria enter the bloodstream and attack the heart. Some surgical procedures (such as tonsillectomies and gastrointestinal tract surgery) and respiratory procedures (such as professional teeth cleaning) briefly cause bacteria to enter the bloodstream and possibly attack the heart (American Heart Association, 2007).

Some medications (such as arthritis medication) and stimulants (such as caffeinated beverages) that individuals consume can cause the heart to race and may trigger heart attacks.

congenital heart disease problems with the structure of the heart resulting from a birth defect

Congenital heart disease is a problem with the structure of the heart as a result of birth defect. The anatomical defects can range from a small hole in one of the inside walls of the heart (septal defects) to defects involving the valves or arteries and veins that carry blood to the heart or the body, respectively. Without surgical intervention in utero or at birth, some congenital heart problems can result in death. Others cause varying degrees of disability and require treatment later in life. About 1 of every 100 babies born has some form of heart defect, representing 1 percent of births. In Canada, there are about 100,000 adults who, as children, had surgery to correct congenital heart defects (HSFC, 2012).

The remainder of this chapter examines four common cardiovascular diseases: arteriosclerosis, coronary heart disease, stroke, and hypertension.

Arteriosclerosis

arteriosclerosis blanket term for a group of ischemic cardiovascular diseases characterized by a narrowing or hardening of the arteries

atherosclerosis a common type of arteriosclerosis; a slow, progressive disease in which arterial blockage results from fatty deposits collecting in the arteries

Arteriosclerosis is not a single disease but a group of ischemic cardiovascular diseases characterized by a narrowing or hardening of the arteries. In these diseases, blood flow to vital organs is restricted by a progressive blockage of the arteries.

Atherosclerosis is a common type of arteriosclerosis, a slow, progressive disease that may start in childhood, in which arterial blockage results from fatty deposits collecting in the arteries. The deposits are typically composed of cholesterol, cellular debris, fibrin (a clotting material in the blood), and calcium. Atherosclerosis is not restricted to one area of the body, although some areas may experience a great-

FIGURE 10.3 Atherosclerosis: Cross-Sectional View of an Artery

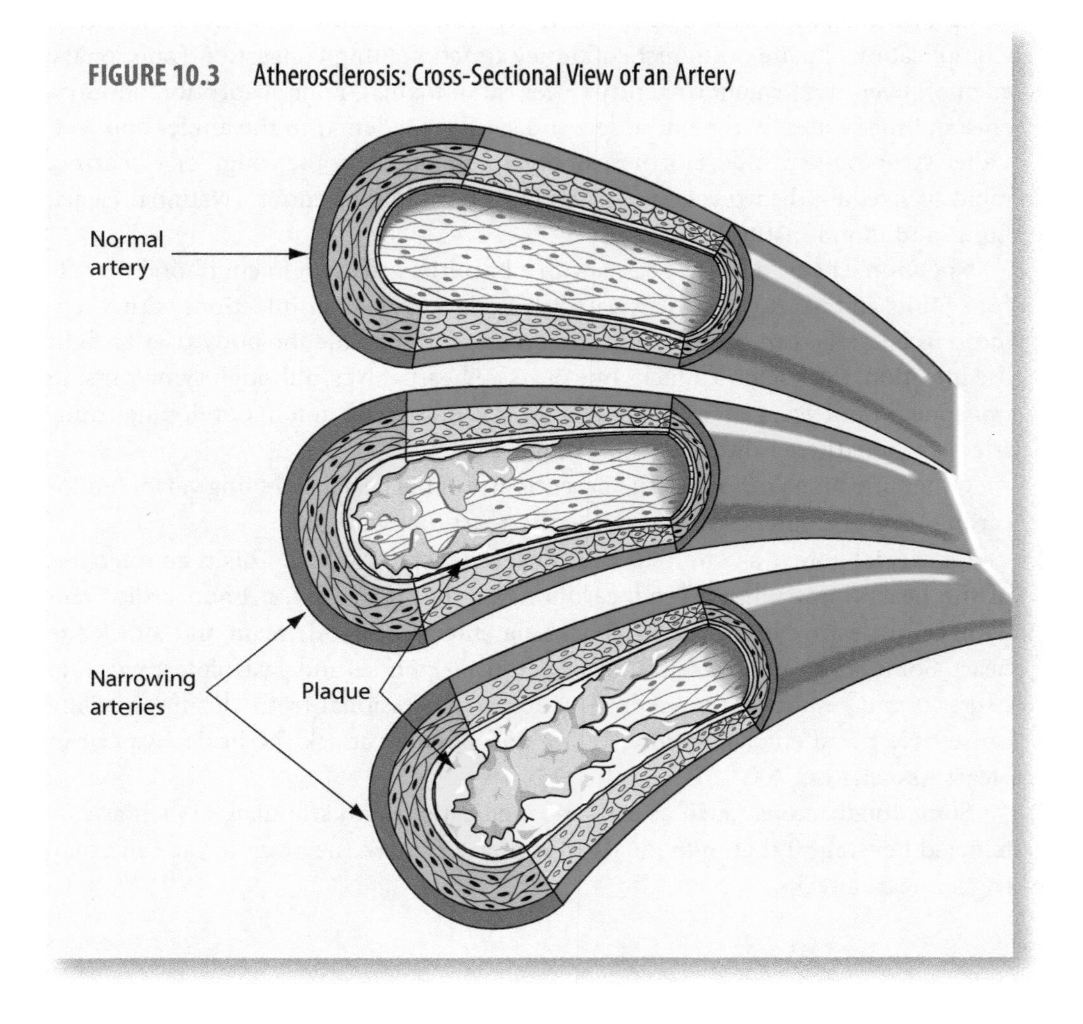

er degree of blockage than others. This buildup of deposits in the arteries is called plaque (see Figure 10.3). There are two types of plaque. Hard plaque causes the artery walls to thicken and harden. Soft plaque is more likely to break apart from the walls and enter the bloodstream, which can cause a blood clot that can partially or totally block the flow of blood in an artery. If this happens, the tissue past the blockage is deprived of blood and oxygen, and it may either die or suffer severe damage.

The causes of atherosclerosis are complicated. It is believed that the inner lining of the arteries becomes damaged and the body reacts by laying down the fatty deposits. Over time, the blood vessels become progressively thicker. High blood pressure, cholesterol, triglycerides in the blood, and smoking can contribute to the development of plaque.

Symptoms may not be apparent until the disease is far enough advanced to block a large part of the vessel. In the arteries of the heart (coronary arteries) it will cause angina (chest pain), which can lead to coronary heart disease. In the brain or carotid arteries (the two large arteries on either side of the head that carry blood to the brain), it can cause a stroke. Narrowed or blocked arteries may also cause problems in your intestines, kidneys, and legs.

Coronary Heart Disease

Coronary heart disease, a type of ischemic cardiovascular disease, occurs when fatty deposits block one or more coronary arteries (arteries supplying the heart). When the blockage becomes severe enough to restrict the blood flow, insufficient oxygen reaches the heart and the person may experience severe chest pains called **angina pectoris**. Angina can be infrequent or constant, depending on the severity of the restriction.

In the most extreme cases, no oxygen can get past the blockage. When this happens, a heart attack (**myocardial infarction**) occurs (see Figure 10.4). The cells past the blockage become damaged or die. The number of damaged and dead cells determines the seriousness of the attack—the greater the damage, the smaller the chance of recovery. Damage to the heart muscle may cause the heart to quiver rapidly (ventricular fibrillation), preventing the heart from delivering oxygenated blood to other organs and tissues, especially the brain. Permanent brain damage can occur within five minutes if the heart does not resume pumping blood to the brain. Myocardial infarction can also lead to **cardiac arrest** (the heart stops pumping).

If emergency medical personnel reach a heart attack victim in time, they can administer medication to limit the damage and open up the coronary artery. If left untreated, the dead or damaged areas of the heart muscle are replaced by scar tissue, which weakens the pumping action of the heart and can lead to heart failure and other complications. The heart may go into arrhythmia (irregular heartbeat or rhythm), causing ventricular fibrillation. Survival rates are highest for those victims able to receive clot-busting medication within an hour of a heart attack.

Sudden cardiac arrest is a major cause of death in Canada. Each year, more than 45,000 Canadians suffer from a sudden cardiac arrest (Heart and Stroke Foundation of Manitoba, 2011). Arrhythmias such as ventricular fibrillation cause most sudden cardiac arrests. The time between the onset of cardiac arrest and the performance of defibrillation is the major determinant for success in any resuscitation attempt. While cardiopulmonary resuscitation (CPR) can support circulation and ventilation for a short period of time, it is unlikely to convert ventricular fibrilla-

coronary heart disease
a type of ischemic heart disease in which fatty deposits block one or more coronary arteries (arteries supplying the heart)

angina pectoris
severe chest pains associated with advanced cases of coronary heart disease

myocardial infarction
a heart attack

cardiac arrest
cessation of the heart's pumping action

FIGURE 10.4 Diagram of Myocardial Infarction (Heart Attack)

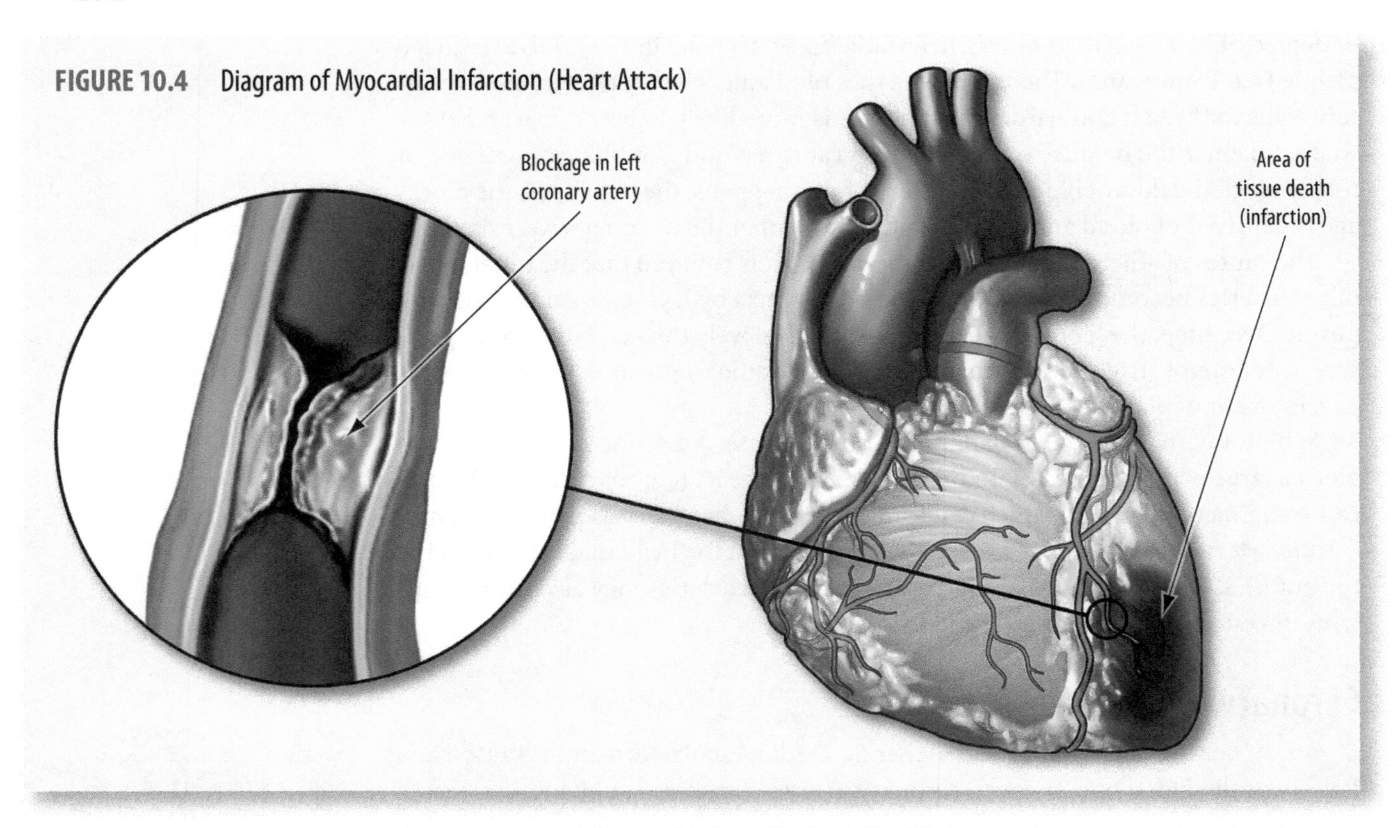

tion to a normal heart rhythm. Early defibrillation is the intervention that is most likely to save lives. If the heart is not restarted within a few minutes, brain damage and death will occur. Of those who suffer a sudden cardiac arrest that happens out of the hospital, fewer than 5 percent survive the trip to hospital because of delays in recognizing the cardiac emergency and gaining access to the appropriate care (Heart and Stroke Foundation of Manitoba, 2011).

An automated external defibrillator (AED) is a portable device the size of a laptop computer (but approximately 13 centimetres thick) that aids in rescuing people having a heart attack. Once the machine's adhesive pads are attached to a victim, the AED analyzes the heart rhythm, advises the rescuer of the need for defibrillation, and prompts the rescuer to press a button to deliver a controlled shock, or series of shocks, as required, or tells the rescuer to keep administering CPR. Restoration of the rhythm requires defibrillation to be administered within a few minutes of the cardiac arrest. The use of external defibrillators with CPR within the first three minutes of cardiac arrest can increase the chance of survival by up to 75 percent (Weisfeldt, Sitlani, Ornato, Rea, Aufderheide, et al., 2010). On average, early use of an AED defibrillation before emergency medical services arrives seems to nearly double a victim's odds of survival. Every minute that passes reduces the chances of survival by 7–10 percent (Heart and Stroke Foundation of Manitoba, 2011). After more than 12 minutes of ventricular fibrillation (irregular, rapid, and chaotic firing of the ventricles), the survival rate is less than 5 percent (Larsen, Eisenberg, Cummins, & Hallstrom, 1993).

Administering CPR before emergency personnel arrive, even in the absence of an AED, also increases the victim's likelihood of survival, and for this reason everyone should know CPR. CPR is the process of externally supporting the circulation and respiration of a person who has had a cardiac arrest. Artificial respiration and chest compression substitute for normal breathing and circulation until advanced life support measures can be taken. The flow of oxygen to the brain can be sustained and the amount of permanent damage can be reduced.

A heart attack victim may need to undergo bypass surgery to restore blood supply.

Recognizing the Signs of a Heart Attack

Thousands of Canadians die from heart attacks each year because they do not recognize the signs and symptoms. These are not always sudden or severe. Quick recognition of the symptoms may reduce the severity of damage and prevent death. For some, a heart attack starts as muscular soreness or flu-like symptoms, but these progress and can include the following:

- prolonged, heavy, squeezing pressure, or squeezing pain, in the centre of the chest, sometimes spreading to the shoulders, arms, neck, jaw, or throat; in women, pain may be a vague chest discomfort or entirely absent
- shortness of breath, paleness, sweating, or weakness
- dizziness, nausea, vomiting, or indigestion
- a feeling of extreme anxiety and fear, or denial that anything is wrong

Signs may be mild or severe. Until the 1980s, it was believed that male and female heart attack victims experienced the same symptoms. We know today that this is not always so. For example, women are more likely to experience unique symptoms, such as:

- vague chest discomfort
- unusual fatigue
- sleep disturbance
- indigestion
- back pain

The majority of women (78 percent) experience at least one symptom for more than one month prior to their heart attack. Only 30 percent report classical symptoms (McSweeney, Cody, O'Sullivan, Elberson, Moser, et al., 2003). As well, some heart attack tests and treatments may not work as well for women as for men.

Research on treating heart attacks has progressed a great deal in the past 40 years. There are now treatments to open blocked arteries while a heart attack is in progress or soon after. One particularly successful process, called reperfusion, uses drugs to restore blood flow to the heart muscle. Once the blocked arteries are opened, the heart attack usually stops. If treatment occurs early enough, damage to the heart muscle is minimized, and the pumping ability of the undamaged tissue is not as greatly impaired, which means that the heart attack survivor is able to enjoy a higher quality of life.

FYI

The Framingham Heart Study

The objective of the Framingham Heart Study, which began in 1948, was to identify the common factors or characteristics that contribute to cardiovascular disease by following its development over a long period of time in a large group of participants who had not yet developed overt symptoms of cardiovascular disease or suffered a heart attack or stroke. Researchers recruited men and women between the ages of 30 and 62 from the town of Framingham, Massachusetts, and began the first round of extensive physical examinations and lifestyle interviews, which they would later analyze for common patterns related to the development of cardiovascular disease.

Since the study's inception, the subjects have continued to return to Framingham every two years for a detailed medical history, physical examination, and laboratory tests. In fact, the third generation of these families is now being recruited and examined to understand how genetic factors relate to cardiovascular disease. This study, which has being going on for over six decades, is viewed throughout the world as pioneering research. It has led to identification of major CVD risk factors, as well as valuable information on blood pressure, blood cholesterol and triglyceride levels, age, gender, and psycho-social issues. For more information about the study, go to www.framinghamheartstudy.org.

Risk Factors Associated with Coronary Heart Disease

Coronary heart disease risk factors are conditions or habits that raise your risk of coronary heart disease and heart attack. There are some risks that you cannot control, while others you can.

Uncontrollable Risk Factors for Coronary Heart Disease

The major uncontrollable risk factors for heart disease are the following:

- *Family history of coronary heart disease* Having a family history of cardiovascular disease appears to increase the risk significantly. If your father or brother had a heart attack before age 55, or if your mother or sister had one before age 65, you are more likely to get heart disease yourself.
- *Ethnicity* South Asians, Aboriginal peoples (First Nations, Inuit, and Métis), and blacks are at greater risk for hypertension and thus are at higher risk for cardiovascular disease than are whites. These groups also have a worse chance of surviving heart attacks (HSFC, 2003).
- *Gender* Men have a greater risk of suffering cardiovascular disease in their younger years. Women catch up to men quickly after reaching menopause because the protection of female hormones is removed. Some women increase their risk before menopause if they smoke and take oral contraceptives.
- *Age* Your risk increases as you get older. The risk of strokes doubles every decade after age 55.

Controllable Risk Factors for Coronary Heart Disease

Many police services now offer educational programs to help officers assess their risk of developing coronary heart disease and to modify risky behaviours. Smoking-cessation programs, cholesterol assessments, blood pressure clinics, and the fitness pin award offered by the Police Fitness Personnel of Ontario are some of the initiatives that have been undertaken.

Here are some of the risk factors for coronary heart disease that you *can* control:

- *Smoking* Smoking poses the greatest risk for heart disease. Smokers increase their risk for cardiovascular disease by 70 percent. Exposure to second-hand smoke may increase the risk of cardiovascular disease by 25–30 percent (US Department of Health and Human Services, 2006a). Although we do not fully understand how cigarettes damage the heart, there are two possible explanations. One is that carbon monoxide in cigarette smoke may cause a deficiency of oxygen in the body, causing the heart to work harder. The other centres on the nicotine and tar released in cigarette smoke, which cause damage to the blood vessel walls and allow cholesterol and plaque to build up. In addition, women who both smoke and use oral contraceptives have an increased risk of stroke (HSFC, 2003).
- *Physical inactivity* Individuals who do not participate in at least moderate physical activity increase their risk for cardiovascular disease. Exercise increases levels of "good" (HDL) cholesterol, improves serum lipids and blood pressure, helps people manage stress, and improves the efficiency of

the heart, lungs, and muscles. Exercise also reduces body weight and improves diabetes. Individuals who are having difficulty becoming physically active should seek professional assistance (such as a certified personal trainer), and those who have been diagnosed with heart disease or who have identified risk factors should seek professionally trained personnel who are familiar with these issues (such as a certified exercise physiologist).

- *High blood cholesterol* Abnormally elevated cholesterol, low-density lipoproteins (LDL), and triglycerides, and low levels of high-density lipoproteins (HDL), are increased risk factors for developing vascular diseases, particularly coronary heart disease. We know that elevated levels of total serum cholesterol and LDL cholesterol are important risk factors for strokes, including carotid artery disease (HSFC, 2003).
- *High blood pressure* Defined as blood pressure greater than 140/90. High blood pressure is a major risk factor for strokes, coronary heart disease, peripheral vascular disease, and congestive heart failure. A great deal of research indicates that lowering blood pressure can reduce the incidence of stroke, myocardial infarction, ischemic heart disease, vascular disease, renal (kidney) disease, heart failure, and overall death rate. We know that those who are overweight, are physically inactive, drink heavily, and consume excessive salt have a higher risk of developing high blood pressure. There is also a higher risk of metabolic cardiovascular risk factors, which include insulin resistance, obesity, hyperuricemia (an excess of uric acid in the blood, often producing gout), and dyslipidemia (an abnormal concentration of lipids or lipoproteins in the blood) (HSFC, 2003). A startling statistic is that 42 percent of us with high blood pressure don't even know that we have it (HSFC, 2007b).
- *Diabetes* People with diabetes tend to have elevated blood fat levels and increased atherosclerosis. Because overweight individuals have an increased risk for diabetes, it becomes more difficult to differentiate the effects on cardiovascular disease. Cardiovascular disease is in fact the leading cause of death in diabetics. Diabetes increases the risk of high blood pressure, strokes, and heart and vascular diseases, particularly in women. There are also added risks of peripheral vascular disease, eye problems, and kidney disease. After the age of 50, the percentage of men with diabetes is higher than the percentage of women (HSFC, 2003).
- *Obesity* Being overweight puts additional strain on your entire body. If you are more than 13.5 kilograms (30 pounds) overweight, you are at higher risk for heart disease and stroke (HSFC, 2001). Your heart must work harder to push blood through extra capillaries that feed the excess fat. This pressure can damage the vessels. People who are overweight or obese are at risk for developing high blood pressure, high blood lipids, and diabetes, all of which put them at a high risk for cardiovascular or heart disease. Among individuals aged 18–64, being overweight—having either excess weight (defined by WHO as a body mass index [BMI] of 25.0–29.9) or obesity (BMI ≥ 30.0)—is one of the most common factors that influences the development of high blood pressure and diabetes, both of which are risk factors for cardiovascular diseases (HSFC, 2003, p. 27).

- *Stress* As discussed in Chapter 12, people who have especially high stress levels are considered time bombs for a heart attack. When under stress, the body produces stress chemicals, which in turn increase blood pressure. Chronic hostility and aggression are two key personality factors related to the greatest risk.
- *Inadequate consumption of fruits and vegetables* As discussed in Chapter 8, Canada's Food Guide (Health Canada, 2012) recommends that everyone eat one dark green and one orange vegetable each day; choose vegetables and fruit prepared with little or no added fat, sugar, or salt; prepare vegetables by steaming, baking, or stir-frying, rather than deep-frying; and consume vegetables and fruit more often than juice. Fruits and vegetables are associated with reduced risk of cardiovascular diseases. They are important for intake of natural vitamins, antioxidants, and fibre. Potassium, which is present in many fruits and vegetables (for example, bananas, tomatoes, and sweet potatoes), has been shown to be protective, particularly against strokes (HSFC, 2003).
- *Poor dental hygiene* Periodontal disease (gum disease) is associated with heart disease, strokes, and diabetes. Good dental hygiene is important for reducing gum disease and the risk of heart disease. With increased risk of endocarditis, police officers who work 12-hour shifts need to be aware of how important it is to brush their teeth regularly and floss daily. This means taking a toothbrush to work. It is also important to avoid food that contains excessive amounts of sugar.
- *Sleep deprivation* Sleep deprivation (less than 5 hours) is now associated with a higher risk of hypertension in middle-aged adults (Cappuccio, Stranges, Kandala, Miller, Taggart, et al., 2007). Studies have shown that if you sleep less than 6 hours per night and have disturbed sleep, you stand a 48 percent greater chance of developing or dying from heart disease and a 15 percent greater chance of developing or dying from a stroke, because of the hormonal and chemical changes that take place in the body in the absence of sleep (Miller & Cappuccio, 2007).

stroke
paralysis and a sudden loss of consciousness caused by an interruption of blood flow to the brain; a thrombotic or thromboembolic stroke occurs when blood flow is interrupted by a blood clot that travels to the brain; a hemorrhagic stroke occurs when very high blood pressure causes a weakened blood vessel near the brain to break

subarachnoid hemorrhage
hemorrhage that occurs when a blood vessel on the surface of the brain bleeds into the space between the brain and the skull

Stroke

Stroke—paralysis and sudden loss of consciousness caused by an interruption of blood flow to the brain—is one of the leading causes of death in Canada. Over 50,000 people suffer a stroke in Canada each year, and 15 of every hundred die (HSFC, 2012). Of the survivors, only a third make a full recovery. Not only elderly people die from a stroke; in 2007, 10.3 percent of all stroke deaths occurred in people under age 65. For every 100,000 Canadian children under the age of 19, there are 6.7 childhood strokes (Statistics Canada, 2011).

A stroke can occur when a blood clot travels to the brain and interrupts the blood supply (and thus the oxygen supply) to the brain. As a result, brain cells die and the parts of the body they control can stop functioning. A thrombotic stroke occurs in about 80 percent of the stroke population (HSFC, 2006b).

A stroke may also occur when very high blood pressure causes a weakened blood vessel near the brain to break. This is called a hemorrhagic stroke, and accounts for 20 percent of strokes (HSFC, 2006e). **Subarachnoid hemorrhage** is uncontrolled bleeding on the surface of the brain, in an area between the brain and the skull. **Intracerebral hemorrhage** occurs when an artery deep within the brain ruptures. Both can be caused by structural problems with the blood vessels in the brain. An **aneurysm** is a weakened area in the blood vessel wall that fills with blood and bulges. As a result of high blood pressure or trauma, the vessel can rupture and cause uncontrolled bleeding in the brain. An **arteriovenous malformation (AVM)** is a malformation of the blood vessels, usually present at birth, that becomes weak and risks hemorrhaging.

A **transient ischemic attack (TIA)** occurs when the blood supply to the brain is temporarily interfered with. About 15,000 Canadians each year suffer a TIA. People who have had a TIA are five times more likely than the general population to have a full-blown stroke within two years (HSFC, 2006a). These attacks can last for seconds or hours and can happen for a variety of reasons. They do not cause permanent neurological damage and are not necessarily a warning sign of an impending stroke.

A stroke damages the brain and causes a sudden loss of brain function. Because your brain is divided into a number of sections, there are different effects for each.

The effects of *left hemisphere strokes* include:

- weakness or paralysis on the right side of the body
- trouble reading, talking, thinking, or doing math
- behaviour that is more slow and cautious than usual
- trouble learning or remembering new information
- requiring frequent instructions and feedback to finish tasks

The effects of *right hemisphere strokes* include:

- weakness or paralysis on the left side of the body
- vision problems
- problems with depth perception, up and down, front and back
- inability to pick up objects, button a shirt, or tie a shoe
- inability to understand a map
- short-term memory loss
- forgetting or ignoring objects or people on your left side
- having difficulty with judgment, including acting impulsively or not realizing your own limitations

Brain stem strokes (at the base of brain), which are uncommon, include the following problems:

- difficulty with breathing and heart function
- body temperature control problems
- difficulties with balance and coordination
- weakness or paralysis of arms and legs on both sides of the body
- difficulty with chewing, swallowing, and speaking
- vision problems

intracerebral hemorrhage
bleeding in the brain resulting from the rupture of a blood vessel

aneurysm
a weak or thin area in a blood vessel that causes it to expand and fill with blood; aneurysms may occur as a result of a disease, an injury, or a congenital abnormality in the vessel

arteriovenous malformation (AVM)
a malformation of the blood vessels of the brain, usually present at birth; an arteriovenous malformation can increase the risk of stroke

transient ischemic attack (TIA)
a temporary interference with the blood supply to the brain

DID YOU KNOW?

For every minute of delay in treating a stroke, the average patient loses 1.9 million brain cells, 13.8 billion synapses, and 12 kilometres of axonal fibres (nerve fibres that conduct electrical impulses). A stroke survivor has a 20 percent chance of having another stroke within two years.

SOURCE: Saver, 2006.

Strokes in the cerebellum are also less common, but they have more severe effects, including:

- ataxia (inability to walk with coordination and balance)
- dizziness
- headache
- nausea and vomiting

Even if these symptoms seem to disappear quickly, one should seek medical attention immediately. More than 40 percent of potential stroke patients who receive medical treatment within the critical three-hour time window will significantly reduce the risk or degree of long-term impairment. Since 1998, mortality rates for patients 30 days after a stroke have decreased 4.5 percent in Ontario (HSFC, 2007c). Between one-third and two-thirds of stroke survivors will experience a loss of function in physical, cognitive, or communication skills that requires some form of rehabilitation (Canadian Institute for Health Information, 2009).

The Risk Factors for Stroke

As with heart attacks, there are risk factors for stroke that you cannot control, and others that you can.

Uncontrollable Risk Factors for Stroke

Risk factors for stroke that you *cannot* control include the following:

- *Age* Although strokes can occur at any age, most strokes occur in persons over 65.
- *Family history of stroke* Those with a parent or sibling who had a stroke before age 65 are at increased risk of having a stroke.
- *Ethnicity* Aboriginal peoples and those of African or South Asian descent are more likely to have high blood pressure and diabetes, putting them at higher risk for strokes.
- *Gender* Until menopause, women have lower risk of stroke than men. After that, women take the lead.
- *Prior stroke or TIA* If you have had a previous stroke or a TIA, your risk is greater for another stroke.
- *Socio-economic status* Lower socio-economic levels increase the risk of poorer nutritional intake.

Controllable Risk Factors for Stroke

Risk factors for stroke that you *can* control include the following:

- *High blood pressure* High blood pressure affects one in five Canadians and is the number one risk factor for stroke. Blood pressure that is consistently more than 140/90 is considered high, but if you are diabetic, 130/80 is high (HSFC, 2007b). With high blood pressure there is an increased risk of burst blood vessels, resulting in a stroke.
- *Smoking* Smoking, whether primary or second-hand, can contribute to plaque buildup in your arteries and increase the risk of blood clots, doubling the risk of an ischemic stroke (HSFC, 2006c).

- *High blood cholesterol* Increased levels of LDL cholesterol build up plaque in your arteries causing atherosclerosis, which can lead to a blockage in the brain.
- *Obesity* Those who carry extra weight are more at risk to suffer from high blood pressure, which places a great strain on the blood vessels of the brain.
- *Physical inactivity* Those who do not stay physically active increase their risk of unhealthy weight, high blood pressure, high cholesterol, and higher stress levels.
- *Excessive alcohol consumption* Those who drink too much alcohol can increase their blood pressure, which can lead to a stroke. A meta-analysis published in the *Journal of the American Medical Association* concluded that heavy alcohol consumption increases the relative risk of stroke, while light or moderate alcohol consumption may be protective against total and ischemic stroke (Reynolds, Lewis, Nolen, Kinney, Sathya, et al., 2003).
- *Stress* Stress releases hormones that increase blood pressure and blood cholesterol, which leads to atherosclerosis.
- *Heart disease—atrial fibrillation* Atrial fibrillation affects approximately 200,000 to 250,000 Canadians. It is estimated that up to 15 percent of all strokes are due to atrial fibrillation. Caused by high blood pressure, atrial fibrillation can cause blood clots to form, leading to strokes (HSFC, 2006d).

Recommendations to Prevent Heart Attacks and Strokes

By taking ownership of your health and well-being, you can significantly reduce your risk of heart attack and stroke.

The Heart and Stroke Foundation (HSFC, 2005, 2010) makes the following recommendations:

- Have your blood pressure taken by a health-care professional at least once every two years and discuss your readings together. You can self-test at your local drug store to monitor your blood pressure on a more regular basis. If it is above the high-normal ranges of between 130/85 and 139/89, make an appointment to talk to your health-care professional. Make sure to bring in the readings that you have been monitoring.
- Lead a healthier lifestyle, including regular physical activity (at least 30 minutes of moderate-intensity activity daily) and appropriate nutrition (enrich your diet with fruits, vegetables, whole grains, nuts, and omega-3 fatty acids).
- Reduce your intake of sugars if you are diabetic.
- Reduce your intake of sodium. The goal of the Sodium Reduction Strategy for Canada (Sodium Working Group, 2010) is to reduce sodium intake to no more than 2,300 milligrams (less than a teaspoon of salt) per day by 2016.
- Make an effort to limit or quit smoking.
- Reduce consumption of alcohol. Follow the Canadian low-risk drinking guidelines (two or fewer standard drinks per day, with consumption not exceeding 14 standard drinks per week for men and nine standard drinks per week for non-pregnant women).

- Avoid medication that increases blood pressure, which may put you at risk for stroke.
- Consider taking medication if you have cardiovascular disease, diabetes, truncal obesity (high amounts of abdominal fat), or abnormally high LDL cholesterol levels.
- Those with symptoms may consider surgical intervention (such as carotid stenting, which is the opening of the carotid arteries to allow better blood flow to the brain).

Turn to **assignment 10.1** (in the appendix) and assess your risk for cardiovascular disease.

Then, turn to **assignment 10.2**. Using your first aid text and Internet sites, research how you as a law enforcement officer should be prepared to deal with heart attacks and strokes.

Hypertension

hypertension high blood pressure—the term "essential hypertension" is used for cases in which the cause is unknown

Hypertension (high blood pressure) is estimated to be the leading risk for death in the world (WHO, 2008, 2009). Known as the "silent killer," this health risk can be prevented by following an appropriate lifestyle that is relatively easy to manage. Nearly 6 million Canadians aged 20 years and older—more than one in five adults—are living with diagnosed hypertension. By 2011/2012, the number diagnosed with hypertension is forecasted to increase to 7.3 million—an estimated increase of 25.5 percent from 2006/2007 (PHAC, 2010a).

Hypertension increases with age. Over a lifetime, 90 percent of middle-aged and older men and women participating in the Framingham Heart Study were likely to develop hypertension (Vasan, Beiser, Seshadri, Larson, Kannel, et al., 2002). It was estimated that by 2011/2012, among all adults with diagnosed hypertension, almost one in two (48.9 percent) would be in the 55- to 74-year age range.

It has been documented that 40 percent of hypertensive adults in Canada are unaware they have hypertension. Of those who are aware, only about two-thirds are being treated pharmacologically, and about 13 percent are being treated and controlled (Joffres, Hamet, MacLean, L'Italien, & Foder, 2001). Unfortunately, the prevalence of hypertension is predicted to rise with an aging, sedentary population that has poor dietary habits and increasing obesity. High blood pressure can double or even triple your risk of heart disease and stroke, and increase your risk of kidney disease.

Approximately 11 percent of the Canadian adult population (3.6 million) has high-normal blood pressure (130/85–139/89 mmHg). In 2006, a trial was conducted to prevent hypertension in overweight adults with high-normal blood pressure with the use of pharmacotherapy (Julius, Nesbitt, Egan, Weber, Michelson,

FYI

The DASH Eating Plan

The DASH (Dietary Approaches to Stop Hypertension) Eating Plan, supported through the National Heart, Lung, and Blood Institute (2012), was developed as an eating plan that is low in sodium, saturated fat, cholesterol, and total fat. It emphasizes fruits, vegetables, whole grain products, fish, poultry, nuts, and fat-free or low-fat milk and milk products that are rich in potassium, magnesium, and calcium, along with protein and fibre. It is a diet that limits the consumption of red meats, sweets, added sugars, and sugar-containing beverages. This diet's emphasis is to lower blood pressure and decrease the risks of cardiovascular disease and diabetes. It also stresses losing weight, exercising regularly, and limiting consumption of alcohol. For more information about this plan, see US Department of Health and Human Services, 2006b (in the References).

et al., 2006). In the participants treated with a placebo, a startling 40.4 percent developed hypertension within two years and 63.0 percent within four years. This very high risk is confirmed by the Framingham study, where 37.3 percent of those aged 35–64 and 49.5 percent of those above age 65 with high-normal blood pressure developed hypertension within four years (Vasan, Larson, Leip, Kannel, & Levy, 2001).

The focus of the Canadian Hypertension Education Program (CHEP, 2007) is to encourage adults to monitor their blood pressure regularly, reassess blood pressure in those with high-normal values, educate on preventable lifestyle risks, and educate to reduce dietary sodium (PHAC, 2010a). Ultimately, these researchers would like Canadians to reduce their dietary intake of sodium to no more than 1,500 milligrams per day. In 2007, additional evidence became available on the antihypertensive effectiveness of soluble fibre, whole grains, and protein from plant sources (Appel, Sacks, Carey, Obarzanek, Swain, et al., 2005; He, Gu, Wu, Chen, Duan, et al., 2005; Rasmussen, Vessby, Uusitupa, Berglund, Pedersen, et al., 2006). This recommendation emphasizes fruits, vegetables, low-fat dairy products, dietary and soluble fibre, and whole grains and protein from plant sources, which reduce saturated fat and cholesterol.

There are two forms of high blood pressure: essential (or primary) and secondary. Essential hypertension is a common condition that accounts for 90–95 percent of hypertension. It originates within the body and is not a result of disease; in fact, no cause for it can be determined. Secondary hypertension develops as the result of disease, such as abnormalities of the kidneys, adrenal gland tumours, and some congenital heart defects, and as a result of taking certain prescription and over-the-counter medications.

Risk factors for essential hypertension include the following:

- family history of hypertension
- gender (men are more likely to have hypertension at a younger age, but women's risk increases significantly after menopause)
- age (more often in people over 35)
- ethnicity (the risk is higher for South Asians, Aboriginal peoples, and blacks than for whites)
- obesity (if you are 20 percent or more above your ideal body weight, your blood must pump through more body tissue to supply necessary oxygen and nutrients)
- smoking (nicotine causes blood vessels to constrict, and other chemicals in burning tobacco damage the lining of the arteries)
- high levels of salt or sodium in your diet
- heavy alcohol consumption (raises blood pressure by interfering with the flow to and from the heart)
- use of oral contraceptives (hormonal supplements may increase blood pressure, and this tendency increases with age if you are over 35, obese, and smoking)
- physical inactivity (the less fit you are, the faster your heart pumps)
- stress (your reaction to stress can cause elevated blood pressure)

Secondary hypertension, which accounts for 5 percent of hypertension cases, is caused by abnormalities in one or more of the organs or systems of the body. Causes of secondary hypertension include:

- narrowing of the renal arteries, which causes hypertension in the kidneys
- tumours of the adrenal glands (glands that sit right on top of the kidneys), which can cause other conditions, such as hyperaldosteronism, Cushing's syndrome, and pheochromocytoma
- coarctation of the aorta (a rare hereditary disorder characterized by the narrowing of the aorta above the renal arteries, causing lack of sufficient blood flow to the kidneys and influencing the release of a number of hormones to boost blood pressure to the kidneys)
- pregnancy and pre-eclampsia (commonly called toxemia), an increase in blood pressure that can lead to kidney damage, convulsions, and coma in the mother, as well as eye or brain damage in the fetus
- metabolic syndrome and obesity

About Blood Pressure

Blood pressure is measured in two parts and is expressed as a fraction—for example, 120/80 or 120 over 80. The first number refers to *systolic pressure*, or the pressure that is applied to the walls of the arteries when the heart contracts. The second value is *diastolic pressure*, or the pressure on the arterial walls during the heart's relaxation phase. This is the phase where the heart refills with blood. The higher your systolic or diastolic pressure, and the length of time during which it stays high, the more damage will occur to your blood vessels. This damage increases the risk for strokes and heart attacks.

Normal blood pressure varies for different individuals based on weight, age, gender, ethnicity, and physical condition. Table 10.1 classifies blood pressure to give you a clearer idea of what your blood pressure reading means.

TABLE 10.1 Classification of Hypertension

CATEGORY	SYSTOLIC	DIASTOLIC
Optimal	< 120	< 80
Normal	< 130	< 85
Pre-hypertension	120–139	80–89
High-normal	130–139	85–89
Grade 1 (mild hypertension)	140–159	90–99
Grade 2 (moderate hypertension)	160–179	100–109
Grade 3 (severe hypertension)	≥ 180	≥ 110
Isolated systolic hypertension (ISH)	≥ 140	< 90
The category pertains to the highest-risk blood pressure		

SOURCE: Chalmers et al., 1999.

For most people, blood pressure should be less than 140/90. It is now recommended that people with diabetes or kidney disease have blood pressure less than 130/80. Blood pressure less than 120/80 is very good unless it causes dizziness (CHEP, 2007).

A physician will diagnose you with hypertension under the following conditions (CHEP, 2007):

- if your blood pressure is extremely high (above 200/120)
- if your blood pressure is higher than 160/100 over three visits
- if your blood pressure is higher than 140/90 over five visits
- if you have diabetes or kidney disease and blood pressure higher than 130/80
- if your blood pressure is higher than 135/85 when measured over a week at home, twice a day, in the morning and evening (go to a doctor to confirm)

It is important to have regular checkups with your doctor to ensure that your blood pressure is normal and your general health is good. If you have high blood pressure, you will not be able to perform a BFOR test (see Chapters 1 and 15) without medical clearance. Because the test is a means of screening for law enforcement recruits, you should be aware of your blood pressure. If you are unsure, consult your instructor or doctor. Some people experience "white coat syndrome"—elevated blood pressure that is caused by anxiety about the tester who is taking your blood pressure or anxiety over the result of the test. For those people, it is important to understand what blood pressure is and to have their blood pressure tested repeatedly. Some individuals who are being tested for a BFOR will bring documentation from a doctor who has diagnosed the syndrome as proof that they have been cleared by their physician for testing.

Prevention of Cardiovascular Diseases

Generally, you can help prevent these diseases if you do the following:

- Exercise. Be physically active for 30–60 minutes every day of the week, five times a week. You need to work at an intensity of 70–85 percent (see Chapter 5 for more information).
- If you are overweight, losing about 5 kilograms (11 pounds) may help you get within a healthy range (see Chapter 7).
- Choose foods such as fruits, vegetables, and whole grains, and those lower in saturated and trans fats and salt, and limit fast foods and prepared foods (see Chapter 8).

FYI

Further Information

Further information on cardiovascular disease is available from the website of the Heart and Stroke Foundation of Canada (www.heartandstroke.ca) and through the local offices of the Ontario Heart and Stroke Foundation. The following topics might be of special interest to you or your family:

- blood clots
- aneurysms
- congestive heart failure
- congenital heart defects
- stress testing
- surgical procedures (including intra-uterine surgery to correct heart defects before birth)
- drug therapy
- pacemakers

KEY TERMS

EXERCISES

Multiple Choice

1. The condition where artery walls become thickened, hard, and non-elastic is
   - **a.** arteriosclerosis
   - **b.** atherosclerosis
   - **c.** coronary embolism
   - **d.** coronary thrombosis
   - **e.** high blood pressure
2. Which of the following are considered controllable risk factors for heart disease?
   - **a.** family history of heart disease, stress, obesity
   - **b.** gender, high blood pressure, obesity
   - **c.** inactivity, gender, high blood pressure
   - **d.** high cholesterol levels, stress, inactivity
   - **e.** diabetes, family history of heart disease, obesity
3. Which of the following is considered a major risk factor for heart disease that you can change?
   - **a.** diabetes
   - **b.** inactivity
   - **c.** high blood lipids
   - **d.** gender
   - **e.** smoking
4. A myocardial infarction is caused by
   - **a.** high blood pressure
   - **b.** diabetes
   - **c.** a clot in the brain
   - **d.** weakness in the heart muscle
   - **e.** a blockage in one of the coronary arteries
5. What is the main benefit of good blood supply and circulation in the coronary arteries?
   - **a.** they strengthen heart valves by moving more blood through the heart
   - **b.** they nourish the heart and reduce the risk of a heart attack
   - **c.** they help to prevent blood pooling in the lower limbs
   - **d.** they increase blood pressure in the heart
6. Which of the following lifestyle practices may help control or prevent hypertension?
   - **a.** maintaining a healthy body weight
   - **b.** exercising regularly
   - **c.** not drinking alcohol, or doing so only in moderation
   - **d.** practising stress management
   - **e.** all of the above
7. A stroke is caused by
   - **a.** a blood clot in the coronary artery
   - **b.** a severe headache
   - **c.** a blood clot in the brain
   - **d.** a blood clot in the leg
   - **e.** hardening of the arteries
8. Arteriosclerosis is a term for
   - **a.** chest pain
   - **b.** myocardial infarction
   - **c.** angina
   - **d.** hardening of the arteries
   - **e.** blood clot

9. High blood pressure is, most directly, a measure of

a. potential pain
b. heart stress
c. pressure within blood vessels
d. cholesterol levels
e. advanced aging

10. AED stands for

a. arterial external defibrillator
b. automated energy device
c. arterial emergency dialysis
d. automated external defibrillator
e. atrial emergency device

11. The two upper chambers of the heart are called the

a. atria
b. ventricles
c. aortic valves
d. sinoatrial nodes
e. aortic branches

12. The two lower chambers of the heart are called the

a. atria
b. ventricles
c. aortic valves
d. sinoatrial nodes
e. aortic branches

13. The general term for the thickening and hardening of arteries is

a. atherosclerosis
b. arteriosclerosis
c. plaque formation
d. myocardial infarction
e. carotid plaque

14. The upper limit of high–normal blood pressure is

a. 120/80
b. 160/110
c. 140/90
d. 139/89
e. 150/100

15. The reduction in oxygen flow to the heart causing chest pain is known as

a. ischemia
b. angina pectoris
c. arrhythmia
d. myocardial infarction
e. atrial fibrillation

16. An irregular heartbeat is called

a. tachycardia
b. fibrillation
c. arrhythmia
d. bradycardia
e. atrial flutter

17. Which of the following risk factors for cardiovascular disease is uncontrollable?

a. heredity
b. smoking
c. physical inactivity
d. drinking
e. consuming large quantities of fat

18. Which of the following risk factors for cardiovascular disease is controllable?

a. gender
b. age
c. high cholesterol level
d. family history
e. ethnicity

19. A mild form of a stroke, leaving only temporary symptoms, is called a(n)

a. embolism
b. thrombosis
c. subarachnoid hematoma
d. transient ischemic attack
e. atrial flutter

20. Premenopausal women may have lower rates of heart attacks compared with men due to

a. pregnancy
b. the ability to cope with stress
c. hormone replacement therapy
d. eating better
e. estrogen

21. Normal blood pressure is considered to be
    a. 120/90
    b. 120/80
    c. 130/90
    d. 130/80
    e. 110/60
22. Hypertension is known as the silent killer because
    a. people don't know how to take their blood pressure
    b. people don't pay attention to the symptoms
    c. people are unaware that they have high blood pressure
    d. people don't understand what their blood pressure means
    e. people ignore their symptoms in order to do things they want to do
23. Peripheral vascular disease affects
    a. the amount of blood to the heart due to arteriosclerosis
    b. the calcium and magnesium concentration in the blood
    c. the blood flow to the brain
    d. the lining of the heart from toxins
    e. the amount of blood to the legs due to arteriosclerosis
24. Heart failure is the result of
    a. a lack of circulation in the extremities
    b. a cerebrovascular thrombosis
    c. the heart pump losing its effectiveness
    d. a septal defect
    e. blockage of coronary arteries

Short Answer

1. What is arteriosclerosis?

2. What is coronary heart disease?

3. What are some possible signs of a heart attack?

4. How does hypertension affect the heart and arteries?

5. What special concerns surround women and cardiovascular disease?

6. Drawing on what you have learned so far, list five ways that people can lower their risk of cardiovascular disease. Include explanations of how these lower the risk.

7. What causes strokes?

8. What are the typical symptoms of an impending stroke?

9. Why is hypertension known as the silent killer?

10. Describe the six different types of cardiovascular disease.

11. Why is it important to learn about CPR and how to use an AED?

REFERENCES

American Heart Association. (2007). Bacterial endocarditis. http://www.americanheart.org.

Appel, L.J., Sacks, F.M., Carey, V.J., Obarzanek, E., Swain, J.F., et al. (2005). Effects of protein, monounsaturated fat, and carbohydrate intake on blood pressure and serum lipids: Results of the OmniHeart randomized trial. *Journal of the American Medical Association, 204*, 2455–2564.

Browarski, S., Stonebridge, C., & Theriault, L. (2010). *The Canadian Heart Health Strategy: Risk factors and future cost implications.* Ottawa: The Conference Board of Canada. http://www.conferenceboard.ca/e-Library/abstract.aspx?did=3447.

Canadian Cancer Society. (2010). *Canadian cancer statistics 2010.* Toronto: Author.

Canadian Hypertension Education Program (CHEP). (2007). Recommendations. http://www.hypertension.ca.

Canadian Institute for Health Information. (2009). *Factors predicting discharge home from inpatient rehabilitation after stroke.* Analysis in brief. https://secure.cihi.ca/estore/productFamily.htm?pf=PFC1334&lang=en&media=0.

Cappuccio, F.P., Stranges, S., Kandala, N., Miller, M.A., Taggart, F.M., et al. (2007). Gender-specific associations of short sleep duration with prevalent and incident hypertension. The Whitehall II study. *Hypertension, 50*, 694–701.

Centers for Disease Control and Prevention. (2011). *National diabetes fact sheet: National estimates and general information on diabetes and prediabetes in the United States, 2011.* Atlanta: US Department of Health and Human Services.

Chalmers, J.P., et al. (1999). World Health Organization, International Society of Hypertension guidelines for the management of hypertension. *Journal of Hypertension, 17*, 151–185.

Connelly, C. (2005). *Interventions related to obesity: A state of the evidence review, 2003.* Ottawa: Report commissioned by the Heart and Stroke Foundation of Canada.

Corrao, J.M., Becker, R.C., Ockene, L.S., & Hamilton, G.A. (1990). Coronary heart disease risk factors in women. *Cardiology, 77*, 8–12.

Creager, M.A., & Libby, P. (2007). Peripheral arterial disease. In P. Libby, R.O. Bonow, D.L. Mann, & D.P. Zipes, *Braunwald's heart disease: A textbook of cardiovascular medicine* (8th ed.) (Chapter 57). Philadelphia: Saunders.

He, J., Gu, D., Wu, X., Chen, J., Duan, X., & Whelton, P.K. (2005). Effect of soybean protein on blood pressure: A randomized controlled trial. *Annals of Internal Medicine, 143*, 1–9.

Health Canada. (2007). Canadian tobacco use monitoring survey 2006. http://www.hc-sc.gc.ca/hc-ps/tobac-tabac/research-recherche/stat/_ctums-esutc_2006/wave-phase-1_summary-sommaire-eng.php.

Health Canada. (2012). Start your new year right by following Canada's food guide. http://www.hc-sc.gc.ca/ahc-asc/media/advisories-avis/_2012/2012_01-eng.php.

Heart and Stroke Foundation of Canada (HSFC). (2001). Risk factors. http://www.heartandstroke.ca.

Heart and Stroke Foundation of Canada (HSFC). (2003, May). *The growing burden of heart disease and stroke in Canada.* Ottawa: Author.

Heart and Stroke Foundation of Canada (HSFC). (2006a). Mini strokes: What you need to know! http://www.heartandstroke.ca.

Heart and Stroke Foundation of Canada (HSFC). (2006b). Ischemic stroke & TIA (mini-stroke). http://www.heartandstroke.ca.

Heart and Stroke Foundation of Canada (HSFC). (2006c). Smoking, heart disease and stroke. http://www.heartandstroke.ca.

Heart and Stroke Foundation of Canada (HSFC). (2006d). Heart disease—Atrial fibrillation. http://www.heartandstroke.ca.

Heart and Stroke Foundation of Canada (HSFC). (2006e). Hemorrhagic stroke. http://www.heartandstroke.ca.

Heart and Stroke Foundation of Canada (HSFC). (2007a). Health dictionary. http://www.heartandstroke.ca.

Heart and Stroke Foundation of Canada (HSFC). (2007b). High blood pressure. http://www.heartandstroke.ca.

Heart and Stroke Foundation of Canada (HSFC). (2007c). Report cards on health: 2007 Report on Canadians' health—Time to bridge the gender gap, says the Heart and Stroke Foundation. http://www.heartandstroke.com/site/apps/nlnet/content2.aspx?c=iklQLcMWJtE&b=4955951&ct=4512811.

Heart and Stroke Foundation of Canada (HSFC). (2010). Taking control: Lower your risk of heart disease and stroke. http://www.heartandstroke.com/site/c.iklQLcMWJtE/b.3751103/k.3C8D/Heart_disease__Taking_Control__Lower_your_risk_of_heart_disease_and_stroke.htm.

Heart and Stroke Foundation of Canada (HSFC). (2012). Statistics. http://www.heartandstroke.com/site/c.iklQLcMWJtE/b.3483991/k.34A8/Statistics.htm.

Heart and Stroke Foundation of Manitoba. (2011, October). Automated external defibrillators (AEDs)—Getting started. http://www.heartandstroke.mb.ca/site/c.lgLSIVOyGpF/b.3674275/k.F274/Automated_External_Defibrillators_AEDs.htm.

Heart and Stroke Foundation of Ontario. (2005). *Coordinated stroke strategy. Working to provide Ontario citizens with the best possible stroke care.* Toronto: Author.

Joffres, M.R., Hamet, P., MacLean, D.R., L'Italien, G.J., & Foder, G. (2001). Distribution of blood pressure and hypertension in Canada and the United States. *American Journal of Hypertension, 14*, 1099–1105.

Julius, S., Nesbitt, S.D., Egan, B.M., Weber, M.A., Michelson, E.L., et al. (2006). Feasibility of treating prehypertension with an angiotensin-receptor blocker. *New England Journal of Medicine, 354*, 1685–1697.

Larsen, M.P., Eisenberg, M.S., Cummins, R.O., & Hallstrom, A.P. (1993). Predicting survival from out-of-hospital cardiac arrest: A graphic model. *Annals of Emergency Medicine, 22*, 1642–1658.

Lee, D.S., Chiu, M., Manuel, D.G., Tu, K., Wang, X. et al. (2009). Trends in risk factors for cardiovascular disease in Canada: Temporal, socio-demographic and geographic factors. *Canadian Medical Association Journal, 181*(3–4). doi:10.1503/cmaj.081629.

McSweeney, J., Cody, M., O'Sullivan, P., Elberson, K., Moser, D., et al. (2003). Women's early warning symptoms of acute myocardial infarction. *Circulation, 108*, 2619–2623.

Miller, M.A., & Cappuccio, F.P. (2007). Inflammation, sleep, obesity and cardiovascular disease. *Current Vascular Pharmacology, 5*(2), 93–102.

National Heart, Lung, and Blood Institute. (2012). What is heart failure? http://www.nhlbi.nih.gov/health/health-topics/topics/hf.

Public Health Agency of Canada (PHAC). (2009). *Tracking heart disease and stroke in Canada.* http://www.phac-aspc.gc.ca/publicat/2009/cvd-avc/index-eng.php.

Public Health Agency of Canada (PHAC). (2010a). *Canadian chronic disease surveillance system: Hypertension in Canada, 2010.* http://www.phac-aspc.gc.ca/cd-mc/cvd-mcv/ccdss-snsmc-2010/index-eng.php.

Public Health Agency of Canada (PHAC). (2010b). *Six types of cardiovascular disease.* http://www.phac-aspc.gc.ca/cd-mc/cvd-mcv/cvd-mcv-eng.php.

Public Health Agency of Canada (PHAC). (2011). Obesity in Canada: A joint report from the Public Health Agency of Canada and the Canadian Institute for Health Information. http://www.phac-aspc.gc.ca/hp-ps/hl-mvs/oic-oac/index-eng.php.

Rasmussen, B.M., Vessby, B., Uusitupa, M., Berglund, L., Pedersen, E., et al. (2006). Effects of dietary saturated, monounsaturated, and n-3 fatty acids on blood pressure in healthy subjects. *American Journal of Clinical Nutrition, 83*, 221–226.

Reynolds, K., Lewis, B., Nolen, J.D.L., Kinney, G.L., Sathya, B., et al. (2003). Alcohol consumption and stroke: A meta-analysis. *Journal of the American Medical Association, 289*, 579–588.

Saver, J.L. (2006). Time is brain—Quantified. *Stroke, 37*, 263–266.

Sodium Working Group. (2010, July). *Sodium reduction strategy for Canada. Recommendations of the Sodium Working Group.* http://www.hc-sc.gc.ca/fn-an/nutrition/sodium/related-info-connexe/strateg/reduct-strat-eng.php.

Stampfer, M.J., Hu, F.B., Manson, J.E., Rimm, E.B., & Willett, W.C. (2003). Primary prevention of coronary heart disease in women through diet and lifestyles. *New England Journal of Medicine, 343*, 16–22.

Statistics Canada. (2011). *Mortality, summary list of causes, 2008.* Catalogue no. 84F0209XWE. http://www.statcan.gc.ca/pub/84f0209x/84f0209x2008000-eng.pdf.

Terry, D.F., Pencina, M.J., Vasan, R.S., Murabito, J.M., Wolf, P.A., et al. (2005). Cardiovascular risk factors predictive for survival and morbidity-free survival in the oldest-old Framingham Heart Study participants. *Journal of the American Geriatric Society, 53*, 1944–1950.

Tjepkema, M. (2005). Measured obesity. Adult obesity in Canada: Measured height and weight. *Nutrition: Findings from the Canadian Community Health Survey.* Issue no. 1. Catalogue no. 82-620-MWE2005001. Ottawa: Statistics Canada.

US Department of Health and Human Services. (2006a). *The health consequences of involuntary exposure to tobacco smoke: A report of the surgeon general.* Atlanta: Centers for Disease Control and Prevention. http://www.surgeongeneral.gov/library/secondhandsmoke/report.

US Department of Health and Human Services. (2006b). *Your guide to lowering your blood pressure with DASH.* NIH publication no. 06-4082. Washington, DC: National Institutes of Health and National Heart, Lung, and Blood Institute. http://www.nhlbi.nih.gov/health/public/heart/hbp/dash/new_dash.pdf.

Vasan, R.S., Beiser, A., Seshadri, S., Larson, M.G., Kannel, W.B., et al. (2002). Residual lifetime risk for developing hypertension in middle-aged women and men. *Journal of the American Medical Association, 287*, 1003–1010.

Vasan, R.S., Larson, M.C., Leip, E.P., Kannel, W.B. & Levy, D. (2001). Assessment of frequency of progression to hypertension in non-hypertensive participants in the Framingham Heart Study: A cohort study. *Lancet, 358*, 1682–1686.

Weisfeldt, M.L., Sitlani, C.M., Ornato, J.P., Rea, T., Aufderheide, T.P., et al. (2010). Survival after application of automatic external defibrillators before arrival of the emergency medical system: Evaluation in the resuscitation outcomes consortium population of 21 million. *Journal of the American College of Cardiology, 55*, 1713–1720.

Women's Heart Foundation. (2007). *Women and heart disease facts.* http://www.womensheart.org/content/HeartDisease/heart_disease_facts.asp.

World Health Organization (WHO). (2008). *The global burden of disease: 2004 update.* Figure 4: Distribution of deaths by leading cause groups, males and females, world, 2004 (p. 10). Geneva: Author. http://www.who.int/healthinfo/global_burden_disease/GBD_report_2004update_full.pdf.

World Health Organization (WHO). (2009). *Global health risks: mortality and burden of disease attributable to selected major risks.* Geneva: Author. http://www.who.int/healthinfo/global_burden_disease/GlobalHealthRisks_report_full.pdf.

11

Back Health

LEARNING OBJECTIVES

After completing this chapter, you should be able to:

- Describe the prevalence of back pain and back injuries in policing.
- Describe the functions of the spine.
- Describe the causes of back pain, and identify the special risks to a healthy back posed by policing.
- Describe how arthritis, osteoporosis, and repetitive strain injuries have a potential impact on a law enforcement officer.
- Describe how to maintain a healthy back.
- Describe how back injuries are treated.

OVERVIEW

Back pain, most of which occurs in the lower back, is one of the most common health complaints among Canadian adults. Almost everyone experiences some type of back pain during the course of their lives. In most cases the pain subsides within a couple of days or weeks. However, for some it may occur repeatedly, and in some cases it may never go away. For some people it has a major impact on their ability to do regular chores around the house and perform simple daily tasks. More than 70 percent of back problems begin during routine daily activities. Accidents and other forms of trauma account for only 30 percent of back problems (Canadian Physiotherapy Association, 2006). Next to the common cold, low-back pain is the most common reason for missing work. On average, 90 percent of people with acute low-back pain will recover within four weeks (Canadian Physiotherapy Association, 2006).

Low-back pain is a disease of inactivity. More than 80 percent of low-back pain problems are caused by inadequate muscular development. Low-back pain usually makes its first appearance between the ages of 30 and 50, at a point in life when people are spending more time on family and job-related activities and are less physically active (National Institute for Neurological Disorders and Stroke, 2003). Routine activities such as housework, taking out the garbage and recycling bins, gardening, or reaching for an object may trigger an episode of acute back pain, which may last for hours, days, or even years.

This chapter looks at the causes of low-back pain, including the special risks faced by law enforcement officers. It also discusses how to prevent and manage back pain.

In the late 1990s, Canadian researchers conducted a survey of a random sample of 1,002 members of the Royal Canadian Mounted Police (RCMP) to determine whether back problems were more common in this group than the general public (Brown, Wells, Trottier, Bonneau, & Ferris, 1998). Researchers found that the general public reported a one-year prevalence rate between 25 and 62 percent, while the RCMP had a one-year prevalence rate between 44 and 62 percent (Brown et al., 1998). The researchers concluded that the prevalence of back problems in the sample of RCMP officers was similar to that of the general public, and that police officers did not have a higher risk of back problems due to certain aspects of their job, such as wearing a seatbelt or riding in a patrol vehicle all day (Brown et al., 1998). However, a later study found that wearing boots had a small effect on posture and the biomechanical load on the spine. In that study, researchers also found that the duty belt did not have any significant effect on an officer's flexibility and range of motion, but it did increase the metabolic cost of wearing the equipment, which could tire constables by the end of the day and predispose them to the onset of low-back pain (Kumar & Narayan, 2001). Another study found that wearing heavy body armour, combined with exposure to vehicle vibration for over two hours per day, did increase the risk of low-back pain (Burton, Tillotson, Symonds, Burke, & Mathewson, 1996), while yet another found that officers who drove and sat in the same vehicle all day were at greater risk than those whose daily tasks were varied, such as officers who spent part of their day walking (Gyi & Porter, 1998; Lis, Black, Korn, & Nordin, 2006).

Wearing a vest and firearms or carrying an overloaded backpack may lead to poor posture, overstretching of the soft tissue of the neck and back, and excessive strain on muscles and joints. Over time, the physical strain of carrying heavy loads may lead to the following problems:

- Harmful strain and fatigue in the muscles and soft tissues of the back from overuse. Constantly carrying the weight on one side may cause the spine to develop an adaptive curve, and leaning forward too much may affect the natural curve of the lower back and increase the curve of the upper back and shoulders.
- Spinal compression, improper alignment, or both may hamper the proper functioning of the discs between the vertebrae that provide shock absorption, which in turn leaves the back more vulnerable to injury.
- Stress to or compression of the shoulders and arms can compress the nerves, resulting in tingling, numbness, or weakness in the arms or hands.

The Spine

To understand back pain, you first need to know something about the spine. The spine has 33 bones, called **vertebrae**. These extend from the base of the skull to the end of the trunk (see Figure 11.1). The spine is naturally curved, which ensures proper balance and weight bearing. The spine has the following functions (Fahey, Insel, & Walton, 1997):

vertebrae
the bones of the spine (singular: vertebra)

- It provides structural support for the body, especially the thorax (chest).
- It surrounds and protects the spinal cord (a column of nervous tissue that acts as a continuation of the brain and connects the brain to the rest of the nervous system).
- It serves as an attachment site for a large number of muscles, tendons, and ligaments. (See Chapter 4 for information on muscles, tendons, and ligaments.)
- It allows movement of the neck and back in all directions.

Each vertebra is made up of a large bone, called the body, and a bony ring. The vertebrae link together to form a "tunnel" that protects the nerves and spinal cord. The lumbar vertebrae are under constant pressure from the weight of the upper body. The wear and tear of this pressure over a period of time may contribute to the development of low-back pain. The vertebrae are separated by flexible, gelatinous, shock-absorbing pads called **intervertebral discs**, which are approximately 90 percent water in young people but only about 70 percent water in older people (we lose the water as we age) (Greenberg & Dintiman, 1997). As a result, in older people the spine is more vulnerable to injury. The discs act as shock absorbers between the vertebrae in the spine.

intervertebral discs
flexible, gelatinous, shock-absorbing pads that separate the vertebrae

As we age or experience disc degeneration (typically, age 40 onward), the normal gelatin-like centre of the discs degenerates and the spaces between the vertebrae narrow. This puts additional stress on the vertebrae, which causes further wearing and may place pressure on the spinal cord or nerve endings. Degeneration of the intervertebral discs, which is often called **degenerative disc disease (DDD)** of the spine, is a common disorder of the lower spine. Disc degeneration may lead to other disorders such as spinal stenosis (narrowing of the spinal canal that houses the spinal cord and nerve roots, which may affect the lumbar or cervical nerves), spondylolisthesis (forward slippage of a disc and vertebra), and retrolisthesis (backward slippage of a disc and vertebra). Disc degeneration in the neck is called

degenerative disc disease (DDD)
degeneration of the intervertebral discs

cervical disc disease; in the mid-back it is known as thoracic disc disease, and in the lumbar spine it is called lumbago.

Cervical disc disease affects the hand, shoulder, and arm, resulting in pain, numbness or tingling, and weakness. Thoracic disc disease affects the area between the end of the neck and just above the waistline, resulting in limited or painful movement of the upper back, numbness or tingling, and weakness in the legs. It can be painful when coughing, sneezing, or taking a deep breath. Lumbago is pain in the lumbar region of the spine that can be caused by factors such as injury, arthritis, back strain, abuse of the back muscles (poor posture, sagging mattress, or ill-fitting shoes), or by a number of disorders (listed above), resulting in numbness and tingling in the lower back and legs, weakness in the legs, loss of bowel or bladder control, fevers or chills, and unexplained weight loss.

Age, repetitive strain, and possibly genetics cause disc wear and tear. Because there is little blood supply to the discs, they cannot repair themselves if injured.

FIGURE 11.1 The Spine

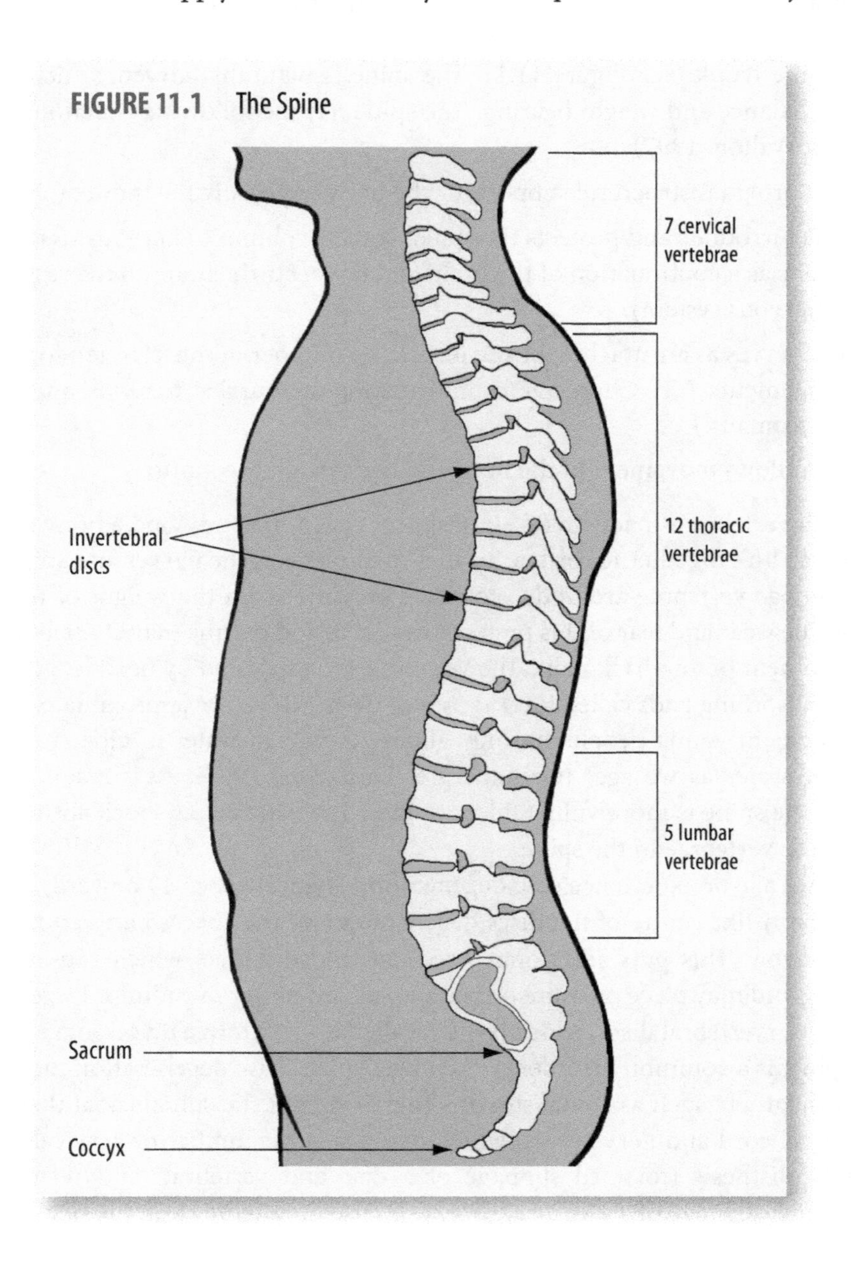

FIGURE 11.2 Process of Herniation of an Intervertebral Disc: Side View

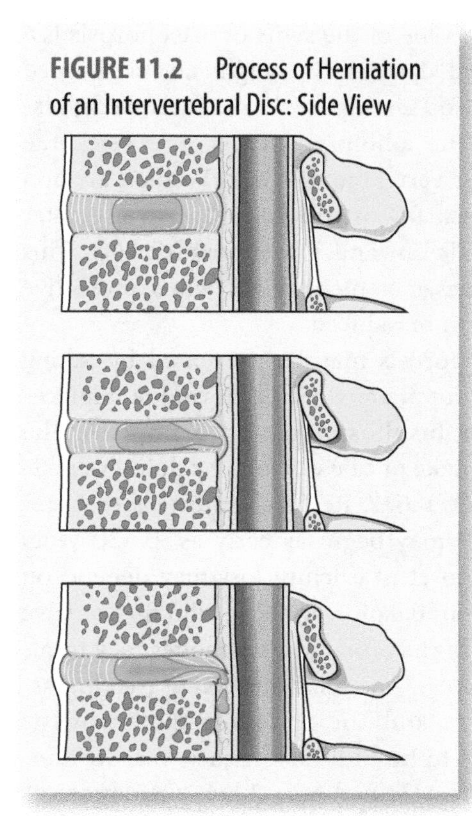

FIGURE 11.3 Herniation and Rupture of an Intervertebral Disc: Top View

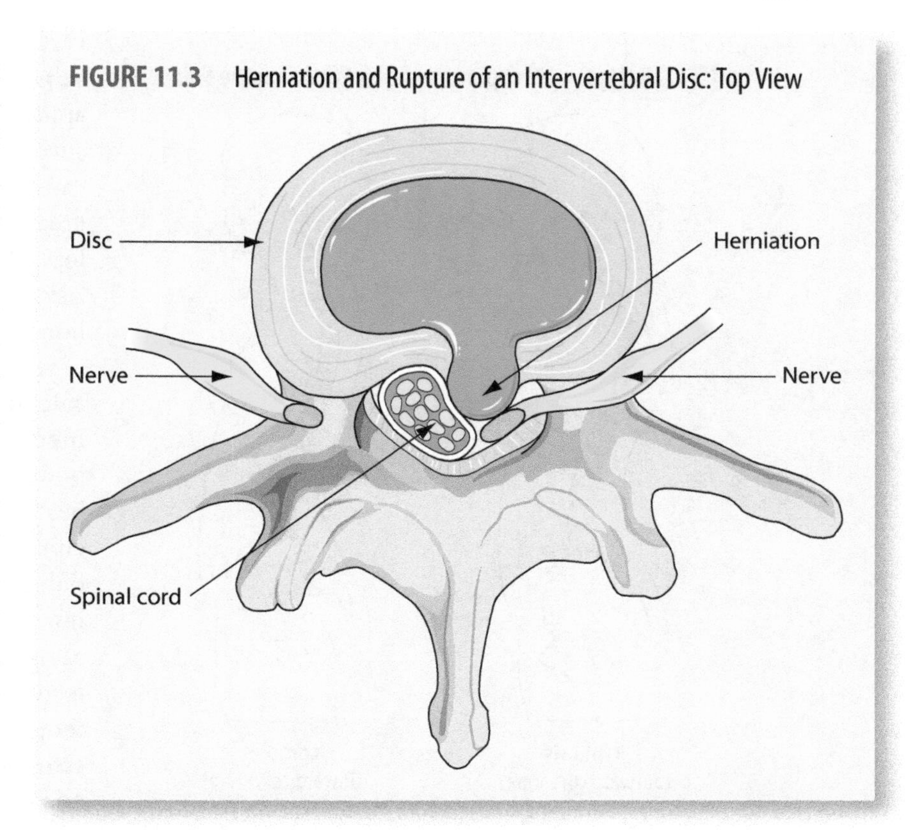

One common injury is a "slipped" or herniated disc, which occurs when sudden pressure causes the disc to rupture and its gelatinous interior to protrude through the outer coating of the disc (see Figures 11.2 and 11.3). The protruding material may put pressure on adjoining nerves, causing considerable low-back pain, which radiates into the legs. However, most back problems involve the muscles, tendons, or ligaments, not the bones. As we grow older, the discs become flatter, and if stressed or weakened, the outer part (annulus) may bulge or tear. The location of the pain depends on where the disc is pressing on the nerve. In the lumbar region it is called sciatica, a condition we will discuss later in this chapter.

Osteoporosis

osteoporosis
a condition common in older people, in whom bones become increasingly soft and porous, thinner, and more brittle, making them susceptible to risk of fracture, particularly of the hip, spine, and wrist

Another problem that occurs in our aging population is an increase in back injuries as a result of osteoporosis. **Osteoporosis** is a bone disease common in older people, in whom the bones become increasingly soft and porous, thinner, and more brittle, making them susceptible to the risk of fracture, particularly of the hip, spine, and wrist. Seventy percent of hip fractures are osteoporosis-related. Hip fractures result in death due to complications (such as pneumonia) in up to 20 percent of cases, and disability in 50 percent of those who survive. Osteoporosis is known as the "silent thief" because bone loss often occurs without symptoms.

Approximately 1.4 million Canadians suffer from osteoporosis (Osteoporosis Canada, 2007). As we age, the discs begin to lose their gelatinous mass, resulting in compression of the

DID YOU KNOW?

A full 25 percent of women over age 50, and 50 percent over age 70, develop osteoporosis. Seven in 10 fractures in those over the age of 45 are due to this disease.

SOURCE: Public Health Agency of Canada (PHAC), 2007.

FIGURE 11.4 Osteoporosis and Its Effects on the Spine

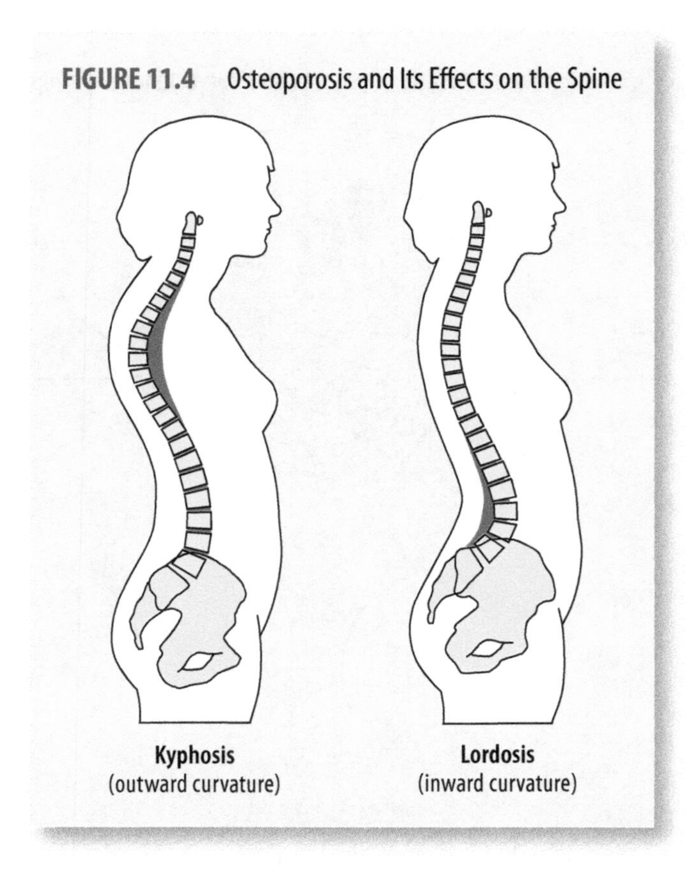

vertebrae. One of the signs of osteoporosis is a substantial decrease in height and a stooped appearance (see Figure 11.4). Increased pressure on the adjoining nerves and vertebrae causes the vertebrae to crack. Women are at a greater risk for osteoporosis due to a greater loss of calcium and lower bone density. This risk increases at menopause, when protective hormones are reduced.

Osteoporosis may be prevented by taking calcium supplements and hormone replacement, or bisphosphonates to improve the body's uptake of calcium, and by doing weight-bearing exercises. Research indicates that calcium loss may begin as early as 25–30 years old; the onset of calcium loss may depend on hormone imbalance, so those who do not have as much of the protective hormones may be affected sooner. The financial cost of treating osteoporosis and the fractures that result is estimated to be $1.9 billion each year in Canada alone (Henneberg, 2006; Osteoporosis Canada, 2011b).

Causes

There are three main factors that are attributed to osteoporosis (National Institutes of Health, 2003; Osteoporosis Canada, 2011b):

1. Suboptimal bone growth during childhood, adolescence, or early adulthood, not allowing for peak bone mass to be achieved. Peak bone mass density is achieved at an early age (16 in girls, 20 in boys). If there are nutritional concerns or lack of physical activity, peak bone mass density will be less.
2. Accelerated bone loss during adulthood, usually due to a drop in sex hormone levels associated with aging (that is, menopause in women, low testosterone levels in men). Women and men alike begin to lose bone in their mid-30s; as they approach menopause, women lose bone at a greater rate, from 2 to 5 percent per year.
3. Bone loss secondary to disease conditions, including eating disorders, medications, and medical treatments.

Risk Factors for Osteoporosis

The risk factors for osteoporosis include (National Institutes of Health, 2003; Osteoporosis Canada, 2011b):

- *Gender* Women are at higher risk.
- *Fracture history* Personal history of fracture after age 50, or a family history of fractures, increases the risk.

- *Race* Asian and Caucasian women are at greater risk.
- *Body frame and weight* Women who have a small frame or who are below 127 pounds are at greater risk.
- *Age* Risk increases with age.
- *Menopause* Women can lose more than 20 percent of their bone mass in the first five to seven years following menopause.
- *Low testosterone in men* Testosterone levels decrease with age.
- *Absence of or abnormal menstruation* Delayed onset of menstruation, absence of menstruation, or an abnormal menstrual cycle can increase the risk.
- *Certain medications and conditions* Medications and conditions that affect vitamin D and calcium absorption increase the risk. Those with celiac and Crohn's disease are especially susceptible.
- *Lack of physical activity* Inadequate weight-bearing activity increases the risk.
- *Lifestyle factors* Cigarette smoking and excessive alcohol use increase the risk.
- *Nutritional factors* Low calcium intake increases the risk of bone loss.

Diagnosis of Osteoporosis

Four major risk factors for fractures are age (over 65 years), low bone mineral density, fragility fractures after age 40, and family history of osteoporosis. Some of the minor risk factors include excessive caffeine and alcohol use, smoking, low calcium intake, early menopause (before age 45), and weight less than 57 kilograms (125 pounds) (Mills, 2006). Osteoporosis Canada has recommended that everyone over the age of 65, and those who are over 50 and have at least one major risk factor or two minor risk factors, should have a bone densitometry test, which assesses density of the hip and spine, on a yearly basis (Mills, 2006). Bone densitometry allows accurate and precise skeletal assessment, and enables detection of osteoporosis prior to actual fractures. It can also determine if there is any onset of fractures in the spine and limbs. With information about a patient's risk factors and the results of bone densitometry, a physician can determine diagnosis of mineral loss in the bone.

The Causes of Back Pain

Although some people have a weak back for genetic reasons, inadequate muscular development is the major cause of back pain. The strength of a muscle is directly related to the amount of work it does. Strength increases the more the muscle is made to work against an opposing force. If the muscle is not worked enough, it loses strength. In physically inactive people, the large muscle groups are not worked enough and therefore lack sufficient strength. For the back, insufficient muscle strength means that correct body alignment is compromised.

The back is supported, and its movement is controlled, by 140 muscles. Typically, a muscle, ligament, or tendon strain or sprain causes nearby muscles to spasm (involuntarily contract) in an attempt to support the back. The most frequently documented cause of low-back pain is muscle strain, with overexertion and irregular (fast, awkward) movements such as lifting, twisting, turning, bending, pushing, and pulling being typical underlying factors (Bonneau, Stevenson, & Gledhill,

2001). It is estimated that 70 percent of back problems are due to improper alignment of the spine and pelvic girdle (hip bones) caused by inflexible and weak muscles (Greenberg & Dintiman, 1997). Poor flexibility and weak muscles in the back, pelvis, and thighs may increase the curve of the lower back and cause the pelvis to tilt too far forward. Good flexibility in these areas, along with good muscle strength and good posture, helps prevent abnormal pressure on sensitive spinal nerves.

Poor abdominal muscle group development is another common cause of low-back pain. If the abdominal muscles are weak, they cannot exert enough pressure to keep the pelvis in place, and it tilts forward. This in turn causes the vertebrae in the lower back to become slightly displaced and press against one another, producing an ache in the lower back.

The hamstring muscles are another muscle group implicated in low-back pain. This group consists of three large muscles, located at the back of each thigh, which are associated with movement at the hip and knee joints. The difficulty most people face in trying to touch their toes with their fingertips without bending their knees is largely due to the hamstrings' inability to stretch far enough. This inability stems from an inflexibility or shortening of the hamstrings caused by physical inactivity or long periods of sitting. The hamstrings' inflexibility or shortening may cause pain in the hamstrings themselves and referred (travelling) pain in the lower back.

Factors that may compound low-back pain include physical injury, hard sneezing or coughing, improper lifting or bending, long hours of sitting or standing, sitting slumped in overstuffed chairs or car seats, anxiety, depression, obesity, and diseases such as arthritis. Vertebral joints may be affected by degenerative arthritis, causing inflammation within the joint. Although back pain may result from sudden, traumatic injuries, in most cases people cannot identify a specific injury as the starting point of their condition.

Risk Factors for Back Pain

Although we know that anyone can experience back pain, there are a number of factors that increase your risk. Several of these factors are not under your control:

- growing older
- having a family history of back pain
- being a man (statistically, more men work in physically demanding careers that increase their risk of injury)
- having children (two or more full-term pregnancies triple a woman's risk of osteoporosis and potential collapse of the vertebrae)
- having a congenital birth defect
- having a degenerative disease of the spine, such as osteoporosis or arthritis

Factors that you *can* control include the following:

- lack of exercise
- sitting for long periods of time, lifting or pulling heavy objects without using proper form (see Figure 11.5), bending or twisting frequently, heavy physical exertion, repetitive motions, and exposure to constant vibration such as when driving

- smoking—you are twice as likely to have low-back pain if you smoke or are exposed to second-hand smoke. Lorentzon and colleagues (2007) have shown that adolescent smokers have significant loss in bone mass density resulting in a lower peak bone mass, mainly as a consequence of reduced cortical thickness (the density of the outer layer of the bone).
- being overweight—weighing more than 20 percent over your ideal body weight increases your risk of back problems. However, Zhao and colleagues (2006) believe that losing weight to reduce back problems may increase the risk of osteoporosis.
- having poor posture
- having an illness or disease that causes chronic coughing
- having a mental health problem, such as severe anxiety or depression
- suffering from a significant amount of stress

There are also several activities that can increase your risk of back pain and injury:

- running or jogging without the proper equipment or on uneven surfaces
- skiing and snowboarding
- sledding, snowmobiling, or tobogganing
- sports that require forceful twisting, like gymnastics, trampolining, and wrestling
- contact sports like football or rugby
- work-related activities that require repeated lifting, bending, or twisting of the back

FIGURE 11.5 Improper and Proper Techniques for Lifting Heavy Objects

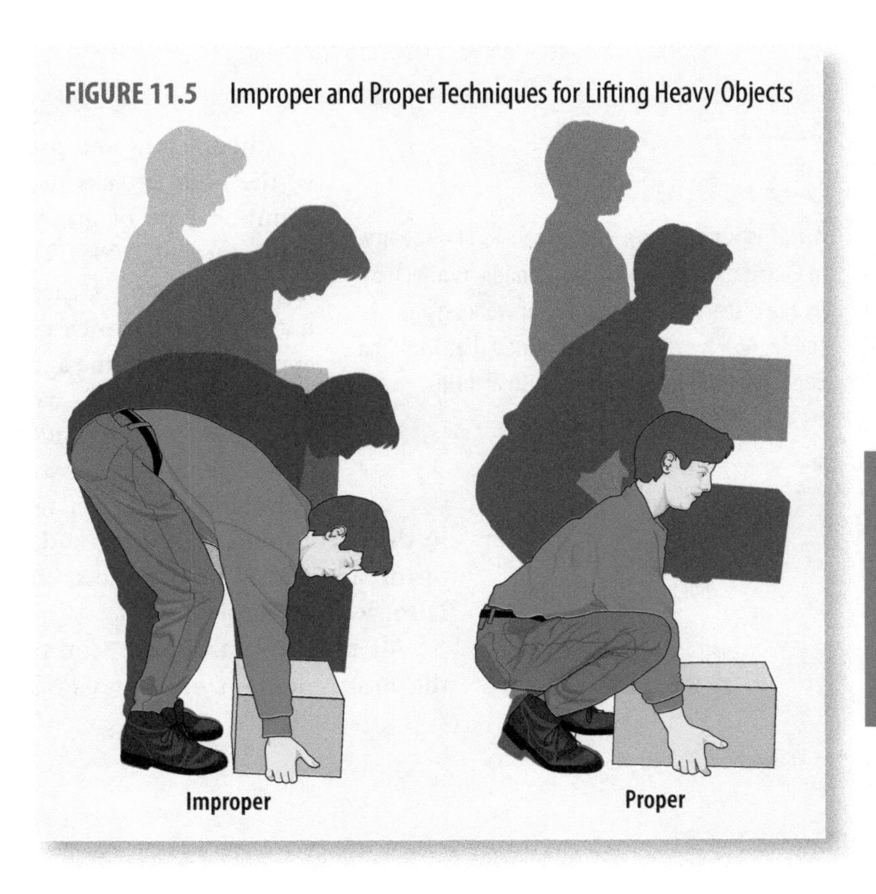

Arthritis

Arthritis is a group of conditions that affect the joints of the body. It comprises more than 100 conditions, including lupus, fibromyalgia, gout, and scleroderma. The most common type of arthritis in Canada is osteoarthritis (degenerative arthritis; see Figure 11.6), which affects 3 million Canadians, or 1 in 10 (Murphy, Spence, McIntosh, & Connor Gorber, 2006). This disease may occur following trauma to a joint as a result of an infection or aging. Osteoarthritis is also sometimes confused with, or may be associated with, degenerative disc disease. This is because osteoarthritis and degenerated discs are commonly found together. However, they are separate conditions. Juvenile arthritis (JA) is one of the most common chronic illnesses in Canada, affecting 1 in 1,000 boys and girls under the age of 16. By 2026, it is estimated that more than 6 million Canadians older than 15 will have arthritis.

arthritis
a group of conditions in which there is a degeneration of a joint following trauma to the joint (as a result of an infection or aging)

FIGURE 11.6 Progression of Osteoarthritis

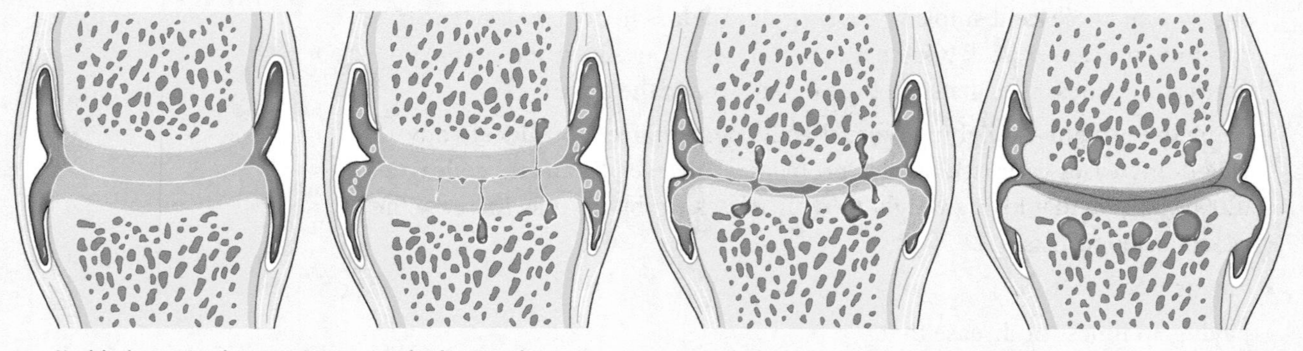

DID YOU KNOW?

Arthritis is one of the leading causes of disability in Canada. Of the 4.5 million Canadians affected by the disease, 60 percent are of working age (under 65). By 2031, it is estimated that 7 million Canadians will be diagnosed with arthritis.

SOURCE: Arthritis Society, 2011a.

fibromyalgia chronic disorder characterized by widespread musculoskeletal pain, fatigue, and multiple "tender points," particularly in the neck, spine, shoulders, and hips

Rheumatoid and psoriatic arthritis are autoimmune diseases (that is, the body attacks itself). Rheumatoid arthritis is the second most common type of arthritis, affecting 300,000 Canadians, or 1 in 100 (Murphy et al., 2006). The immune system attacks healthy joints, resulting in damage to cartilage, bone, tendons, and ligaments. Three times as many women as men get rheumatoid arthritis, and it most commonly appears between the ages of 25 and 50 (Arthritis Society, 2011b).

Septic arthritis is caused by joint infection. Gouty arthritis occurs when uric acid deposits build up in the joints, causing joint inflammation. **Fibromyalgia** is a chronic disorder characterized by widespread musculoskeletal pain, fatigue, and multiple "tender points," particularly in the neck, spine, shoulders, and hips. Additional symptoms may include sleep disturbances, morning stiffness, and anxiety (National Institute for Neurological Disorders and Stroke, 2003).

All arthritis causes pain. Chronic pain and reduced mobility and function are the most common outcomes of long-term arthritis. Osteoarthritis is typically

FACTS ABOUT . . .

The Costs of Arthritis in Canada

- In 2000, the total cost associated with arthritis was $6.4 billion. This represents one-third the total costs attributed to musculoskeletal diseases, the most costly group of diseases in Canada.
- Indirect costs associated with arthritis accounted for twice the direct costs ($4.3 billion and $2.1 billion, respectively).
- With respect to direct costs, arthritis accounted for over one-half of hospital care expenditures for all musculoskeletal diseases, nearly three-fifths of drug expenditures, and approximately one-half of physician care expenditures.
- In indirect costs, arthritis accounted for more than 80 percent of all musculoskeletal mortality costs and over one-quarter of morbidity costs due to long-term disability.
- Total costs were greater in women ($4.1 billion) than men ($2.3 billion) because of the higher prevalence of arthritis among women.
- Those in the labour force (35–64 years of age) account for over two times the cost incurred by the elderly (65 years and over)—$4.1 billion and $1.7 billion, respectively.

SOURCE: PHAC, 2010.

worse at night or following rest. Rheumatoid arthritis, on the other hand, is usually worse in the mornings. Warm showers or baths seem to relieve the symptoms, but many who experience this pain are less likely to use the affected joint.

Treatment depends on the history of the pain, such as when it started, how many joints are affected, how long the pain lasts, what aggravates the inflammation, and what helps to relieve the pain. Physical examinations and X-rays confirm the state of the condition, and blood tests confirm the diagnosis. There are medications that you may discuss with your doctor regarding treatment. Early diagnosis of arthritis may help prevent irreversible joint damage (see Figure 11.7).

FIGURE 11.7 Effect of Arthritis on the Hip Joint

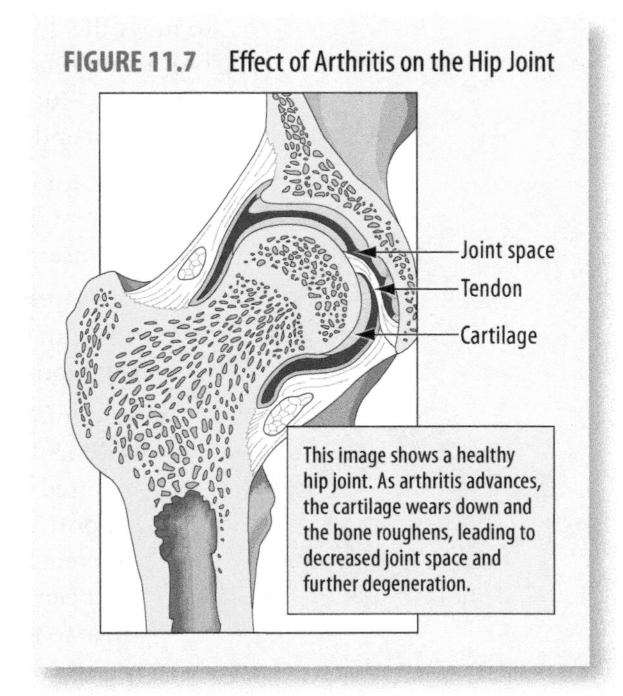

Repetitive Strain Injury

Repetitive strain injury (RSI) is associated with back pain. RSI arises when soft tissue is subjected to repeated trauma (such as typing or using a computer mouse) without the chance to recover from each trauma. In the upper body it results in injuries such as tendinitis, carpal tunnel syndrome, DeQuervain's disease (a painful disorder affecting the tendons at the base of the thumb), epicondylitis (tennis elbow or golfer's elbow), thoracic outlet syndrome, and tension neck syndrome.

repetitive strain injury (RSI)
an injury that arises when soft tissue is subjected to repeated trauma (such as may be caused by typing or using a computer mouse) without the chance to recover from each trauma

Repetitive activity damages tendons, affects circulation, and causes biomechanical stresses on soft tissue by not allowing enough recovery time between movements. Symptoms include pain, numbness, and tingling in the affected body parts (Tjepkema, 2003). Repetitive strain injuries take a toll not only physically but mentally. An RSI may affect work with functional and activity limitations, and may cause sleep disturbances. In 2001, 10 percent of Canadians aged 20 or older reported having an RSI serious enough to have limited their usual activities at some point in the previous 12 months (Tjepkema, 2003). Most RSIs affect the upper body—specifically, 25 percent of cases occur in the neck and shoulders, 23 percent in the wrists or hands, 19 percent in the upper or lower back, 16 percent in the elbows or lower arms, and 17 percent in a lower extremity or unspecified body part.

There are two broad groupings of repetitive strain injuries: tendon-related disorders and peripheral nerve entrapment disorders. *Tendon-related disorders*, which involve the inflammation of the tendon and sheath or injuries to them, include tendinitis (inflammation of the tendon), tenosynovitis (inflammation of the tendon sheath), epicondylitis, and rotator cuff tendinitis. *Peripheral nerve entrapment disorders* involve compression of a nerve. The most common is carpal tunnel syndrome (compression of the medial nerve), and the second most common is cubital tunnel syndrome (compression of the ulnar nerve) (Tjepkema, 2003).

Many workers have jobs in which they have little or no control over how the job is done or the rate at which the job must be completed. Often these jobs involve rapid, repetitive tasks. Law enforcement officers, for example, are often required to perform repetitive tasks that adversely affect their back and shoulder muscles and tendons. Altercations and repetitive movements such as use of force or firearms training may cause inflammation. With the introduction of computers into vehicles and poor ergonomic conditions (such as the location of the computer, inability to move the display, vest and belt hampering movement to face the display, and so on), many officers complain about shoulder and wrist pain. Ranney (1995) and Anderson, Zutz, and Plecas (2011) identify several features of law enforcement equipment and tasks that are conducive to RSI and back problems generally:

- Law enforcement may require officers to perform the same task for a long time without a chance to rest or exercise a different set of muscles. Sitting in a cruiser for hours is an example.
- Law enforcement may require substantial muscular force—for example, when an officer must restrain a person or remove him or her from a volatile situation.
- Law enforcement may require officers to maintain an awkward posture that is difficult to hold for even a short time. For example, officers are sometimes required to stand for long periods in boots that provide inadequate foot support. Similarly, cruiser seat design does not address the needs of different body types. If a seat has been damaged by excessive use and has not been repaired, officers are forced to sit in a position that does not allow them to maintain proper posture, which puts additional strain on the back.
- The equipment belt that uniformed officers wear weighs 5–9 kilograms (10–20 pounds) or more and puts strain on the lower back whether one is sitting or standing. Most duty belts are typically 5.5–5.7 centimetres (2.25 inches) wide. Slowly, services are replacing leather ones (which were stiff and inflexible) with nylon ones. However, with the addition of a radio, flashlight, latex gloves, baton, pepper spray canister, handcuffs, handgun, and spare magazines, this can place uncommon pressure on the front of the pelvis and abdomen. In addition, the equipment attached to the belt may cause an officer to sit in an awkward position. Patrol vehicle seats can be another factor in belt discomfort. Raised sides on seats can produce pressure on the sidearm and radio, causing the officer to push forward to reduce the amount of low back support. Worn seats cause officers to sink lower in the middle of the seat, causing additional discomfort.
- Officers who work outdoors in winter face a higher risk of back injuries. If they have to respond quickly to an altercation or other incident, their cold, stiff muscles and joints are more likely to suffer damage.

Sciatica

sciatica
pain anywhere along the sciatic nerve as the result of compression, inflammation, or irritation; generally, the pain travels from the back of the thigh to the back of the calf, and also may extend upwards, to the hip

Sciatica, or sciatic neuritis, is a common back condition. The sciatic nerve exits the spinal column between the lowest vertebrae and the sacrum (see Figure 11.1). This nerve supplies sensation to the back of the thighs and buttocks, knee flexors, and foot muscles. When it is compressed, inflamed, or irritated anywhere along its length, pain may result. Sciatica may result in wasting of the muscles of the lower leg. It may result from poor posture, disc degeneration, a bulging disc, or pregnancy where the fetus is pushing on the nerves. Symptoms range from a sensation of "pins and needles" or numbness to a burning feeling in the leg or foot. The pain from a bulging disc is usually worse when you are active, and feels better when you are resting. Coughing, sneezing, sitting, driving, and bending forward may make the pain worse because these movements put more pressure on the nerve.

This problem is especially hard on officers who must sit in their cruisers for long periods of time. With extended sitting in a vehicle, many people feel their legs burn or go numb, making it very difficult to get out of the cruiser quickly and respond to emergencies.

Preventing Back Pain

Physical conditioning is the key to preventing back injury. In addition to getting regular aerobic exercise, officers need to develop strong back and stomach muscles, which are necessary to support the spine. Law enforcement personnel also need to learn the proper ways to stand, bend, lift, sit, rest, and sleep. They must regularly perform exercises that stretch and strengthen the major muscles affecting the back, and be as active as possible. Flexibility is a major factor in back health. Without it, many individuals suffer back strain.

Both abdominal and back muscles require adequate exercise to maintain strength and tone. Although we use our thigh muscles whenever we walk or climb stairs, deep abdominal and back muscles are usually left unconditioned and inactive. It is important to strengthen the flexor, extensor, and oblique muscles to support the spine. Lack of such exercises can lead to muscle atrophy (wasting), which can cause back pain from the inability of the muscles to hold up the spine. Under stress, our muscles tighten. This means that when we have a physical altercation or fight-or-flight response, we tighten and may injure the lower back. Tight hamstrings can result in straining of the lower back, while weak abdominal muscles cause hip flexors to tighten, resulting in an increase in the curve of the lower back.

Exercises for a Healthy Back

Flexion and extension exercises will help you maintain a healthy back and are also used to recover from low-back injuries.

Flexion Exercises

- *Cat back* Kneel on the floor, resting on your hands and knees. Allow your spine to sag slightly. Then arch your back like a cat as high as possible. Try to hold this position for a few seconds. Performing this exercise is often easier if you lower your head as you arch your back.
- *Pelvic tilt* Lie on your back with knees bent and feet flat on the floor. Press the small of your back against the floor and tighten your stomach and buttock muscles. Do not push with your feet. Performing this exercise correctly should cause the lower part of your pelvis to rotate forward and flatten your back against the floor. Hold for six seconds, and then relax the muscles for six seconds. Repeat six times. When learning this exercise, it is often helpful to put one of your hands in the hollow of your back so that you can feel the small of your back pressing down toward the floor.

Extension Exercises

When used to alleviate low-back pain, these exercises should be repeated at two-hour intervals six to eight times a day. For prevention, these exercises may be done as part of your daily workout.

TOP TEN...

Tips for a Healthy Back

In addition to exercising, the following tips will help you keep your back strong and flexible and prevent low-back pain.

1. To warm up for an activity, swing any tool you will be using (such as an adze, rake, shovel, axe, or golf club) lazily back and forth around your head and shoulders in different positions, gradually working up to a full range of motion. Work your way up to the effort required to do the activity.
2. When lifting an object, warm up the muscles first. Then stand close to the load, facing the direction you want to go. Bend at the knees and hips rather than keeping your legs straight and bending at the waist (see Figure 11.5). Your feet should be shoulder-width apart. Ensure that you have a good grip on the load. Lift gradually, keeping your arms straight and pushing up with your leg muscles. Keep the object close to your body. If you must turn, do not twist at the waist; ensure that you have enough space for your entire body to turn before lifting. Also, be aware that lowering objects causes less strain than lifting; pulling them is easier than carrying; and pushing is less demanding than pulling.
3. When standing, make sure most of your weight is on the balls of your feet and not on your heels. Your feet should be shoulder-width apart, your knees should be slightly bent, and your arms should fall naturally to your sides. Periodically, shift your weight from one foot to the other.
4. Keep your body aligned. When you stand up against a wall, the back of your head, shoulders, and buttocks should touch the wall. When sitting, keep your knees slightly higher than your hips. Sit upright rather than with your shoulders forward by placing your feet on a footrest (or use books, pillows, or a cardboard box). If you use a back support, make sure it fits you.
5. Do not sit in the same position for a long period of time. Get up and move around. This reduces the strain on your back muscles and ligaments and helps improve circulation to relieve muscle fatigue and discomfort.
6. Leaning against a solid support when you are sitting, such as sitting on a chair rather than a bench with no back, helps reduce fatigue.
7. When sitting at a desk or in front of a computer, place your chair as close as possible to the desk or computer so that you are sitting in an upright position. If your back flattens when you sit, try putting a lumbar roll (a low-back pillow, often sold in drugstores) behind your lower back. Your feet should be flat on the floor and your knees higher than your hips.
8. Once a day, lie on your back with your feet up on a couch at a 90-degree angle. This straightens the lower back. Doing the pelvic tilt on the floor also reduces the strain on your lower back.
9. Try sleeping on your side with your knees and hips bent. If you lie on your back, place a pillow under your knees. Do not lie on your stomach; this hyperextends the back. Your mattress should be firm enough to support your spine in its neutral position. The mattress should not sag. Consider adding a layer of foam for extra support.
10. When walking, keep your toes pointed straight ahead. Keep your back flat, your head up, and your chin in.

- *Lower-back relaxing* Lie on the floor on your stomach, arms at your sides, and head turned to one side. Now, try to relax the muscles in your lower back. Hold for a few minutes.
- *Upper-back lift (modified)* Lie on your stomach with your chin resting on the floor. Put your elbows under your shoulders on your chest and support your body on your forearms. Keep your neck in a straight line. If you notice a re-

duction in pain, hold this position for up to five minutes. If the pain increases, discontinue immediately. If this exercise helps, move on to the next one.

- *Upper-back lift* Lie on your stomach with your chin resting on the floor. Put your hands under your shoulders with forearms flat on the floor. Straighten (extend) your elbows as you tighten your back muscles to lift your body up without triggering pain. Keep the pelvis, hips, and legs completely relaxed. Try to extend your back as much as possible, but do not push with your arms. Hold this position for two seconds and then return to the starting position. Repeat 10 times.

Exercises to Avoid

A number of exercises that were popular in the 1960s and 1970s and are still recommended by some people put too much strain on the spine and should be avoided. Here are a few examples:

- standing toe touch while keeping the legs straight with knees locked
- standing hamstring stretch with legs straight and knees locked (which puts excessive strain on the knees and lower back)
- prone arch—lying on your stomach and trying to bring your head to your feet
- yoga plough—lying on your back and trying to put your feet up behind your head (which strains the neck and back)
- sit-ups, especially where you put your hands behind your head and pull on your neck to assist the sit-up (which may pull your vertebrae out of alignment)

If you are involved in a fitness program and believe an exercise you are asked to do may harm your back, speak to the instructor and ask for an alternative. Do not do anything that causes pain. Protecting your back is more important than adhering strictly to a fitness program, and you are the person most aware of your body's limitations.

Proper Sitting in a Vehicle

It is essential to sit properly, especially when driving. Because law enforcement officers may spend a great deal of time in vehicles, it is important that they look after their backs. Officers complain of low-back pain and general backaches as the result of sitting in cruisers that are damaged and uncomfortable. Whether you are on the job or enjoying a drive, here are some guidelines to assist you in sitting correctly (Mack, 2002):

- When adjusting your seat, begin by sitting with your buttocks as far back in the seat as possible. Make sure that your lower back is pressing firmly against the back of the seat. Then, move your seat forward until your right foot is on the floorboards behind the pedal with your knee slightly bent (this will ensure maximum pressure when you are braking in an emergency).
- Your backrest should be near the upright position to place less pressure on the lower back. Your chest should be at least 20–25 centimetres (8–10 inches) from the centre of the steering wheel. Your wrists should be able to reach

over the wheel when the car is stopped, and your elbows should be slightly bent when your arms are placed in the normal driving position. Shorter individuals may require seat cushions and pedal extenders to accomplish this. When driving, officers are encouraged to sit back with their torsos at an approximate 100-degree angle or more (Kumar & Narayan, 2001).

- Your head restraint is important for preventing whiplash. The middle of the back of your head should come in full contact with the restraint.
- Your rear-view mirror should be positioned so that you can see the two rear pillars as well as the roofline and bottom of the rear window. Your side mirrors should be positioned so that you can see the adjacent lane rather than the side of the vehicle.
- Seatbelt position is very important. The lap portion should be pulled down snugly over the hipbones to prevent the belt from riding up in a crash (which could cause internal injuries). The shoulder belt should be high enough to ensure that the belt does not fall off your shoulder (to prevent your hitting the steering wheel or windshield).
- When getting into the vehicle, first sit on the seat, and then rotate your legs in as one unit to prevent twisting of the spine. When exiting the vehicle, make sure to rotate your legs as one unit to the door, place your feet on the ground, and then stand up. If you have spent a long time in the vehicle, this will prevent excessive twisting of the spine, which has lost mobility from sitting in one position.
- Redistribution of the components in your duty belt can help you sit properly. Kumar and Narayan's (2001) study proposed that the minimal amount of equipment be attached to an officer's duty belt. They suggested that the baton be moved to a pocket on the thigh and the radio to a pocket on the chest in a designed uniform. Many police services are now issuing phones to their officers, and even BlackBerry devices in order to supply a lightweight phone and computer in a single piece of equipment. The bullet magazine, handcuffs, and pepper spray should all be placed on the front of the duty belt to ensure that the back is fully supported by the car's backrest. A soft pouch like the one containing latex gloves could be placed on the lumbar spine.
- During normal policing when emergencies are not expected, officers should consciously and periodically change their posture, move around, or change physical activity. It is recommended that every 50 minutes of continuous work of one type should be followed by a 10-minute period of another activity (Kumar & Narayan, 2001).
- When sitting in a vehicle, do not keep your legs fully extended. Your knees should be bent to prevent back strain and shortening of the hamstring muscles. Push the front seat of your vehicle forward so that your knees will be higher than your hips. This will reduce the strain on your back and shoulder muscles.
- An added seat cushion with upholstered memory foam and a rubber layer underneath will decrease the tendency to slide as you get in and out of the car.
- Strapping a lumbar cushion to the seat will provide additional lumbar support.

Nutritional Considerations for a Healthier Back

When an excess amount of protein, refined carbohydrates, and fats are consumed over a period of time, the body becomes more acidic. Because the body prefers alkaline minerals, calcium in particular is removed from bones and transported to the rest of the body to neutralize the acidic environment. Some goes into the kidneys and is excreted. In addition, phosphorus—found in high-protein foods such as meat, poultry, fish, eggs, and dairy products—competes with calcium for absorption in the intestines. The more phosphorus there is, the less calcium will be absorbed, and as we age, this becomes a concern.

Chapter 8 discusses the body's need for calcium and its best food sources. The points that follow here are a useful review.

How Much Calcium Do You Need?

Calcium requirements are age-related. As we get older, we lose our ability to absorb calcium and so require more of it in our diet. We need to maximize our intake in order to continue to have calcium-dense bones. Table 11.1 outlines calcium requirements by age.

TABLE 11.1
Daily Calcium Requirements

AGE	DAILY CALCIUM REQUIREMENT
0–6 months	210 mg
7–12 months	270 mg
1–3 years	500 mg
4–8 years	800 mg
9–18 years	1,300 mg
19–50 years	1,000 mg
51+ years	1,200 mg

SOURCE: Adapted from Health Canada, 2005.

How to Maximize Your Calcium Intake Through Diet

By consulting a reliable food chart, such as the one found at the Canada's Food Guide website (Health Canada, 2011), you can calculate your daily calcium intake. Osteoporosis Canada (2011a) has a calculator that can help you find out whether you are getting the recommended levels. (See References for both.)

Foods Containing Easily Absorbed Calcium

Excellent sources of calcium include milk, cheese, and yogurt. Skim milk has the same amount of calcium as whole milk, with less fat and cholesterol. The calcium in soy beverages is absorbed at 75 percent the rate of milk. Some soy beverages and orange juices are fortified with calcium (check their labels). Some vegetables and fish (canned salmon and sardines), and meat alternatives such as lentils and beans, are rich in calcium. If you cannot consume or do not like dairy products, make sure you are eating calcium-rich alternatives. If you are unsure, consult a dietitian.

Foods That Cause Calcium Loss Through Urination

Over 90 percent of sodium comes from processed food rather than table salt. Because salt acts as a diuretic, you should read labels to ensure that your sodium intake from packaged foods is kept to a minimum.

Caffeine is also a diuretic. If you consume more than four cups of coffee a day, you should drink one glass of milk for every cup of caffeine-containing beverage, or avoid caffeinated beverages altogether. Of particular note, energy drinks and carbonated beverages can be higher in caffeine than coffee or tea, resulting in detrimental effects such as irritability, sleep disturbance, and diarrhea, besides calcium depletion.

Vitamin D and Calcium

Vitamin D, the "sunshine vitamin," is also necessary to bone health. It helps maintain serum calcium (the amount of calcium found in the bloodstream) and phosphate concentrations in the body (Institute of Medicine, 1997). It improves muscle strength, and reduces fracture rates and rates of falling (Bischoff-Ferrari, Dawson-Hughes, Willett, Staehelin, Bazemore, et al., 2004; Bischoff-Ferrari, Dietrich, Orav, Hu, Zhang, et al., 2004; Bischoff-Ferrari, Willett, Wong, Giovannucci, Dietrich, et al., 2005). In some cases, it plays a role in the prevention of certain cancers and protection against autoimmune diseases (Garland, Garland, Gorham, Lipkin, Newmark, et al., 2006).

Although exposure to sunlight helps the body produce vitamin D, increased sun exposure is not recommended because it increases the risk for skin cancer (Health Canada, 2012). Many people (particularly those over 50) do not get enough vitamin D from food sources alone. Health Canada recommends that everyone between the ages of 9 and 70 take a daily 15-μg (600-IU) supplement of vitamin D (Health Canada, 2012). Sources include fortified cow and goat's milk, margarine, fruit and vegetable juices, cheeses, and yogurts. The only natural dietary sources of vitamin D include oily fish (salmon, mackerel) and egg yolks.

Treating Back Injuries

Although prevention is the key to keeping your back healthy, almost everyone will experience low-back pain at some point. Treatment usually involves the following:

- one to three days of bedrest on a firm mattress supported by plywood
- moderate application of heat and cold; a prolonged bath may relax a strained back, but make sure the water is not too hot (a warm bath with Epsom salts relaxes muscles)
- gentle massage until muscle spasms are eliminated or significantly reduced
- after recovery, daily exercises to strengthen the back and abdominal muscles

In the longer term, you are encouraged to do the following:

- Exercise aerobically for 30 minutes three or four times a week, working toward 30 minutes every day.
- Reduce abdominal fat by changing your dietary habits. Abdominal fat strains the lower back.
- Continue your daily back and abdominal exercises.

For patients with a new episode of low-back pain, prompt access to physiotherapy is cost- and time-effective. More than 70 percent of patients require only a single clinic visit, and less than 5 percent need to be referred to a specialist (Pinnington, Miller, & Stanley, 2004).

Surgery is rarely needed to correct low-back problems, but be sure to consult a physician for diagnosis and treatment in all cases of back pain. Do not take your back's health lightly.

Turn to **assignment 11.1** (in the appendix) to complete an assessment of your own back health.

KEY TERMS

arthritis, 261
degenerative disc disease (DDD), 255
fibromyalgia, 262
intervertebral discs, 255
osteoporosis, 257
repetitive strain injury (RSI), 263
sciatica, 264
vertebrae, 255

EXERCISES

True or False?

1. Back flexibility and strengthening exercises should be done daily to maintain a healthy back.
2. When lifting the 80-lb. (36-kg) bag in the PARE test, it is best to keep your knees straight and lift primarily with your arms to prevent back strain.
3. Sharp muscle pain in the back is an indication that you should stop the activity you are engaged in.
4. Numbness, tingling, or burning in your legs can be a symptom of a cervical injury.
5. Lumbago is a term used for low-back pain.

Multiple Choice

1. The solution for reducing muscular imbalances is to ________________ tight back muscles and ________________ weak abdominal muscles.
   a. strengthen, stretch
   b. strengthen, rest
   c. stretch, strengthen
   d. shorten, strengthen
   e. rest, exercise
2. Which of the following is true of posture?
   a. a rigid posture is desirable
   b. muscle weakness does not influence posture
   c. alignment of one body part may affect another
   d. good posture requires additional muscular effort
   e. poor posture has not been linked to any health problems
3. The most common health complaint in people under the age of 50 is
   a. headache
   b. neckache
   c. backache
   d. leg problems
   e. foot problems
4. Which of the following is recommended for lifting a heavy load?
   a. lift with the leg muscles
   b. push or pull an object instead of carrying it
   c. carry the load in one arm to keep the other arm free
   d. let the arm muscles do most of the work
   e. bend over the object with a straight back and lift up with your arms
5. What is least likely to lead to back problems?
   a. aging
   b. lack of strength
   c. poor flexibility
   d. poor coordination
   e. protruding abdomen
6. When directing traffic, what standing position should you avoid?
   a. back arched
   b. knees locked
   c. knees bent
   d. one foot forward
   e. back straight
7. The most common cause of low-back pain is
   a. a slipped disc
   b. a herniated disc
   c. weak back muscles and strong stomach muscles
   d. weak stomach muscles
   e. weak stomach muscles and lack of back flexibility

8. Which of the following factors can contribute to low-back pain or increase the risk for low-back pain?
   a. being between the ages of 50 and 64
   b. depression, apathy, inattentiveness, boredom, emotional upsets, and lack of focus when doing your job
   c. tight muscles due to stress
   d. all of the above put an individual at higher risk for low-back pain
   e. there are no known factors that contribute to back pain
9. Pain that radiates down the back of the leg is known as
   a. osteoarthritis
   b. sciatica
   c. osteoporosis
   d. fibromyalgia
   e. repetitive strain injury
10. Which statement is true of arthritis?
   a. it is a rare condition
   b. it includes a variety of joint problems
   c. flexibility makes arthritis worse
   d. it is typically better at night
   e. it is characterized by good range of motion of a joint
11. If you lift an object, you should
   a. bend forward from the waist
   b. bend to the side
   c. lift as heavy a weight as you can
   d. bend at the knees and hips
   e. pay someone to do it for you

Short Answer

1. Describe the functions of the spine.
2. Summarize the causes of low-back pain.
3. What is a herniated disc? What are some of the causes of this type of injury?
4. What is arthritis and what impact does it have on your joints?
5. What is an RSI? What are some of the symptoms associated with RSI?

6. What is osteoporosis and what can you do to prevent the disease?

7. What special risks to a healthy back do law enforcement officers' duties create?

8. Describe some techniques for preventing low-back pain.

9. How are back injuries treated?

REFERENCES

Anderson, G.S., Zutz, A., & Plecas, D.B. (2011). Police officer back health. *Journal of Criminal Justice Research*, *2*(1), 1–17.

Arthritis Society. (2011a). Arthritis in the workplace. Toronto: Author. http://www.arthritis.ca.

Arthritis Society. (2011b). Rheumatoid arthritis—Know your options. http://www.arthritis.ca/document.doc?id=87.

Bischoff-Ferrari, H.A., Dawson-Hughes, B., Willett, W.C., Staehelin, H.B., Bazemore, M.G., et al. (2004). Effect of vitamin D on falls: A meta-analysis. *Journal of the American Medical Association*, *291*, 1999–2006.

Bischoff-Ferrari, H.A., Dietrich, T., Orav, J., Hu, F.B., Zhang, Y., et al. (2004). Higher 25-hydroxyvitamin D concentrations are associated with better lower-extremity function in both active and inactive persons aged 60 years. *American Journal of Clinical Nutrition*, *80*, 752–758.

Bischoff-Ferrari, H.A., Willett, W.C., Wong, J.B., Giovannucci, E., Dietrich, T., et al. (2005). Fracture prevention with vitamin D supplementation: A meta-analysis of randomized control trials. *Journal of the American Medical Association*, *295*, 2257–2264.

Bonneau, A., Stevenson, J.M., & Gledhill, N. (2001). Back fitness and back health assessment considerations for the Canadian physical activity, fitness and lifestyle appraisal. *Canadian Journal of Applied Physiology*, *26*(3), 291–317.

Brown, J.J., Wells, G.A., Trottier, A.J., Bonneau, J., & Ferris, B. (1998). Back pain in a large Canadian police force. *Spine*, *23*, 821–827.

Burton, A.K., Tillotson, K.M., Symonds, T.L., Burke, C., & Mathewson, T. (1996). Occupational risk factors for the first-onset and subsequent course of low back trouble: A study of serving police officers. *Spine*, *21*(22), 2612–2620.

Canadian Physiotherapy Association. (2006). Back pain: "Oh, my aching back!" http://www.physiotherapy.ca/PublicUploads/222460BackPainInfo.pdf.

Fahey, T.D., Insel, P.M., & Walton, T.R. (1997). *Fit and well: Core concepts and labs in physical fitness and wellness* (2nd ed.). Mountain View, CA: Mayfield.

Garland, C.F., Garland, F.C., Gorham, E.D., Lipkin, M., Newmark, H., et al. (2006). The role of vitamin D in cancer prevention. *American Journal of Public Health, 96*, 252–261.

Greenberg, J.S., & Dintiman, G.B. (1997). *Wellness: Creating a life of health and fitness*. Needham Heights, MA: Allyn and Bacon.

Gyi, D.E., & Porter, J.M. (1998). Musculoskeletal problems and driving in police officers. *Occupational Medicine (London), 48*(3), 153–160.

Health Canada. (2005). Dietary reference intakes. http://www.hc-sc.gc.ca/fn-an/nutrition/reference/table/ref_elements_tbl-eng.php.

Health Canada. (2011, September 1). Eating well with Canada's food guide. http://www.hc-sc.gc.ca/fn-an/food-guide-aliment/index_e.html.

Health Canada. (2012, March 22). Vitamin D and calcium: Updated dietary reference intakes. http://www.hc-sc.gc.ca/fn-an/nutrition/vitamin/vita-d-eng.php.

Henneberg, E. (2006). Canadian research contributions are front and centre. IOF World Congress on Osteoporosis, Toronto 2006. *Osteoporosis Update, 10*(3).

Institute of Medicine (IOM). (1997). *Dietary reference intakes for calcium, phosphorus, magnesium, vitamin D, and fluoride*. Washington, DC: National Academy Press.

Kumar, S., & Narayan, Y. (2001). Low back pain among RCMP officers: An investigation into vehicles, duty belts, and boots. *Canadian Police Research Centre (CPRC) Technical Report*, September, 1999. TR-01-99.

Lis, A.M., Black, K.M., Korn, H., & Nordin, M. (2006). Association between sitting and occupational LBP. *European Spine Journal, 16*(2), 283–298.

Lorentzon, M., Mellstrom, D., Haug, E., & Ohlsson, C. (2007). Smoking is associated with lower peak bone mineral density mainly as a result of reduced cortical thickness in young adult men. *Journal of Clinical Endocrinology & Metabolism, 92*(2), 428–429.

Mack, T. (2002, February–March). Health news: Just sit right here. *Leisureways*. Oakville, ON: Formula.

Mills, K. (2006). Standards for bone mineral density testing. http://www.osteoporosis.ca.

Murphy, K.A., Spence, S.T., McIntosh, C.N., & Connor Gorber, S.K., for the Population Health Impact of Disease in Canada (PHI). (2006). *Health state descriptions for Canadians: Musculoskeletal diseases*. Catalogue no. 82-619-MIE2006003. Ottawa: Statistics Canada.

National Institute for Neurological Disorders and Stroke. (2003). Low-back pain fact sheet. http://www.ninds.nih.gov/disorders/backpain/detail_backpain.htm.

National Institutes of Health. (2003). What is osteoporosis? http://www.niams.nih.gov.

Osteoporosis Canada. (2007). What is osteoporosis? http://www.osteoporosis.ca.

Osteoporosis Canada. (2011a). Calculate my calcium. http://www.osteoporosis.ca/index.php/ci_id/5355/la_id/1.htm.

Osteoporosis Canada. (2011b). Facts and statistics. http://www.osteoporosis.ca/index.php/ci_id/8867/la_id/1.htm.

Pinnington, M.A., Miller, J., & Stanley, I. (2004). An evaluation of prompt access to physiotherapy in the management of low back pain in primary care. *Family Practice, 21*(4), 372–380.

Public Health Agency of Canada (PHAC). (2007). Trends and impact: The basis for investment decisions. Trends related to health spending and prevention strategies. http://www.phac-aspc.gc.ca/alw-vat/trends-tendances/index-eng.php.

Public Health Agency of Canada (PHAC). (2010). Economic burden of arthritis. In *Life with arthritis in Canada: A personal and public health challenge* (chapter 6). http://www.phac-aspc.gc.ca/cd-mc/arthritis-arthrite/lwaic-vaaac-10/8-eng.php#Cos.

Ranney, D. (1995). *Pain at work and what to do about it*. Waterloo, ON: Department of Kinesiology, University of Waterloo.

Tjepkema, M. (2003). Repetitive strain injury. Ministry of Industry. *Health Reports, 14*(4). Statistics Canada Catalogue no. 0040282-003-XIE. Ottawa: Statistics Canada.

Zhao, L.J., Liu, Y.J., Hamilton, J., Recker, R.R., & Deng, H.W. (2006). Interventions decreasing obesity risk tend to be beneficial for decreasing risk to osteoporosis: A challenge to the current dogma. *Osteoporosis International, 17*(Suppl. 2), S37 (Abstract P152SU).

12

Stress

LEARNING OBJECTIVES

After completing this chapter, you should be able to:

- Explain the differences among neutral, good, and bad stress.
- Describe the health effects of stress.
- Describe the kinds of stress that law enforcement personnel face.
- Explain what a critical incident is, how it can cause stress for law enforcement personnel, and how the stress should be handled.
- Explain what post-traumatic stress disorder is, how to recognize someone suffering from it, and what you can do to help an individual.
- Describe the characteristics of type A, type B, and type C personalities.
- Develop and implement stress management techniques.

OVERVIEW

Many officers view stress as a normal part of their career. Others, who have been on the service for 10 to 20 years, report feeling considerably more pressure than when they began working in law enforcement. Their stress levels continue to increase because, in spite of statistics indicating a general decline in violent crime in Canada since 1991, public perception, public scrutiny, and adverse media publicity suggest otherwise. Among the offences that have increased in recent years are homicides, sexual offences against children, and child pornography, including exploitation of children over the Internet (Statistics Canada, 2012).

Officers in the field today are at increased risk of contracting air- and blood-borne diseases such as tuberculosis and HIV/AIDS. Added to these stressors are the issues of dealing with ever-changing technology, cultural diversity, and the imperative of "political correctness." Family-related stresses can further affect job performance and concentration on the job.

Changing Roles in Law Enforcement and the Impact on Officers

Community policing has come to the forefront of the job in policing. Working directly with the community can provide job satisfaction and overall departmental efficiency. However, the transition to community policing has caused apprehension on the part of officers who must implement this fundamental shift in policing philosophy on a day-to-day basis. At times, the stress to perform to both service and community standards can be overwhelming.

Everyone lives with stress; it is an equal-opportunity destroyer, affecting people in all demographics. The World Health Organization has described stress as "a global epidemic" (WHO, 2003, p. 7). Stress itself is neither positive nor negative. How you handle or react to what you perceive as stress is what determines its effect on your life. This chapter examines what stress is; its causes, effects, and symptoms; and how it can be managed. More specifically, it looks at stress in law enforcement, with a special focus on critical incidents and post-traumatic stress disorder. We will also look at strategies for managing stress.

DID YOU KNOW?

In a 2010 survey, 27 percent of Canadian workers aged 20 to 64 described themselves as being "quite a bit" or "extremely" stressed on a regular basis. The identified causes of stress were work (62 percent), finances (12 percent), time (12 percent), family (8 percent), and personal/other (6 percent).

SOURCE: Crompton, 2011.

Defining Stress

stress
a "non-specific response of the body to any demands made upon it" (Selye, 1974)

Dr. Hans Selye (1974) was the first to define **stress**, which in his words is the "non-specific response of the body to any demands made upon it." Shafer (1996) explains stress as the arousal of the mind and body in response to demands made on them. Experts in the field of psycho-neuro-immunology (PNI) suggest that as much as 85 percent of all disease and illness—from the common cold to cancer—can be linked to stress (Kiecolt-Glaser, 1999; Seaward, 2005).

Stress is a reaction to a stimulus or demand that produces an elevated state of readiness or arousal. The greater the stimulus, the greater the stress reaction. Emergency personnel benefit from a moderate amount of stress arousal, which makes a person more alert to his or her surroundings and helps the individual respond to the stress.

The Types of Stress

There are three types of stress:

1. *Neutral stress (neustress)* With this kind of stress, the mind and body are aroused but the stress is neither harmful nor helpful (Morse & Furst, 1979). An example is observing that traffic is slowing down in front of you.
2. *Good stress (eustress)* This kind of stress is caused by the factors that initiate emotional and psychological growth. Eustress provides pleasure, adds meaning to life, and fosters an attitude that tries to find positive solutions to problems. It encourages optimal performance and can improve health. An example is competing with classmates to win a race.
3. *Bad stress (distress)* This kind of stress results in negative responses both in a person's career and in life. Unchecked negative stress can interfere with the physiological and psychological functioning of the body and may ultimately give rise to a hypokinetic disease or disability (Selye, 1974). Examples are being faced with a physical challenge you cannot accomplish (such as performing a run within a certain time) or not having enough money to pay for next month's rent.

Turn to **assignment 12.1** (in the appendix) to fill out a life experience survey.

The Stress Response

Hans Selye concluded that the body reacts to good and bad stress in the same way. He labelled the stress response—the body's reaction to stress—the **general adaptation syndrome (GAS)**. It includes three stages: the fight-or-flight response, the stage of resistance, and the stage of exhaustion (Selye, 1956).

general adaptation syndrome (GAS)
the body's reaction to stress

The *fight-or-flight response* (or alarm stage) is the stage when the body prepares itself to cope with a stressor. The response is a warning signal that a stressor is present (whether real or imagined). This is a primitive survival mechanism that is rarely triggered today. As the body prepares for fight or flight, powerful stress hormones and steroids are pumped into the bloodstream, senses become more acute, muscles tense, digestion ceases, breathing and blood pressure rates increase, and there is an urge to empty the bladder or bowels. If the stressor is only imagined, over time we suffer the ill effects of chronic arousal, leading to excessive wear and tear on the body. So, we need to avoid those triggers that elicit the stress response.

In the *stage of resistance*, the body actively resists and attempts to cope with the stressor. If you are able to channel that energy, your body returns to normal. However, being aroused for too long and too often may lead to fatigue. Headaches, forgetfulness, constipation, diarrhea, asthma, anxiety attacks, and high blood pressure are all signs of prolonged arousal.

The *stage of exhaustion* can result in illness and, ultimately, death. During this phase, the body is subjected to repeated stress response breakdowns. If you are healthy enough, you will succeed in resisting stress. However, if the body cannot cope, disease and malfunction of organ systems result. For example, chronic high blood pressure can lead to kidney and heart disease, which can result in premature death.

The Effects of Stress

Most people look after their cars better than their bodies. While they may watch what they put in their gas tanks, they have little regard for what they eat. Under stress, most people tend to lose their appetite; they eat less, eat irregularly, and eat poorer-quality food. This usually means a decrease in energy intake to levels too low to sustain normal activities, let alone cope with stressful situations.

Stress combined with poor eating habits can wear your body down. Stress can have short- or long-term effects on your body. When your body responds negatively to stress, such responses often manifest as **psychosomatic symptoms** (physical symptoms resulting from mental conflict).

psychosomatic symptoms
physical symptoms resulting from mental conflict

Turn to **assignment 12.2** (in the appendix) to take a test to determine whether you recognize stress in your life and your level of fitness in managing stress.

Next, let's look at some of the short- and long-term effects of stress and their physical consequences.

Short-Term Effects of Stress

Short-term effects are seen soon after stress is experienced and can be corrected with proper stress management. The effects are as follows:

- less energy and more fatigue (a result of lower blood sugar levels)
- paleness
- slowing down of bodily functions, such as digestion and wound healing (a result of loss of important minerals and reduced absorption of nutrients from food)
- higher blood pressure and heart rate
- loss of appetite and decreased taste for food
- depression
- more susceptibility to infections
- impairment in performance of job- or family-related responsibilities

Under these conditions, some people resort to artificial means to regain normal function. They consume over-the-counter stimulants or caffeine to remain alert and large doses of vitamins to replace depleted resources. They also resort to concoctions such as condensed-liquid vitamin supplements and "power bars." But these simply put additional stress on the body. Caffeine, for example, increases irritability, interferes with sleep, and, by destroying stomach enzymes, weakens the stomach lining. If left untreated, these short-term effects will slowly or quickly wear away at your physical and mental health, with serious ramifications.

Long-Term Effects of Stress

The possible long-term effects of stress include:

- nervous stomach and stomach aches
- constipation or diarrhea
- ulcers
- inflammation of the digestive system
- indigestion

- headaches
- high blood pressure
- allergic reactions such as asthma, eczema, and hives
- an inability to function under normal circumstances, including loss of concentration and an inability to focus

Chronic Exposure to Stress

Without proper stress management, constant or chronic exposure to stress—sometimes bottled up over several years—can lead to long-term or continual effects, such as:

- elevation of heart rate and blood pressure
- weakening of the immune system
- inflammation of the stomach lining
- allergic reactions such as hives, hay fever, asthma, and congested breathing
- muscle-tension and migraine headaches
- muscle stiffness, aches, cramps, and backaches
- hypokinetic diseases (diseases brought on by partial or complete lack of physical activity, including cardiovascular and digestive diseases, diabetes, excess fat, and lower-back pain)

Emotional Effects of Chronic Stress

Chronic stress can also have emotional consequences, including:

- depression, leading to an inability to function normally at work and at home
- cynicism and suspiciousness
- emotional detachment from daily life
- excessive aggressiveness (which may trigger citizen complaints)
- marital or family problems
- alcoholism and other substance abuse
- suicide

Stressors

A **stressor** is any physical, psychological, or environmental event or condition that initiates the stress response. However, what is stressful for one person may not be stressful for another. Also, what is stressful for someone at a certain time may not be stressful for that same person at another time.

stressor
any physical, psychological, or environmental event or condition that initiates the stress response

Stressors in Daily Life

Some common stressors in daily life include:

- changes and transitions (marriage, separation, divorce, death of a loved one, moving, job change or loss, going to school away from home or for the first time in a number of years)
- relationships (continued conflicts, lack of support)

- lifestyle (inconsistent with values, too committed to a particular lifestyle)
- money problems (economic recession, credit card debt, financial losses)
- loss of self-esteem (falling behind academically or professionally, failing to meet personal standards and goals or others' expectations)
- fatigue or illness (poor diet, lack of sleep, lack of exercise)
- attempting to juggle family, academic, and career demands

Unresolved stress can sometimes lead to suicide. In Canada, suicide is the second highest cause of death for youths aged 10–24, following motor vehicle collisions. Each year, on average, 294 youths die from suicide, while more attempt it (Statistics Canada, 2011). Aboriginal teens and gay and lesbian teens may be at particularly high risk, depending on the community in which they live, family support, and their own self-esteem. Although suicidal youth give signs of distress, the warning signs may be few or unclear. To learn more about this topic, see the Canadian Children's Rights Council (2012) (in References).

Stressors in Law Enforcement

Finn (1997) identified five main categories of stress in law enforcement:

1. *Problems in the officer's personal life* The divorce rate for officers is five times that of the general population. Some officers' significant others must assume the role of both parents, rearrange their agendas to fit duty schedules (especially in specialized units), or simply learn to function independently. This can sometimes result in a breakdown in communication. Family members may be affected by an officer's passive coolness or anger from the stress of his or her exposure to conflict, causing them to feel alienated or frightened. An officer's children may react to concerns over their parent's safety with nightmares, regressive behaviour, lack of emotion, anxiety, and aggressive and inappropriate outbursts.
2. *Pressure of law enforcement work* This stress is produced by real threats and dangers, such as entering a dark and unfamiliar building, responding to a weapons call, pursuing lawbreakers at high speeds, or responding to a prison inmate disturbance. It also is influenced by the need to keep current with technology as well as the workload (a shortage of personnel can affect the workload of individuals). For those in isolated communities, time spent away from family and boredom may also cause stress. For others, personal beliefs may conflict with the reality of their job. High standards may conflict with the demands of getting the job done. Some officers have a strong need to be in control, to do something exciting, and to help and rescue others, and these issues may conflict with the performance of more mundane day-to-day responsibilities.
3. *Organizational stress* The paramilitary nature of public (and some private) policing and corrections work has particular stressors. Examples include constant adjustment to changing schedules, working at odd hours, work overload, uncertainty about job requirements, and complying with detailed rules and procedures.

4. *Stress caused by public attitudes toward police work and officers* Expectations of the general public—and even of other police—can produce tensions in community policing, such as when an officer's gender or race is not accepted. Difficulties "fitting in," perceptions of bias, and social isolation can all lead to stress.
5. *Operational stress* This is produced by the realities of modern policing, such as understaffing, constantly having to adopt a "band-aid" approach to problems, lack of equipment, and dealing with criminals, homeless people, and people in distress. It also has to do with police bureaucracy and the feeling of not being supported by one's bosses. Other stress-creating situations include being lied to often, being required to put oneself in dangerous situations to protect the public, the seeming injustice of some of our laws, and the constant awareness that one may be held legally liable for one's actions. In addition, there are issues around promotional opportunities, lack of support, poor communication, and top-down decisions made by high-ranking police administrators.

Stressors from Workplace Health and Safety Hazards

Police officers encounter many occupational health and safety risks on a daily basis or at some point in their career. These are grouped into five categories (Parsons, 2004):

1. *Physical hazards*, such as a criminal with a (visible) weapon, or the possibility of (invisible) radiation. Ellis and colleagues (1993) found that police officers were at greatest risk for assault when arresting and transporting suspects and prisoners. One Canadian study indicated that police officers are at greatest risk for loss of work time due to violence (Boyd, 1995).
2. *Chemical hazards*, including furnace fumes, car exhaust, or, in a situation like 9/11, clouds of carcinogens. There has been some research around exposure to radio frequencies, the use of police traffic radar, and sunshine being linked to cancer, including testicular, cervical, colon, and skin cancer (melanoma) (Van Netten, Brands, Hoption Cann, Spinelli, & Sheps, 2003).
3. *Biological hazards*, including micro-organisms in the air or communicable diseases like HIV/AIDS, tuberculosis, and hepatitis A, B, or C.
4. *Ergonomic hazards*, including injuries to the musculoskeletal system from uncomfortable working positions, heavy physical tasks, or altercations with and handcuffing of suspects. A study of RCMP officers found the main source of back problems to be seatbelt use and riding in a patrol car all day (Brown, Wells, Trottier, Bonneau, & Ferris, 1998; Czarnecki & Janowitz, 2003); however, other research took issue with vibrations (such as from motorcycles), wearing body armour, and working on a computer terminal in a confined space (such as car computers) (Gyi & Porter, 1998).
5. *Psycho-social hazards*, including difficulties with supervisors or fellow workers, sexual harassment, discrimination, or dealing with issues like suicide. One study found that after dealing with lying, cheating, and hostile people on the street, officers can start mistrusting friends and even family, or develop a negative attitude toward their work (Kohan & O'Connor, 2002). Police suicides can result from the stressful nature of

law enforcement work in terms of overload shiftwork and exposure to violent and life-threatening situations. Departmental politics, inadequate resources to do the job, and lack of support and recognition from management also increase the stressful nature of police work (Loo, 2003).

These are just some of the stressors that may affect your future work in law enforcement. Remember that some individuals perceive particular stressors as positive, while others perceive the same stressors as negative. As a result, the impact of particular stressors varies from person to person.

Critical Incidents

critical incident
a situation faced by police and other emergency service personnel that causes them to experience unusually strong emotional reactions that have the potential to interfere with their ability to function at the scene (current stress) or later (residual stress)

A **critical incident** is a situation faced by police and other emergency services personnel that causes unusually strong emotional reactions, which may interfere with their ability to function at the scene (current stress) or later (residual stress). Critical incidents are sudden and unexpected; disrupt one's sense of control; disrupt beliefs and values, as well as assumptions about the world in which we live, the people in it, and the work we do; involve the perception of a life-damaging threat; and may involve emotional or physical loss. How a given person will react to a particular event on a particular day cannot be predicted. For officers who are used to being in control of their emotions and their surroundings (type A personality), the debilitation caused by a critical incident may be surprising, embarrassing, frustrating, or overwhelming.

Most officers recover from critical incident stress and remain healthy and productive. But symptoms that last for more than four weeks may indicate a much more serious problem. The intensity of such an experience takes time to subside. If vivid "flashbacks" or nightmares haunt you, make you feel emotionally numb or overwhelmed, and you are losing sleep, it is possible that you are suffering from post-traumatic stress disorder (PTSD) (see below).

This trauma is stress run amok. Typically, stress deregulates the nervous system for a short period of time; within days or weeks, we return to equilibrium as the nervous system calms down. But when we are severely traumatized, the residual effects compromise our lives, relationships, and overall ability to function.

Types of Critical Incidents

Law enforcement personnel are often faced with critical incidents related to life and death. The following are some examples and the kinds of feelings they cause:

- *Death/injury/shooting in the line of duty* The myth of invulnerability is shattered.
- *Suicide of a co-worker* Job and personal life pressures, and the pressure of balancing the two, come into focus. Colleagues also experience guilt over not being there to help.
- *Death of a child* The innocence represented by children can have a profound impact on officers, sometimes pushing them over the edge. Officers may feel that what they stand for is useless. Should an officer have a family of his or her own, factors of identification can add even more stress.

- *Prolonged but failed rescue attempt* If the officer has come to know the victim, the officer may exhibit symptoms of stress arising from a deep sense of personal failure.
- *Mass-casualty incidents* Incidents involving carnage or mass fatalities—such as the attack on New York City's World Trade Center in September 2001, the Hurricane Katrina disaster in 2005, the 2005 murder of four RCMP officers in Mayerthorpe, Alberta, the 2010 earthquake in Haiti, or the 2011 earthquake, tsunami, and ensuing nuclear meltdowns in Japan—can compromise an officer's ability to cope. This reaction may be intensified when compounded by mass confusion and shortages of staff and resources.
- *Officer's safety is unusually jeopardized* Daily exposure to potential danger, combined with a specific situation in which an officer becomes unusually vulnerable and lacks control, can trigger a stress reaction. An example is the York Regional Police officer who died during a routine traffic stop in 2011.
- *Responding officer knows the victim* Arriving on the scene and discovering that you know the victim can trigger a critical stress reaction of the "if only I had driven faster" variety.
- *Officer responding to an abused individual* Officers must respond to incidents involving serious physical assault, including sexual assault, incest, molestation, and gang assaults that go beyond comprehension of human decency.
- *Events with excessive media coverage* In addition to dealing with the situation, officers must deal with crowd control and onlookers' morbid interest in seeing what has happened.

Factors Affecting Responses to Critical Incidents

Some officers are better able than others to cope with the stress of critical incidents. The following are some factors that affect coping (Connor & Butterfield, 2003):

- *Nature of the event* Has the officer witnessed this type of incident before? How severe is the incident?
- *Degree of warning* Was the officer dispatched to the scene with an appropriate warning, or did the officer happen upon the scene?
- *Ego strength/coping style* Does the officer cope with tragic situations more easily than others do by accepting those situations as "fate"?
- *Prior mastery of the experience* How many times has the officer been exposed to a similar situation?
- *Proximity* How close does the officer feel to the person or incident? For example, if a child is involved, has the officer a child of the same age?
- *The amount of stress in the officer's life at the time* Is there already a great deal of stress in the officer's life, either at work or at home? If so, the incident may have a stronger impact.
- *The nature and degree of social support available to the officer after the critical incident* The more support an officer receives, the better are his or her chances of coping with the stress of a critical incident. The reactions of those supporting the officer may or may not be appropriate, and thus may further affect the individual.

Symptoms of Stress Arising out of Critical Incidents

Critical incidents can be overwhelming. We have to remember that the personnel who respond to them are human. Each officer will respond differently, and what may be easy to cope with one day is impossible to cope with the next. Most people are resilient enough to move through an incident, while others will never be the same. We have to be sensitive to the pressures faced by people who confront extreme situations every day. Recognizing the symptoms of stress can allow us to help them. Developing symptoms is never a sign of weakness. Symptoms should be taken seriously.

For some, symptoms can be overwhelming to every part of their being. For others, the effect takes weeks, months, or possibly years to be totally felt. These overwhelming responses to stress can result in **post-traumatic stress disorder (PTSD)**. This disorder changes the way the body responds to stress, probably as a result of chemical imbalances that increase the levels of stress hormones and alter the reactions of the nervous system. For example, trauma victims may have recurring images of the critical incident and respond in a distressful way to similar situations.

post-traumatic stress disorder (PTSD) disorder that changes the way the body responds to stress, probably as a result of chemical imbalances that increase the levels of stress hormones and alter the reaction of the nervous system

The symptoms of stress exhibited after a critical incident can be divided into four kinds: physical, cognitive, emotional, and behavioural (American Psychiatric Association, 2000, pp. 429–484).

1. *Physical symptoms*
   - aches, pains, muscle tension, trembling, and poor coordination
   - jumpiness and being startled by sudden sounds or movements
   - cold sweats, dry mouth, pale skin, and difficulty focusing the eyes
   - feeling out of breath, hyperventilating until the fingers and toes cramp or go numb
   - upset stomach, vomiting, diarrhea, constipation, and frequent urination
   - chronic fatigue and pain—every movement requires a great deal of effort
   - a distant, haunted, faraway stare
   - substance abuse
   - sexual dysfunction
   - insomnia
2. *Cognitive symptoms*
   - difficulty making decisions
   - confusion
   - detachment and withdrawal
   - disorientation
   - poor concentration and loss of interest in activities
   - memory loss, especially with respect to recent events or the trauma itself
   - inability to perform multiple tasks
   - flashbacks (visual or auditory)
   - daydreams, nightmares, and bad dreams
   - avoidance of reminders of the event

- contemplation of suicide
- compulsive behavioural patterns
- symptoms of attention deficit hyperactivity disorder (ADHD)

3. *Emotional symptoms*
   - grief, including spontaneous crying
   - numbness
   - guilt
   - feelings of hopelessness and being overwhelmed
   - depression, extended periods of sadness
   - anxiety, fear, and edginess
   - panic attacks
   - self-doubt
   - irritability, anger, and resentment
   - hyper-startled responses
   - feeling detached from reality
   - vigilance to the point of paranoia
   - intrusive thoughts
   - flashbacks or nightmares
   - sudden floods of emotions or images related to the initial event
   - a loss of previously sustained beliefs
4. *Behavioural symptoms*
   - decreased job performance and increased absenteeism
   - detachment and increased isolation from friends, colleagues, and family
   - increased premature departure from work or social gatherings
   - outbursts of laughter or tears
   - changes in normal humour patterns
   - excessive talkativeness or silence
   - low morale
   - hostile tone of voice
   - destructive changes in relationships with family, friends, and colleagues
   - hypervigilance, jumpiness, or an extreme sense of being "on guard"
   - curling up and rocking continuously
   - body tremors, hand-wringing, and facial tics
   - running without purpose
   - substance abuse
   - acting like an adolescent and taking up reckless, sometimes life-threatening hobbies
   - avoidance of situations that resemble the initial event
   - obsession with death

FACTS ABOUT . . .

Debriefing

- People with high levels of disaster exposure are 3.1 times more likely to attend a debriefing than those with low levels of exposure.
- Females are 2.7 times more likely to attend a debriefing than males.
- Those with previous disaster experience are 2.7 times more likely to attend a debriefing than those without prior experience.
- Older subjects are more likely than young subjects to talk about the critical incident with their spouse/significant other, a co-worker, or another person.
- People with higher education are more likely than those with lower education to talk about the critical incident with their spouse/significant other, co-worker, or another person.

SOURCE: Fullerton, Ursano, Vance, & Wang, 2000.

Helping a Colleague Cope with a Critical Incident

The police subculture holds on to many myths that can lessen an officer's ability to cope with the aftermath of a critical incident. An officer's recovery can be hampered by beliefs such as "If you can't deal with it, you need to find a new line of work" and "Officers should keep their problems to themselves." Attempting to deny their reactions to stress can cause officers to suffer in silence and not seek help, and in some instances to disrupt their lives and the lives of their families. It is important that officers cope with their stress and come to terms with stressful incidents. It is also important for colleagues to help officers cope with the stress of critical incidents.

The process of debriefing officers has advanced in the last 20 years. Debriefing involves the provision of assistance by a qualified mental health professional to officers who have been involved in a traumatic incident. Although many police services take officers who have been involved in traumatic incidents off duty to deal with the situation, depending on staffing issues, the process may be delayed for up to 72 hours. Debriefing is intended to help alleviate the trauma felt by the officers and to help speed up the recovery process. The point is not to deal with blame or the cause of the incident, but rather its emotional and psychological consequences, such as guilt, sadness, or anger. This is no substitute for therapy. Whether debriefing is done in an individual or platoon setting, it is important that supervisors ensure it is done in a timely fashion (Everly & Mitchell, 2000).

In addition to debriefing, awareness of the initial psychological and physiological responses to traumatic events may also be reassuring when adverse responses occur. Such education can more readily identify individuals who are at risk and provide earlier intervention (Ghahramanlou & Broadbeck, 2000; Figley, 1995). This approach isn't perfect, however. According to the Ontario Ombudsman's report, *In the Line of Duty* (Marin, 2012), police services are far from providing what current and former officers and their families need today to deal with operational stress injuries and prevent suicide. Time will tell whether police services can implement these initiatives.

Here are some ways you can help others when you see that they are suffering the effects of stress after a critical incident:

1. *Manage the situation*
   - Maintain a calm and reassuring presence.
   - Remove the officer from the scene as soon as possible.
   - Facilitate the officer's understanding of the situation. Encourage him or her to talk. Let the officer tell and retell the story. Asking, "Are you okay with this?" is better than saying nothing.
   - Encourage the officer to talk about his or her feelings. Acknowledge that reactions of grief and fear are normal. Let the person know that you are there and that you care.
   - Normalize the officer's reactions as much as possible. Reassure the officer that his or her symptoms are not unusual.

2. *Mobilize support*
   - Assess the social, familial, and community resources and supports available. Help the officer notify family members that he or she is safe. Encourage the officer's family and friends to listen to his or her story. Encourage family and friends to share their feelings.
   - Give the officer plenty of fluids (but no alcohol or caffeine).
   - Encourage the officer to engage in physical activity as soon as he or she is able.
   - Provide phone numbers or help the officer access employee assistance programs, chaplaincy services, and family counselling.
   - If the officer experiences chest pain, hyperventilates, has an elevated heart rate, or exhibits other serious physical symptoms, have him or her seek immediate medical attention.
3. *Follow up*
   - Keep the officer informed about the facts surrounding the incident and any ongoing investigations.
   - Check back with the officer to see how he or she is coping and whether available resources and supports are being used. Encourage others to check as well.
   - Offer to support the officer at court hearings, community meetings, meetings with insurance companies—any event that directly relates to the trauma.
   - If necessary, initiate referrals for outside agencies or participation in counselling (including family) and psychotherapy.
   - Post-traumatic stress disorder may actually alter the way the brain functions. Serotonin, a chemical in the brain, is drastically affected by stress. Encouraging the officer to seek medical intervention may be necessary.

Research (Brown, 2003) indicates that officers should be followed up for at least two years after a critical incident, because the individual often does not recognize the symptoms of stress. For many, the symptoms generally subside and normal function gradually returns. For some, symptoms may appear to be gone, but can surface again in another stressful situation.

Do *not* do the following:

- Second-guess the officer.
- Say, "I understand how you feel." (You may think you do, but to a victim, his or her pain is unique.)
- Say, "Everything is going to be fine." Acknowledge that things may never be the same but they will get better over time.
- Try to protect the officer by withholding information (but use your judgment in this regard, and seek legal advice if necessary).

FYI

Police Suicide

Twice as many police officers die by their own hand as do in the line of duty. Suicide among police officers occurs at a rate of almost twice that of the general population. Officers going through a divorce are five times more likely to commit suicide, and if they are in serious trouble on the job, suspended, or facing termination, they are seven times more likely to commit suicide.

According to 2008 statistics, officers between the ages of 35 and 39 years old were at the highest risk of suicide during that year, as were officers with 10–14 years in law enforcement. Of greater concern was the finding that police work provides a fertile ground for suicide-precipitating factors, including relationship problems, culturally approved alcohol use, and maladaptive coping mechanisms. In addition, the availability of firearms and exposure to psychologically adverse incidents may contribute to this causal chain of suicide.

SOURCE: Goldfarb, 1999; O'Hara & Violanti, 2009.

- Say things like, "It could have been worse," "You can always get another (pet, house, car)," "It's best if you just stay busy," and "You need to get on with your life."
- Say, "When this happened to me ..." Even if you had an identical experience, the victim's need to talk about his or her own trauma is probably greater than the need to listen to another person's experience.
- Give too much advice.
- Make promises and not come through.

Some officers will find that moving on to another career is appropriate, but law enforcement is as much of a calling as medicine or the clergy, as suggested by the large number of students who have known since they were five or six years old that all they ever wanted to be was a police officer. Make sure you have exhausted all methods of support before letting someone—possibly yourself—make such a monumental decision.

If you are helping a child through a critical incident, here are some additional points to consider:

- Answer questions honestly but without frightening details.
- Don't be afraid to admit that you don't have all the answers.
- Allow the child to express his or her feelings so that you have a starting point for talking about the situation.

Developing Critical Incident Survival Skills

It is important to prepare for and deal with critical incident stress before, during, and after an event. The more prepared you are for stress, the better you may deal with it.

In the case of a short-term event, you can do the following:

- Prepare for emergencies by training and drilling.
- Prepare and maintain equipment.
- Gather information before deployment.
- Update information frequently.
- Follow legitimate directions of knowledgeable leaders.
- Take rest breaks and nourishment.
- Do not take on personal blame for tragedies that befall others.
- Maintain a positive attitude.

After the event:

- Ensure that your equipment is ready for the next call.
- Avoid alcohol, as it worsens stress reactions.
- Eat nutritious foods and get plenty of fluids.
- Avoid or limit caffeine intake.
- Exercise to reduce stress reactions.
- Participate in operational reviews.
- Talk about the incident with trusted friends, colleagues, or leaders.

In the case of a prolonged event:

- Orient crews to the time every 20 minutes. Time awareness reduces fatigue, mistakes, and injuries.
- Let emergency crews know approximately how long they will work, and provide the objectives of their mission.
- Rotate crews when possible. A rule of thumb is to provide 30 minutes of rest for every two hours of work.
- Take more frequent breaks in extremely hot or cold conditions.
- Take more frequent breaks if encountering extremely stressful stimuli.
- When dealing with a critical incident, four 12-hour shifts should be the maximum, because fatigue and injuries are a major risk to individuals.
- Avoid or limit caffeine (coffee, tea, chocolate).
- Avoid fatty foods, salt, white bread, and soft drinks (sugary products). Water is better.
- Avoid alcohol for at least three days after a traumatic experience.
- Do not use salt tablets, as they irritate the stomach.

Additional Stress in Your Teens into Adulthood

As you prepare for your career in law enforcement, you too may be faced with additional stress while you gain experience through education, volunteering, and everyday life. Teen stress is similar to adult stress in terms of signs and symptoms. However, adolescents have unique stressors that they face, such as the following:

- physical changes, including an increase in weight and height, menarche (onset of menstruation), and pubertal changes
- mental changes, including issues with independence, sexual attraction, aggressive behaviour, and exposure to experimenting with new things (such as substance abuse)
- emotional issues, which include changing relationships with peers, responsibilities to family, academic demands, financial issues, separation or divorce of parents, romantic relationships, and getting along with siblings and other family members

Behavioural Types

Why do different people respond differently to stress? The theory of behavioural types offers some answers.

Type A Behaviour

First identified in the late 1950s by Drs. Meyer Friedman and Ray Rosenman (1994), type A behaviour describes a person who is competitive, impatient, and a polyphasic thinker (thinks of two or more things at once). A type A personality also experiences an intense sense of urgency, is aggressive and frequently hostile, is intensely driven toward achievement but frequently lacks properly defined goals, and is unable to concentrate on work because distracting thoughts intrude.

Type A personalities are likely to be highly stressed. Recent research indicates that people who are hostile, cynical, and angry a great deal of the time face a higher risk of heart disease, atherosclerosis, and hypertension (Myrtek, 2001). They are very competitive and tend to be tense and agitated when it comes to work. They have poor impulse control and always need to be active. Type A personalities have a mixture of right- and left-brain dominance. They express their anger with verbal outbursts, and experience negative emotions. They like to have control over everything, so they tend to be leaders. In addition, they often react in a hostile manner when criticized, and they tend to be risk takers. Many law enforcement officers are type A personalities.

Type B Behaviour

In type B behaviour, a person takes things one at a time; concentrates effectively; is flexible, unaggressive, and patient; and does not get upset if daily tasks are not completed. A type B personality takes life as it comes, living in the "here and now"; does not get extremely upset at failing to achieve a goal; usually sets more realistic goals than a type A person; makes time for activities such as exercise, hobbies, and seeing friends; and handles stressful situations more effectively. Type B personalities are intuitive and spontaneous. They are right-brained dominant and non-judgmental. They are open to criticism and use humour to make their point. When they are angry, their anger is directed at the problem, not the person. They support others, are adaptable and flexible, express positive feelings, and generally believe that everyone can get along.

Type C Behaviour

Some people who resemble type A personalities may actually use their type A behaviours to resist stress. These hardy people have been characterized as type C (Kobasa, 1982). They are able to channel their energies into creative endeavours or physical fitness without suffering the effects of high stress. Type C personalities take as much time as they need and want; they are future-oriented. They like to weigh pros and cons before making a decision. They tend to be left-brain dominant and more patient than type A personalities. They analyze and try to figure out what to expect. Type C personalities, however, can be more sensitive to criticism. Thus, they can be resentful and more likely to give the "silent treatment" to a person with whom they are angry. Overall, they have a higher risk of cancer, and have a tendency to be inflexible.

Go to **assignment 12.3** (in the appendix) and assess your behavioural type. After you have done the survey, answer the questions.

Coping with Stress

Police officers tend to believe that the emotions and stress reactions arising from critical incidents must be hidden. But this way of coping with stress is unhealthy. Once we recognize that we are under stress, we find that the skills to cope with that stress are right at our fingertips. Many stress management programs now include cognitive aspects (for example, time management, social engineering), but few address the spiritual issues of stress: values, relationships, and even the purpose of life.

Here are some strategies for coping with stress:

1. Exercise—aerobic exercise releases chemical compounds in the body, called endorphins, that combat stress.
   - Exercise lowers blood pressure and improves sleep. It can lower weight and cholesterol levels as well.
   - Exercise can reduce the potential for injury during emergency situations and the severity of injuries if they occur.
2. Make better nutritional decisions to keep your body healthy and fight infections.
   - Eat a balanced diet of fresh food including fruits, vegetables, and grains, as set out in *Eating Well with Canada's Food Guide* (Health Canada, 2012).
   - Drink plenty of water every day (at least eight glasses).
   - Avoid overeating.
   - Decrease your intake of artificial sweeteners.
   - Limit your salt intake to prevent hypertension.
   - Limit your caffeine intake.
3. Avoid alcohol and drug abuse (including cigarette smoking, as nicotine depletes vitamins C and E and thus increases your vulnerability to stress-related diseases).
4. Manage self-talk (how you perceive and express yourself).
   - Reframe your point of view and accentuate the positive.
   - Stress is a challenge. Learn to control and overcome it.
   - Perceive adverse situations as opportunities rather than setbacks.
   - Emotions should serve us, not dominate us. Self-blame and guilt distort reality. Do not jump to conclusions. Think clearly and review facts.
   - Stop blaming others.
   - See adverse situations as temporarily bearable. Categorize, remember, visualize, and anticipate situations. Then you can make decisions about what to do.
   - Take things less seriously. Find humour where you can every day. Sometimes it is present even in difficult situations. Learn to laugh at yourself.
5. Manage your actions.
   - Decide which battles are worth fighting. Don't stress over issues that are relatively unimportant. Learn to take a stand, or learn to decline—and stick by it.
   - Be assertive.
   - Learn to listen to people.
   - Use more appropriate communication styles.

6. Use appropriate time-management skills.
   - Balance work and play; set aside time for recreational activities. Do not try to cram 80 years of life experience into 20 years.
   - Set aside time for idleness each day (without guilt).
   - Set realistic goals.
7. Develop a support group.
   - Learn to ask for help. Call a friend.
   - Communicate with trusted people. Contact can lower tension and help you think more clearly to make decisions.
   - Spend quality time with family and friends who have a positive outlook on life.
   - Develop satisfying relationships.
   - Have friends who do not do emergency work. People outside of the job can offer support, a different perspective, security, nourishment, and new energy.
8. Control physical stress responses. Biofeedback, meditation, and self-hypnosis are excellent stress reduction tools, but they require some training.
   - Use breathing exercises.
   - Use muscle relaxation and visual imagery exercises.
   - Use yoga.
9. Remember to take the time to laugh at yourself.
10. Resolve issues of anger and fear.
11. Engage in hobbies like drawing, writing, singing, or playing with pets.
12. Watch stress-relieving programs such as comedies or cartoons.

Relaxation Techniques

Let's look at how stress responses can be controlled by relaxation techniques. To benefit from these techniques, you must prepare by not drinking caffeinated beverages, eating, or smoking for at least an hour beforehand, and by not exercising for at least two hours beforehand.

Breathing

Breathing is affected by the stress response. When you are stressed, your breathing becomes more rapid and shallow, and your heart rate increases. To elicit a relaxation response, you must slow down your breathing and learn to take deeper breaths. By breathing correctly, you will oxygenate your blood more efficiently, and this will trigger the parasympathetic "quieting response" (a sense of control over the body and its reactions to stressors).

Try the following breathing exercise:

1. Monitor your heart rate for 15 seconds and then multiply by 4 to obtain beats per minute.

2. Sit up straight with your spine against a chair back.
3. Put your left hand over your chest and your right hand over your abdomen.
4. Breathe normally. You will probably notice that your chest expands more than your abdomen.
5. Now practise a new way of breathing by briefly holding in your breath and then slowly releasing the air. To do this most effectively, breathe through your nose. When you take a deep breath, you should feel your diaphragm (the muscle that separates the thoracic cavity from the abdominal cavity) push down and your abdomen expand outward as you get oxygen into the lower third of the lungs.
6. Continue to breathe slowly for about five minutes while attempting to relax and slow your breathing. At the end of five minutes, you should feel relaxed and be able to resume normal activities.
7. Monitor your heart rate again. If you are more relaxed, your heart rate should be lower than when you started.

Diaphragmatic breathing is a skill that takes practice. Once you become familiar with the technique, you will be able to do it almost anywhere you are, at any time.

Meditation

Meditation can involve focusing the mind, and thereby quieting the body, by sitting or lying down comfortably and quietly with eyes closed for 10–20 minutes once or twice a day. It does not involve thinking, though you will probably find that turning off thoughts is almost impossible. Rather than fight your thoughts, simply try not to get caught up in them. Some people find that listening to the sound of the wind or ocean waves helps them to quiet their thinking. Ideally, you should not fall asleep when you meditate, although this may happen if you are extremely tired.

Meditation methods include the following:

- Mindful meditation is simply noting internal thoughts and bodily processes, such as your breathing (Kabat-Zinn, 1991).
- Transcendental meditation involves inducing a meditative state twice a day by closing your eyes and repeating a mantra (a sound without meaning).
- Zen meditation focuses on breathing.
- Benson's (1975) meditation technique for relaxation involves focusing on a word or phrase associated with your beliefs. The idea is to turn to your inner self to find harmony.

Autogenic Feedback

Through passive suggestion, you practise focusing on the heaviness, warmth, and relaxed state of your muscles. The following is an autogenic (self-generated) feedback exercise. Begin by lying or sitting in a comfortable position, and say each phrase to yourself slowly and distinctly several times. All four stages in this exercise can be completed in five minutes, or you can take as long as you want.

STAGE 1	• "My legs feel heavy." • "My arms feel heavy." • "My shoulders feel heavy." • "My head feels heavy." • "I can no longer lift my limbs off the ground."
STAGE 2	• "My legs feel warm." • "My arms feel warm." • "My shoulders feel warm." • "My face feels warm." • "My entire body feels warm and comfortable." (Some people imagine putting a blanket on to add to the sense of warmth.)
STAGE 3	• "My heartbeat is slowing and I am becoming calm."
STAGE 4	• "My breathing is slowing and I am relaxed."

Progressive Muscle Relaxation

This technique requires you to alternately tense and relax your muscles.

1. While lying on your back or sitting in a comfortable position, monitor your heart rate for 15 seconds and then multiply by 4 to obtain beats per minute. Concentrate on relaxing and slowing your breathing.
2. Do each of the following exercises twice. Hold for 10 seconds each time.
   a. Curl your toes and hold. Release.
   b. Pull your toes up toward your head and hold. Release. Then take a deep breath and slowly exhale.
   c. Tighten your calf muscles. Release.
   d. Tighten your thigh muscles. Release. Then take a deep breath and slowly exhale.
   e. Tighten your abdominal muscles. Release.
   f. Do a pelvic tilt (described in Chapter 11). Release. Take a deep breath and slowly exhale.
   g. Tighten your back muscles to bring your shoulder blades together. Relax.
   h. Make a fist with both hands. Release.
   i. Tighten your shoulders. Release.
   j. Gently tighten your neck muscles. Release.
   k. Scrunch up your face by tightening your facial muscles. Release. Take a deep breath and slowly exhale.
3. Ensure that your muscles are relaxed. You may have to tense and relax them again.
4. Monitor your heart rate again to see whether it has gone down.

Visualization

Also called mental imagery, guided imagery, or guided daydreaming (Samuels & Samuels, 1975), this technique involves imagining yourself in a quiet and peaceful place, usually a natural setting. Known as Jacobson's method of relaxation, the objective of this technique is to work on the peripheral nervous system to reduce the physiological symptoms of anxiety (Jacobson, 1938) by progressive relaxation of the body and the use of mental imagery to achieve relaxation. It can be done entirely on your own or with the help of instructors or recordings (such as CDs of ocean wave or bird sounds). In a recent cardiology study, Paul-Labrador and colleagues (2006) found that patients who used visualization improved their blood pressure and insulin-resistance components of metabolic syndrome, as well as cardiac autonomic nervous system tone (including heart rate, the heart's ability to contract, and tolerance to physical activity), thereby reducing the physiological response to stress and improving coronary heart disease risk factors.

PERSONAL PERSPECTIVE

Nancy's Beach

The following exercise is based on memories of locations that have had special meaning for me. Feel free to visualize a setting of your own once you have tried this technique.

You will probably need someone to read these instructions to you the first time you try this. I usually do this exercise immediately after doing the progressive muscle relaxation technique described above.

Find a quiet, comfortable spot in which to sit or lie down. Begin by monitoring your heart rate for 15 seconds.

> Take a deep breath and relax. Concentrate on how relaxed you are becoming and how comfortable you are. Close your eyes and concentrate on your breathing. Relax your back, arms, and legs. Concentrate on releasing the tension stored in your body. Feel your chest go up and down with your breathing. Relax and concentrate on your breathing.
>
> Now imagine that you are getting up from your spot to walk down a corridor toward a door. Open that door and walk through it to an escalator. Together, let's go down the escalator: 1, 2, 3, 4, 5, 6, 7, 8, 9, 10. Now step off the escalator and go to the door.
>
> When you reach that door, imagine that you are taking off your shoes, picking up a towel lying beside the door, and then walking through the door. On the other side of the door is a beach and you can feel the warmth of the sun on your body and the white sand under your feet. Close the door behind you.
>
> As you walk toward the dark blue ocean on the right, you can feel the sun on your face and back. You are able to hear the waves and feel a slight breeze on your face. You can feel the cool sand under your feet. Above you, the sky is a clear blue. Find a place to sit or lie down. Remember that you have a towel to use if you need it. You will continue to feel the warmth of the sand and sun. You will hear the waves and the birds in the distance. You are relaxed and quiet. For the next several minutes, allow your mind to relax and continue to enjoy the beach. Enjoy the stillness, warmth, and quiet you are experiencing.
>
> Next, imagine that you are getting up and walking to the water's edge. Dip your hand in the water and splash it on your face. You can now return to the door, feeling refreshed, alert, and at peace. Open the door and take one last look at the beach. Close the door. Lock the door with the key that's hanging by the door, and put the key in your pocket. Know that the imaginary key to this location is yours alone, so that no one but you can gain access to this special place.
>
> You are now going back up the escalator to the first door. Together, let's go back up the escalator: 10, 9, 8, 7, 6, 5, 4, 3, 2, 1. Step off the escalator. Open the door, walk down the corridor, and return to the spot where you began your journey. Take a moment to remember the peaceful time you spent at the beach.
>
> Bring your attention back to the here and now.

Take a deep breath. Before you get up, check whether you were able to slow your heart rate. You should feel refreshed and alert.

Other Relaxation Techniques

Self-Hypnosis

Self-hypnosis acts as a stress reducer by having you concentrate on key words and images. It is a scientifically verified and effective technique that can promote accelerated human change.

With self-hypnosis, you can create desired changes in behaviour and encourage mental and physical well-being. People use it to lose weight, quit smoking, reduce physical pain, and deal with traumatic events. Consultation with a clinical hypnotherapist can help individualize goals and specific techniques.

Biofeedback

Biofeedback is a form of alternative medicine that assesses bodily processes such as blood pressure, heart rate, skin temperature, galvanic skin response (sweating), and muscle tension to raise a person's awareness and conscious control over physiological responses. It involves a physiological feedback monitor such as an electrocardiograph for monitoring heart activity. It allows you to learn appropriate relaxation responses (Choe, Townsend, Blount, Lo, Sadowski, et al., 2007).

Music

Music conjures up images and memories, and can be relaxing and renewing. The music you choose will depend on your own preferences, although quiet, slower music is usually more relaxing.

Yoga

Yoga is a discipline that seeks to unite the mind, body, and soul (Seaward, 2005). The practice of hatha yoga combines breathing, stretching, and balance exercises to achieve a spiritual focus.

T'ai Chi Ch'uan

Known as the "softest" martial art (Seaward, 2005), this discipline brings the body and mind together through the *chi*, or life force, when you do a series of graceful martial arts movements. T'ai chi ch'uan attempts to achieve deep relaxation and as much softness in the musculature as possible. It is characterized by the leverage through the joints based on relaxing the muscles to enhance and increase breathing, body heat, the lymph system, and peristalsis, working toward homeostasis (returning your internal circulation to a healthier, balanced state). This discipline can help you keep calm and steady under pressure. Many community centres offer programs in t'ai chi ch'uan.

Massage

Massage stimulates blood flow and improves muscle tone. It relaxes the muscles and thereby creates a calming effect. Now more popular than ever, massage can be performed by registered massage therapists, chiropractors, physiotherapists, reflexologists, acupuncturists, and other professionals. Non-professionals can also learn massage. Some types of therapies include:

- *Deep tissue massage*, which focuses on deeper layers of muscle tissue in an attempt to release chronic patterns of tension in the body through slow strokes and deep pressure.
- *Swedish massage* is a superficial, gentle message that is designed to relax muscles and increase circulation.
- *Lymphatic massage* is a light-touch technique used to promote health and aid recovery from illness by removing toxic metabolic waste.
- *Cranial massage* is a delicate technique that relaxes the muscles around the neck, jaw, and skull. This method is used to help temporal-mandibular joint (TMJ) dysfunction.
- *Reflexology massage* helps bring about balance, ease, and soundness of mind, body, and spirit by massaging the feet and hands.
- *Aromatherapy* uses essential oils, combined with massage, to provide a powerful calming and energizing effect.
- *Acupuncture* is the technique of placing needles at key points on the body to unblock and redirect energy flow to relieve tension and pain.

Hydrotherapy

Hydrotherapy—soaking in a hot tub, warm bath, or hot shower—is a great way to relax at the end of the day. Warm water (about 38 °C) appears to quiet and soothe the body while slowing down the activity of internal organs. Water seems to have the ability to get rid of stress and rejuvenate the body. Whirlpool baths appear to have higher stress-relief benefits, including reducing anxiety. Herbal baths scented with lavender, linden, passionflower, and chamomile also appear to be effective.

Ultimately, it is up to you to discover what helps you relax and brings your stress levels down. You may need to try several methods, or a particular method a few times, before you find something that suits your needs and personality.

A parting thought: Recognize that if you do not allow time for yourself, mentally and physically, you will begin to experience symptoms of stress. I wish you luck in developing your stress survival skills.

> “It is not the stress that kills us, it is our reaction to it.”
>
> — Hans Selye

KEY TERMS

critical incident, 282
general adaptation syndrome (GAS), 277
post-traumatic stress disorder (PTSD), 284
psychosomatic symptoms, 278
stress, 276
stressor, 279

EXERCISES

Multiple Choice

1. Which of these statements about stress is *incorrect*?
   - **a.** Stress can be self-induced.
   - **b.** Stress can be pleasurable.
   - **c.** Stress can cause psychological disorders.
   - **d.** Individuals differ in what they find stressful.
   - **e.** Your ability to handle stress is hereditary and fixed.
2. A technique of relaxation that uses a machine to monitor body processes is called
   - **a.** yoga
   - **b.** autogenic feedback
   - **c.** biofeedback
   - **d.** transcendental meditation
   - **e.** progressive relaxation
3. Which of the following is *least* likely to be helpful in relieving tension?
   - **a.** taking a brisk walk after sitting for a long time
   - **b.** doing slow stretching exercises
   - **c.** doing rhythmical exercises
   - **d.** drinking alcohol
   - **e.** getting a massage
4. How did Selye label the negative level of stress?
   - **a.** hyperstress
   - **b.** distress
   - **c.** eustress
   - **d.** burnout
   - **e.** neustress
5. What is the first step in managing stress?
   - **a.** Use a relaxation technique.
   - **b.** Recognize symptoms and causes.
   - **c.** Be as fit and healthy as possible.
   - **d.** Get eight hours of sleep a night.
   - **e.** Control lifestyle and avoid stressors.
6. Which is a good way to manage stress?
   - **a.** Allow more time for work.
   - **b.** Avoid talking about your problems.
   - **c.** Think positively.
   - **d.** Insist that things should go your way.
   - **e.** Pretend that the problem will just go away.
7. Why might those in law enforcement be more likely to suffer from critical incident stress?
   - **a.** Their type A personalities predispose them to PTSD.
   - **b.** Jumping in front of traffic causes problems.
   - **c.** Their job involves facing dangerous situations.
   - **d.** They are more sensitive than the general population.
   - **e.** They enjoy the "buzz" of constant stress.
8. Which behaviour type is characterized by an angry, hostile, and impatient personality?
   - **a.** type A
   - **b.** type B
   - **c.** type C
   - **d.** type E
   - **e.** type AB
9. Jacobson's method of relaxation emphasizes
   - **a.** imagery
   - **b.** visualization
   - **c.** autogenic training
   - **d.** meditation
   - **e.** progressive relaxation
10. Post-traumatic stress disorder refers to
    - **a.** a positive ability to handle stress
    - **b.** the result of completing all your credits in first year
    - **c.** an overwhelming response to stress
    - **d.** the response to completing an assignment on time
    - **e.** none of the above

11. Any physical, social, or psychological event or condition that causes our body to have to adjust to a specific situation is known as:
    a. an obstacle
    b. PTSD
    c. a stressor
    d. a strain
    e. a road block
12. During which phase of general adaptation syndrome does the brain prepare the body for the fight-or-flight response?
    a. resistance
    b. adaptation
    c. exhaustion
    d. alarm
    e. homeostasis
13. Working out when stressed can help by:
    a. increasing energy
    b. improving mental alertness
    c. allowing you to step back from the situation to view it in a different way
    d. reducing hostility
    e. all of the above
14. General adaptation syndrome explains
    a. the pattern followed by our physiological responses to stress
    b. the path of our autonomic nervous system when we are aroused by a stressful situation
    c. a means of dealing with post-traumatic stress disorder
    d. how to achieve homeostasis
    e. how well we adapt to new situations
15. With a full load of college courses and a part-time job, Steve suffers from excessive time pressure, excessive responsibility, and excessive expectations to succeed. Steve is suffering from
    a. neustress
    b. burnout
    c. eustress
    d. overload
    e. inconsistent goals and behaviours
16. The physiological arousal response in which the body prepares to combat a real or perceived threat is called
    a. the response phase
    b. the resistance phase
    c. homeostasis
    d. the fight-or-flight response
    e. distress response
17. The characteristics that have been associated with an increased risk for heart disease in a type A personality are
    a. compulsiveness and impatience
    b. competitiveness and fastidiousness
    c. hostility, anger, and cynicism
    d. perfectionism, impatience, and hostility
    e. competitiveness and introversion

Short Answer

1. Define stress.

2. What are the differences among neustress, eustress, and distress?

3. What are some of the general symptoms of stress?

4. List five stressors associated with law enforcement work.

5. What is a critical incident?

6. Describe post-traumatic stress disorder (PTSD).

7. What are some of the signs and symptoms of PTSD?

8. What can you do for a colleague who is suffering from critical incident stress or PTSD?

9. Explain how type A, B, and C personalities cope with stress.

10. Briefly explain five relaxation techniques for coping with stress.

REFERENCES

American Psychiatric Association (APA). (2000). *Diagnostic and statistical manual of mental disorders* (4th ed.). Washington, DC: Author.

Benson, H. (1975). *The relaxation response.* New York: Morrow.

Boyd, N. (1995). Violence in the workplace in British Columbia: A preliminary investigation. *Canadian Journal of Criminology, 37*(4), 491–519.

Brown, H. (2003). The effects of post-traumatic stress disorder (PTSD) on the officer and the family. *Police Stressline.* http://www.geocities.com/stressline_com/ptsd-family.html.

Brown, J.J., Wells, G.A., Trottier, A.J., Bonneau, J., & Ferris, B. (1998). Back pain in a large Canadian police force. *Spine, 23*, 821–827.

Canadian Children's Rights Council. (2012). Child and teen suicides in Canada. http://www.canadiancrc.com/Youth_Suicide_in_Canada.aspx.

Choe, H.M., Townsend, K.A., Blount, G., Lo, C.H., Sadowski, L., et al. (2007). Treatment and control of blood pressure in patients with diabetes mellitus. *American Journal of Health System Pharmacy, 64*(1), 97–103.

Connor, K.M., & Butterfield, M.I. (2003). Posttraumatic stress disorder. *Focus, 1*(30), 247–263.

Crompton, S. (2011). *What's stressing the stressed? Main sources of stress among workers.* Statistics Canada Catalogue no. 11-008-X. http://www.statcan.gc.ca/pub/11-008-x/2011002/article/11562-eng.htm.

Czarnecki, F., & Janowitz, I. (2003). Ergonomics and safety in law enforcement. *Clinics in Occupational and Environmental Medicine, 3*(3), 399–417. http://www.theppsc.org/Staff_Views/Czarnecki/ergonomics_and_safety_in_law_enforcement.htm.

Ellis, D., Choi, A., & Blaus, C. (1993). Injuries to police officers attending domestic disturbances: An empirical study. *Canadian Journal of Criminology, 35*(2), 149–168.

Everly, G.S., & Mitchell, J.T. (2000). The debriefing "controversy" and crisis intervention: A review of lexical and substantive issues. *International Journal of Emergency Mental Health, 2*(4), 211–225.

Figley, C. (Ed). (1995). *Compassion fatigue: Coping with secondary traumatic stress disorders in those who treat the traumatized.* New York: Brunner–Routledge.

Finn, P. (1997, August). Reducing stress: An organization-centered approach. *Law Enforcement Bulletin*, *66*(8), 20–26. Washington, DC: Department of Justice, Federal Bureau of Investigation.

Friedman, M., & Rosenman, R.H. (1994). *Type A behavior and your heart.* New York: Knopf.

Fullerton, C., Ursano, R.J., Vance, K., & Wang, L. (2000). Debriefing following trauma. *Psychiatric Quarterly*, *71*(3), 259–276.

Ghahramanlou, M., & Broadbeck, C. (2000). Predictors of secondary trauma in sexual assault counselors. *International Journal of Emergency Mental Health*, *4*, 229–240.

Goldfarb, D.A. (1999). The effects of stress on police officers. http://www.heavybadge.com/efstress.htm.

Gyi, D.E., & Porter, J.M. (1998). Musculoskeletal problems and driving in police officers. *Occupational Medicine (London)*, *48*(3), 152–160.

Health Canada. (2012). *Eating Well with Canada's Food Guide.* http://www.hc-sc.gc.ca/fn-an/food-guide-aliment/order-commander/index-eng.php.

Jacobson, E. (1938). *Progressive relaxation.* Chicago: Chicago University Press.

Kabat-Zinn, J. (1991). *Full catastrophe living.* New York: Delacorte.

Kiecolt-Glaser, J.K. (1999). Stress, personal relationships and immune function: Health implications. *Brain Behavior Immunology*, *13*, 61–72.

Kobasa, S.C. (1982). The hardy personality: Toward a social psychology of stress and health. In R.S. Sanders and J. Suls (Eds.), *Social psychology of health and illness* (pp. 3–32). Hillsdale, NJ: Erlbaum.

Kohan, A., & O'Connor, B.P. (2002). Police officer job satisfaction in relation to mood, well-being and alcohol consumption. *Journal of Psychology*, *136*, 307–318.

Loo, R. (2003). A meta-analysis of police suicide rates: Findings and issues. *Suicide and Life Threatening Behaviour*, *33*(3), 313–325.

Marin, A. (2012). *In the line of duty: Investigation into how the Ontario Provincial Police and the Ministry of Community Safety and Correctional Services have addressed operational stress injuries affecting police officers.* Ombudsman Report. http://www.ombudsman.on.ca/Resources/Reports/In-the-Line-of-Duty.aspx.

Morse, D.R., & Furst, M.L. (1979). *Stress for success: A holistic approach to stress and its management.* New York: Van Nostrand Reinhold.

Myrtek, M. (2001). Meta-analyses of prospective studies on coronary heart disease, type A personality, and hostility. *International Journal of Cardiology*, *79*, 245–251.

O'Hara, A.F., & Violanti, J.M. (2009). Police suicide—A web surveillance of national data. *International Journal of Emergency Mental Health*, *11*(1), 17–23.

Parsons, J. (2004). *Occupational health and safety issues of police officers in Canada, the United States and Europe: A review essay.* International Council of Police Representative Associations. http://www.safetynet.mun.ca/pdfs/Occupational%20H&S.pdf.

Paul-Labrador, M., Polk, D., Dwyer, J.H., Velasquez, I., Nidich, S., et al. (2006). Effects of a randomized controlled trial of transcendental meditation on components of the metabolic syndrome in subjects with coronary heart disease. *Archives of Internal Medicine*, *166*(11), 1218–1224.

Samuels, M., & Samuels, N. (1975). *Seeing with the mind's eye: The history, techniques, and uses of visualization.* New York: Random House.

Seaward, B.L. (2005). *Managing stress* (5th ed.). Sudbury, MA: Jones and Bartlett Publishers.

Selye, H. (1956). *The stress of life.* New York: McGraw-Hill.

Selye, H. (1974). *Stress without distress.* Philadelphia: Lippincott.

Shafer, W. (1996). *Stress management for wellness* (3rd ed.). Fort Worth, TX: Holt, Rinehart, and Winston.

Statistics Canada. (2011). *Mortality, summary list of causes 2008.* http://www.statcan.gc.ca/pub/84f0209x/84f0209x2008000-eng.pdf.

Statistics Canada. (2012). *Police reported crime statistics in Canada, 2011.* http://www.statcan.gc.ca/pub/85-002-x/2012001/article/11692-eng.pdf.

Van Netten, C., Brands, R.H., Hoption Cann, S.A., Spinelli, J.J., & Sheps, S.B. (2003). Cancer cluster among police detachment personnel. *Environment International*, *28*, 567–572.

World Health Organization (WHO). (2003). *The solid facts: The social determinants of health.* http://www.euro.who.int/__data/assets/pdf_file/0005/98438/e81384.pdf.

13

Shiftwork

LEARNING OBJECTIVES

After completing this chapter, you should be able to:

- Identify the physiological, psychological, and social effects of shiftwork.
- Identify the physiological stages of sleep.
- Explain the importance of proper sleep for shiftworkers.
- Develop shiftwork coping strategies.

OVERVIEW

It is estimated that 25 to 43 percent of all workers work non-traditional hours. Emergency service and crisis intervention workers, especially, have chosen careers tied to round-the-clock availability. This non-standard schedule includes evening or night shifts, rotating shifts, and extended hours on the job. The mental, physical, and social implications are very challenging. You must learn to cope with shiftwork in order to ensure a safe work environment for you and your co-workers.

This chapter looks at shiftwork and its effects. It also considers the importance of sleep and ways to get better-quality sleep, as well as strategies to alleviate the stress caused by shiftwork.

Some young people entering into policing find the idea of working late into the night appealing. Many become "night owls" in their teenage years, finding it easier to do homework and study at night, sometimes into the early morning hours, and perhaps working nights at part-time jobs. Shiftwork allows individuals to do things during the day when conventional workers are working, such as doctor's appointments, shopping without long line-ups, or playing sports. Once an officer is on the job, however, the routines of daytime court appearances, family commitments, and rotating shifts pose a challenge to getting good-quality sleep.

FACTS ABOUT . . .

Shiftwork

- Some 60 to 70 percent of shiftworkers experience sleep disruption, including activity in the home, phone calls, social life away from work, court appearances, appointments that can only be made during the day, and so on.
- Approximately 20 percent of shiftworkers quit their job because they cannot adapt to the demands of shiftwork. Those who persevere even though they cannot adjust suffer the effects of ill health long after they stop working shifts.
- The demands and risks of shiftwork limit socialization with people outside the job. The shiftworker's job therefore becomes his or her life. Further, the unique demands of policing increase the need for collegial support, as other officers are the only ones who can relate to the stresses of the work.
- Law enforcement personnel who work the night shift have more accidents. The mental and physical effects of night work have been shown to affect a worker's concentration, alertness, motivation, and memory. These factors can slow a person's reaction time. Fatigue also increases the risk of driver inattention, speeding, and running off the road.
- Car crashes are the top cause of occupational fatalities, accounting for 22 percent of work-related deaths between 1992 and 2001. In 7 percent of those cases, drowsiness or falling asleep while driving was cited as a primary factor in the crash.
- A higher incidence of serious illness, including heart disease and cancer, is found among police officers and correctional workers who work rotating shifts. Night shifts increase the risk of strokes and heart attacks, regardless of age.
- As officers age, their ability to cope with shift changes diminishes. They find it more difficult to fall asleep and are less able to sleep without interruption.
- A study of 4,000 police officers found that 6.8 percent had chronic insomnia (the inability to obtain an adequate amount or quality of sleep) and 2 percent exhibited shiftwork sleep disorder (a variety of mental and physical ailments associated with disturbed circadian rhythm (discussed later in this chapter).
- Sleep debt has been shown to have a harmful impact on carbohydrate metabolism and endocrine function, which can contribute to metabolic disorders. Officers working the night shift had elevated waist circumferences compared to those who worked non-midnight shifts.
- Shiftwork may cause fatigue and somatic anxiety, which are independent predictors of cardiovascular and digestive symptoms.

SOURCES: International Association for Human Values, 2004; NIOSH, 2004; American Academy of Sleep Medicine, 2007; Waters & Ussery, 2007; Violanti, Andrew, Burchfiel, Hartley, Charles, et al., 2007; Violanti, Burchfiel, Hartley, Mnatsakanova, Fekedulegn, et al., 2009; Brinkley, 2010; Violanti, 2011.

Shift Schedules

Police work typically involves two types of shift schedules (although there are many variations):

- Three eight-hour shifts, usually beginning at 7 a.m. (the day shift), 3 p.m. (the afternoon shift), and 11 p.m. (the night or "graveyard" shift).
- Two 12-hour shifts, usually beginning at 7 a.m. and 7 p.m.

Most shiftwork schedules involve four to seven days on and two to four days off. Each police service has its own arrangement. Some arrangements are tailored to times of peak demand for police services (such as rush hour).

Research has resulted in recommendations for devising healthier shiftwork routines (Wedderburn & King, 1996):

- Minimize permanent nights.
- Minimize the sequence of nights: only two to four night shifts in succession should be worked. Weekly rotating shifts provide insufficient time for the **circadian rhythm**—the 24-hour cycle on which the human biological clock is based—to adjust and enough time for a sizable "sleep debt" to accumulate. Working four to seven night shifts in a row has been condemned by experts.
- Consider shorter night shifts (a maximum of seven or eight hours will minimize errors and accidents).
- Plan rotations with some free weekends.
- Avoid overlong work sequences.
- Avoid early starts (reduced sleep leads to fatigue and increased risk of errors and accidents on morning shifts).
- Rotate forward (clockwise rotation from mornings to afternoons to nights).

circadian rhythm
the 24-hour cycle on which the human biological clock is based

Which shifts are best?

- Fixed shifts offer the least amount of disruption to the circadian rhythm; however, shiftworkers have difficulty reverting to normal hours to participate in family or social activities.
- Working rapidly rotating shifts (two days/two nights) keeps the circadian rhythm day-oriented, because there is insufficient time to adjust and there is less sleep debt; however, individuals may feel "out of sync," and their alertness may be affected.

Ultimately, it is up to the individual agency, in consultation with the professional associations, to address what works most effectively for employees.

Your task is to determine how you will cope with the effects of shiftwork and rotating shifts. Turn to **assignment 13.1** (in the appendix) to assess your **chronotype** —your individual circadian rhythm—and understand its effect on your sleep patterns.

chronotype
a person's individual circadian rhythms, including body temperature, cognitive faculties, and eating and sleeping patterns

Understanding the Importance of Sleep

We need sufficient sleep to work effectively, sustain emotional health, and resist stress. We spend a third of our lives sleeping. Sleep experts say the average amount of sleep we need is 8 hours a night, although some individuals require 10 hours while others seem to get by on 6 hours.

Think of sleep as a slow elevator ride down to the bottom floor. At the bottom is where you sleep deeply, and halfway up is where you take side trips to have dreams. Usually, we ride the elevator about five times each night—every 70 to 90 minutes—as we cycle through the four ever-deeper stages of non-dreaming sleep, then shift into **rapid-eye movement (REM) sleep**. This is the stage of sleep during which we dream. In this intensely cerebral stage, muscle paralysis keeps the body from acting out the dreams that occur.

rapid-eye movement (REM) sleep
a stage of sleep that allows your body to recover from mental fatigue and helps to store memories and consolidate learning

Each of the five stages of sleep provides different resources for recovery from the day's demands. Each night you typically go through the same sequence of sleep stages. Your body begins to slow down and muscle tension decreases. As you enter stage 1 of non-REM sleep, mundane thoughts go through your head. If you are awakened at this stage, you may not know you were asleep. Your brain waves at this stage are smaller and irregular. As you enter stage 2, your brain waves become larger. There is an occasional burst of electrical energy. At this stage your eyes become unresponsive. In stage 3, your brain waves are about five times larger and much slower, and in stage 4, your brain waves form jagged patterns and you are in such a profound state of unconsciousness that it is very difficult to wake you. Then you shift to stage 5 REM sleep, where your pulse and breathing quicken, your face and limbs go slack, and your brain temperature and blood flow increase. Your eyes dart back and forth.

Stages 3 and 4, the two deeper stages of sleep, are necessary for recovery from physical fatigue. It is believed that non-REM sleep helps repair cells, rests the body and mind, and boosts the immune system. Stage 5 REM sleep allows the body to recover from mental fatigue. It also helps to store memories and consolidate learning.

Because the hours that shiftworkers have for sleep do not coincide with natural and social rhythms, they must make a special effort to ensure that they get enough uninterrupted sleep. If their sleep is interrupted, they may not pass through all five stages of sleep and may suffer health problems as a result.

If a new afternoon or night shiftworker adheres strictly to a set sleep pattern, his or her body can usually adjust to shiftwork in about a month. Unfortunately, most of the world adheres to a different schedule. Socially, night shift routines affect dating opportunities, marriage, child care, and dining routines.

Moreover, most courts are open only during the day. This means that a night shift officer must come to court during his or her days off or has to work a night shift and then stay awake to go to court, getting as little as four hours' sleep before being required to go in for the next night shift. Inevitably, night shift officers reduce their sleep time to take advantage of daytime activities on the days they are off duty. This throws the body's sleep adjustment processes into disorder, and the readjustment period must start all over again.

The Effects of Shiftwork

Let's look more closely at some effects of shiftwork and lack of sleep.

Physiological and Psychological Effects

The human biological clock is based on a 24-hour circadian rhythm. (Other organisms also have a biological clock that regulates their periods of activity and inactivity.)

Exposure to light and dark helps establish physiological cycles. The organ that appears to be responsible for this is the suprachiasmatic nuclei (SCN), a small cluster of nerve tissue connected to the point where the optic nerves meet the brain. Stimulated by nerve impulses triggered by exposure to light and dark, this photosensitive nerve centre sets and resets the biological clock. At regular intervals each day, the body becomes hungry and tired, active or lethargic. Body temperature, blood pressure, heartbeat, glandular activity, digestion, brain waves, and so on, rise and fall in a rhythmic pattern. Interference with this cycle reduces mental alertness, elevates the heart rate, upsets the stomach, and causes impatience.

Melatonin is a natural hormone made by the pineal gland (located in the midbrain). Darkness stimulates the pineal gland to secrete melatonin, which promotes sleep by making you feel less alert. This usually happens around 9 p.m., when natural light is gone. Unless an individual is subjected to bright artificial indoor lighting, melatonin is generally released for approximately 12 hours. As you age, the amount secreted decreases. People with flexible biorhythms are more adaptable to shiftwork when young, but are more likely to develop intolerance to shiftwork later in life (Arendt, 2010).

Shiftwork interferes with the circadian rhythm, which is why people who start working new shifts, especially night shifts, need a period of adjustment. If they do not get the necessary uninterrupted sleep between shifts, they will always experience problems. One of the serious results of rotating shiftwork is that 30–50 percent of these shiftworkers report falling asleep on the job at least once a week.

Tied to our circadian rhythm, our body becomes used to metabolizing foods (especially carbohydrates) during the day. At night, our digestive system slows down. Officers tend to eat too fast (based on call volume) and rely on fast foods or snacks, which contain a high percentage of sugars and fat. A growing trend for police is drinking "energy drinks." These are loaded with caffeine and sugars. Enlarged waist circumferences are a direct result. Gastrointestinal and digestive problems such as indigestion, heartburn, stomachache and loss of appetite are more common among rotation shiftworkers and night workers than among day workers (CCOHS, 2010).

Officers who work 3 p.m. to 11 p.m. and 7 p.m. to 3 a.m. shifts generally find it very difficult to fall asleep right away (Akerstedt, Nordin, Alfredsson, Westerholm, & Kecklund, 2010). Many are still alert after hours of trying to fall asleep.

DID YOU KNOW?

Shiftwork causes many of the same effects as jet lag. Jet lag can occur when you cross three or more time zones, with the result that your circadian rhythm is no longer synchronized with periods of light and dark. The consequences of jet lag, which can last for days or even weeks, include sleep problems, irritability, loss of appetite, fatigue, and poor memory. Some people are very severely affected.

When dayworkers move to the night shift, they sleep an average of 5.5 hours a day, not the 7 or 8 hours required. As the sleep deficit builds, we see indications of decreased efficiency in reasoning and reaction time. The sleep deficit can lead to brief periods of dozing or "micro-sleeping," where you fall in and out of sleep for only seconds at a time. The symptoms experienced by the sleep-deprived are similar to those of jet lag. Police officers in this situation report decreased appetite, poor attitude, and general fatigue (Choy & Salbu, 2011).

Some police officers affected by sleep disruptions due to shiftwork have experienced temporary partial paralysis and temporary memory loss. Some experience peripheral hallucinations and see phantom runners out of the corners of their eyes. Others find it hard to keep their thoughts straight and difficult to speak in complete sentences. It is almost as if they are sleep-drunk. These symptoms usually occur during the early morning hours. Individuals may be too sleep-impaired to drive, putting themselves and others at risk. Some may actually drive faster to try to compensate for their sleepiness by doing riskier, more stimulating things. This is when more accidents happen.

For those driving or carrying firearms, fatigue and reduced alertness can become a life-threatening problem (Vila, 2000). The constant disruption of hormonal balances from shiftwork may cause elevated reproductive risks (Nurmine, 1998), including spontaneous premature births and lower birth weights, as well as infertility issues. There is also a link between the disruption of the circadian rhythm and poorer survival rates among patients with breast cancer (Filipski, 2002).

Just turning clocks forward by one hour in the spring can disrupt chronobiological rhythms and influence the duration and quality of sleep, and the effects can last for several days after the time change. This transition has been statistically shown to increase the incidence of acute myocardial infarction (Janszky & Ljung, 2008). Consideration must be made when officers have to rotate shifts or wake up early to go to court or work, thus depriving themselves of necessary sleep.

Sleep Disorders

There are a number of sleep disorders that can be triggered by lack of sleep. These conditions must be assessed and treated. For more information, see National Sleep Foundation (2012) (in References).

narcolepsy
a disorder that causes brain malfunction, leading to one's falling asleep without warning

Narcolepsy is a disorder that affects one in 2,000 people. It is a malfunction in the part of the brain that decides whether you're awake or asleep. People with narcolepsy suddenly fall asleep without warning while carrying on their usual daytime activities. They may experience sudden loss of muscle control, and this may be triggered by strong emotions and vivid dreams. Some of the symptoms include the following (National Sleep Foundation, 2011a):

- *Excessive sleepiness.*
- *Cataplexy*, which is a sudden loss in muscle tone and deep tendon reflexes, leading to muscle weakness, temporary paralysis, or a complete postural collapse. Cataplexy is usually brought on by an outburst of emotion—notably laughter, anger, or being startled.
- *Sleep paralysis*, which is the temporary inability to move or talk during the episode.
- *Hypnagogic hallucinations*, which are sensory dream-like experiences during the transition from wakefulness to sleep. These can be vivid, bizarre, and frightening to the individual.
- *Disrupted major sleep episodes* (disruption of the longest sleep episode that occurs on a daily basis), which involve frequent awakening and increased body movement.
- *Automatic behaviour*, which is unaware behaviour when fluctuating between sleep and wakefulness, such as irrelevant words, lapses in speech, and being unable to explain how you got somewhere.

restless legs syndrome (RLS)
a condition characterized by an overwhelming urge to move the legs when they are at rest

Restless legs syndrome (RLS) is a common and distressing condition that is characterized by an overwhelming urge to move the legs when they are at rest. Symptoms are more profound at night and during sleep (National Sleep Foundation, 2011b), and include:

- uncomfortable feeling in the legs (such as tingling, creeping, itching, or aching)
- involuntary jerking of limbs that is relieved by movement
- difficulty falling or staying asleep due to the symptoms

sleep apnea
a breathing-related sleep disorder in which inappropriate brain signals do not tell the breathing muscles to initiate respiration

Sleep apnea is a breathing-related sleep disorder that is potentially life-threatening. *Central sleep apnea* occurs when the brain fails to send the appropriate signals to the breathing muscles to initiate respiration. *Obstructive sleep apnea*, which is far more common, occurs when the air cannot flow into or out of the person's nose or mouth, although efforts to breathe continue. Sleep apnea is associated with cardiovascular problems. Risk factors include snoring, obesity, smoking, and a small upper airway (National Sleep Foundation, 2011c). Symptoms include:

- breathing pauses, which can happen as often as 20 to 60 times per hour
- breathing pauses accompanied by snoring between the episodes
- gasping or choking sensations
- being awakened just enough to inhale and resume breathing
- excessive daytime sleepiness
- early morning headaches

Social Effects

As mentioned earlier, most of the world operates during daytime hours. Society disregards shiftworkers in planning its schedules. This, of course, poses special problems for shiftworkers, especially those who work only at night. Most shiftworkers restrict their workweek non-work activities to sleeping and eating, and do everything else on their days off. This affects leisure activities, volunteer work, and time with family and friends. Thirty percent of police divorces are related to shiftwork stress. Reduced family time, mismatched energy levels for intimacy, and domestic violence are spillovers from the effects of the stress of working in law enforcement (Anderson, 2011).

Scheduling is a must if spouses are to cope with shiftwork. Planning your days and keeping each other informed of family activities are very important. The parent who works shifts misses school functions, birthday parties, sporting events, and family outings. It becomes difficult to explain to a child why you are constantly missing his or her soccer games but are able to attend your other child's games. Young children find it difficult to understand why a parent has to sleep during the day and why they must play quietly in the house; similarly, they cannot understand why a parent must work weekends. The parent who is not a shiftworker has to compensate for the other, and at times feels overloaded.

Single officers find the social aspect difficult. They have a hard time meeting people during their off hours. Because of the time spent at work, shiftworkers as a whole fall into the trap of socializing only with their own. They tend to lose touch with dayworkers, who in turn have a difficult time understanding shiftworkers. However, with the trend

PERSONAL PERSPECTIVE

Challenges and Opportunities

Shiftwork can offer opportunities that those working day shifts can't enjoy. One of the perks that my husband enjoyed was walking our children to school on the first day of school. I shared the moment only through pictures, because it was always the first day of classes at Georgian College. However, there were many times I had to juggle two soccer or hockey games alone.

Shiftwork not only robs the officer of precious family moments, it also affects his or her family. When my husband was called away for a homicide, instead of enjoying our 20th anniversary trip, I spent the day picking out a ring for myself, by myself. We laugh about it now, and I have a ring to explain the trip that never happened. We had to reschedule our 25th anniversary because of the 2010 G8 conference in Huntsville, when no officers were given time off.

Interestingly enough, when we discussed this issue in class, I was surprised by the number of my students who had had similar experiences yet never discussed the situation as a family.

Feeling robbed of special moments and memories can be hard for all concerned. It is really important to maintain open dialogue about the challenges and to set time aside for both your significant other and family in order to ensure that all feel included.

toward service industries' offering more hours (for example, fitness facilities that are open 24 hours), shiftworkers today may not miss out as much.

There can be a positive side to shiftwork. Law enforcement officers who get four consecutive days off have time for chores and activities around the house that a dayworker may not have. Having days off during the week allows you to go shopping without having to stand in line, to play a round of golf in short order, to walk your child to school and to bring school-aged children home for lunch. Some weekends can be extended to four days, and during the week you can go to a fitness facility during off-peak hours. Those officers with hectic family schedules get some quiet time for themselves while their children are at school.

Coping Strategies

The following suggestions will help you cope with the stress of shiftwork in your professional and personal life.

Eating Nutritious Food

Following *Eating Well with Canada's Food Guide* (Health Canada, 2012) is very important (see Chapter 8). Fruits and vegetables should replace chocolate bars, chips, and candy, which are high in fat and sugar. Consuming light to moderate amounts of protein (meat, fish, low-fat dairy products) is recommended for the beginning of the shift, and complex carbohydrates (whole grains, fruits, vegetables, and legumes) can help get you through the shift.

Try to have your main meal of the day in the middle of your awake period and a couple of hours before starting night duty. Having a regular eating schedule for the shift you are on will reduce the risk of developing gastrointestinal disorders and diabetes.

Don't go to bed hungry or overly full. Have a light snack about one hour before you hit the pillow. Snacks such as cheese, milk, a banana, slices of turkey, and tuna contain the amino acid tryptophan, which helps you fall asleep. Avoid sugary snacks, which may cause your blood sugar to plummet later, causing you to wake up. Excessive drinking of liquids may increase the need to go to the bathroom during your sleep time.

Avoid caffeinated soft drinks, tea, coffee, chocolate, and ASA (Aspirin®, Entrophen®) within five hours of going to sleep. Caffeine affects some people for up to 12 hours. Tobacco should also be avoided because nicotine acts as a stimulant. Alcohol and so-called sleep aids interfere with the depth and quality of sleep. Stimulants to counter listlessness and sleepiness create an unhealthy stimulant–depressant cycle. Recreational drugs can cause restlessness and interfere with sleep. Most sleeping pills contain antihistamines, which have a sedative side effect, inducing light sleep but robbing you of deep sleep.

The Role of Light

When you do paperwork, make sure your workspace is well lit. On patrol, take frequent breaks outside the car to stimulate your biological clock.

Some people are prone to depression in winter, when natural light levels are low. *Seasonal affective disorder* (SAD) is a syndrome associated with decreased light due to climate, latitude, and changes in neurotransmitter function as a result of seasonal changes. If you experience moodiness or depression during winter, getting some sunlight (for example, by taking brisk walks on sunny days, or going south for a holiday) could get you back on track. Artificial light—through the use of full-spectrum lighting in your home or office, or with a phototherapy light box—can replicate the effects of sunlight.

Darkness, on the other hand, is conducive to promoting sleep. When you have to sleep during the day, reduce as much of the light coming into your room as possible. Use dark blinds for your windows, or sleep in a room without windows.

To help you wake up, use a bright lamp with a timer. Set the timer to go off about half an hour before you need to wake up. The light from the lamp will help you wake up by stimulating your body, and is more effective than waking up to the blare of a radio. This should help trick your body into resetting its wake–sleep cycle so you can better cope with changing shifts.

PERSONAL PERSPECTIVE

Letter from a Former Student

Hey Nancy,

It has been just over 3.5 years since I graduated from the police studies degree program at Georgian, and since then I have enjoyed a career with the OPP. Policing and shiftwork have been everything that you promised they would be: long, drawn-out hours followed by minutes of heart-pumping adrenaline rushes. The work has been difficult, yet rewarding. And it has challenged me both mentally and physically.

The fitness aspect is what I wanted to write to you about. Since joining the force, I have had first-hand experience with the challenges of maintaining a healthy lifestyle while working bizarre hours. I had no idea how draining shiftwork and poor nutrition can be on a person's physical and mental health. Strangely, in my first year on the force, the motivation and pleasure that I once had in hitting the gym waned drastically. And it was all too easy to buy a sub or a slice of pizza every day for lunch.

But your lessons reinforced the importance of fitness and nutrition, even when maintaining these is not convenient. And am I ever grateful to you. Not only has my fitness helped me in physical confrontations on the job, but it has also helped me to deal effectively with the many stresses of policing and shiftwork.

Today I am still leading an active, healthy lifestyle, enjoying sports like hockey, baseball, and mountain biking, on top of weight training 3–5 times a week with my wife. Also, I am watching my nutrition, always trying to pack and buy healthy options. All of this contributes to a much happier life off the job.

So here I am, sitting in my cruiser under an overpass running some radar, thinking about how grateful I am for the dedication of teachers such as yourself, and the great example you set for your students.

I hope all is well with you. I will have to stop by one day to catch up over a cup of green tea.

Take care,

Dave

Relaxation Techniques

Meditation and other relaxation techniques (see Chapter 12) help combat high blood pressure (Dickinson, Campbell, Beyer, Nicolson, Cook, et al., 2008), asthma, high cholesterol, sleep disturbances, irritability, and muscle jumpiness (Gooneratne, 2008).

It is also important for shiftworkers to "leave work at work." All too often, an officer takes unresolved issues home.

Add a relaxing bath to your routine. Going from a warm (not hot) bath to a cool room will cause you to release heat, lowering your internal body temperature, which is a key step in inducing sleep.

Have a cup of hot milk. Milk contains tryptophan, an amino acid that helps promote sleep. Milk's carbohydrate mix also helps settle your stomach. It is important not to have your stomach overfull or empty so you can get to sleep.

Using Your Circadian Rhythm to Your Advantage

Shiftworkers need to monitor their body temperature. When your body temperature is rising, you are primed for complex thinking; routine tasks and paperwork are best done when body temperature is falling.

Body temperature passes through two cycles a day. From about 3 a.m. to 6 a.m. there is a trough, or low point. Body temperature rises from 8 a.m. to 10 a.m., when it reaches a peak. After that it falls until reaching a trough around 2 p.m. to 4 p.m., followed by a steady rise until reaching another peak between 7 p.m. and 9 p.m. If you can determine your peaks and troughs, you may be able to cope better with shiftwork. Do highly skilled tasks when your body temperature reaches its peak and menial tasks when it is in its trough.

Ways to help you stay alert include exercise, walking outside in the cold air, putting on a bright light, splashing your face with cold water, having an interesting conversation, and singing.

Physical Activity

Increase your physical activity to increase energy, alertness, balance, appetite, and stamina, and to facilitate sleeping. Beware of prolonged or high-exertion exercise, which can actually increase fatigue. You should engage in physical activity at least three times a week.

For those working afternoon shifts, it may be effective to work out at the end of the shift, when you are still keyed up. Make sure that you have a warm (not hot) shower and a light meal to help relax you when you are done working out.

Most graveyard shiftworkers find it extremely difficult to work out in the morning. A more appropriate time for them is the evening, before beginning a shift, or if the employer allows it, during a lunch period. The only difficulty with an early evening workout is that it can interfere with family time, including meals and children's activities.

Power Napping

Learn to nap effectively. The goal is a nap of 10–20 minutes at least 8 hours before going to bed (any longer can make you more tired and interfere with REM sleep).

FYI

Sleep Issues

For more information on sleep issues, including sleep disorders and treatments, try the following websites:

- National Sleep Foundation.......................... www.sleepfoundation.org
- National Center on Sleep Disorders Research (National Heart, Lung, and Blood Institute)............ www.nhlbi.nih.gov/about/ncsdr
- Canadian Sleep Society (CSS)........................ www.canadiansleepsociety.com
- Institute of Circulatory and Respiratory Health (ICRH)... www.cihr-irsc.gc.ca/e/8663.html

Coping with Noise During Sleep Time

Moderate levels of noise sustain arousal and partially counter the effects of sleep loss. Too much noise, however, can be counterproductive. Ways to reduce noise during the day include adding sound barriers to your bedroom and building a sleeping area in the basement that keeps you secluded from the rest of the family. An alternative is to create white noise. A fan can mask noises inside and outside the house and should help you fall asleep. Sleeping masks and ear plugs may also help.

Sleeping Effectively

It is important to keep to a strict sleep schedule. Keep noises to a minimum, make sure the bedroom is dark enough, ask others to respect your sleep time, and use your bedroom only for sleep and intimacy so that other things, such as television, do not distract you. If you have problems falling asleep after 20 minutes, get up and do something mundane so that you have a better chance of falling asleep when you try again. If you can't fall asleep in the morning, wait until early afternoon, when there's a natural energy dip.

Developing New Friendships

Cultivate friendships with other shiftworker families for social enjoyment as well as for a support system to help you cope with the unique stresses of shiftwork.

Remember that shiftwork will become a part of your life. You will have to make an effort not to let its physical impact interfere with your quality of life. Be aware of what your body is telling you, and learn to take care of yourself.

Turn to **assignment 13.2** (in the appendix) to devise some strategies for coping with shiftwork.

KEY TERMS

chronotype, 305
circadian rhythm, 305
narcolepsy, 308
rapid-eye movement (REM) sleep, 306
restless legs syndrome (RLS), 308
sleep apnea, 309

EXERCISES

Multiple Choice

1. What amount of sleep do shiftworkers get compared with non-shiftworkers?
- **a.** the same
- **b.** more
- **c.** less
- **d.** none of the above

2. How does the most effective shiftwork rotate?
- **a.** from days to nights to afternoons
- **b.** from days to afternoons to nights
- **c.** from afternoons to days to nights
- **d.** from nights to afternoons to days
- **e.** from nights to days to afternoons

3. Which of the following happens during REM sleep?
- **a.** Your body repairs cells and boosts your immune system.
- **b.** You don't get a restful sleep.
- **c.** You recover from mental fatigue.
- **d.** You can easily wake up.
- **e.** Your brain waves become larger.

4. The long-term effects of shiftwork can include
- **a.** problems with sleep
- **b.** eating disorders
- **c.** cardiovascular disorders
- **d.** reproductive disorders
- **e.** all of the above

5. Circadian rhythm refers to
- **a.** your heartbeat
- **b.** your biological clock
- **c.** your reproductive clock
- **d.** a method of birth control
- **e.** the amount of blood flowing through your heart

6. The possible symptoms experienced by sleep-deprived shiftworkers do *not* include
- **a.** temporary partial paralysis
- **b.** poor appetite
- **c.** peripheral hallucination
- **d.** difficulty speaking
- **e.** staying awake easily around sunrise

7. Coping strategies for shiftwork include
- **a.** eating healthy foods
- **b.** getting regular exercise
- **c.** avoiding caffeine
- **d.** not drinking alcohol to fall asleep
- **e.** all of the above

8. To try to sleep during the day with other people around, *avoid*
- **a.** putting sound barriers around your bedroom to keep noise out
- **b.** using white noise to reduce sounds
- **c.** sleeping in the basement when kids are playing in the house
- **d.** using relaxation techniques to fall asleep
- **e.** consuming coffee or chocolate before going to sleep

9. The hormone that helps you feel tired is
- **a.** serotonin
- **b.** melatonin
- **c.** tyroxine
- **d.** adenosine
- **e.** cryprochrome

10. Many people have a clear reduction in task performance around which time of day?
- **a.** midday
- **b.** early morning
- **c.** post-lunch
- **d.** late afternoon
- **e.** early evening

11. Which type of work is most disruptive in terms of causing harmful effects through major changes to the circadian rhythm?
    a. permanent night work
    b. slowly rotating shiftwork
    c. rapidly rotating shiftwork
    d. non-rotating shiftwork
    e. permanent day work

12. In which stage of sleep does REM sleep occur?
    a. stage 3
    b. stage 2
    c. stage 5
    d. stage 1
    e. stage 4

13. Under which condition is melatonin released, and what is the effect of the release of this hormone?
    a. Melatonin is released when light levels are high, making a person feel sleepy.
    b. Melatonin is released when light levels are high, making a person feel awake.
    c. Melatonin is released when light levels are low, making a person feel sleepy.
    d. Melatonin is released when light levels are low, making a person feel awake.
    e. Melatonin is released when a person wakes up, making a person feel sleepy.

Short Answer

1. List five negative physiological effects of shiftwork.

2. List some positive aspects of shiftwork.

3. How can shiftwork affect your social life?

4. List six ways to cope with shiftwork.

REFERENCES

Akerstedt, T., Nordin, M., Alfredsson, L., Westerholm, P., & Kecklund, G. (2010). Sleep and sleepiness: Impact of entering or leaving shiftwork—A prospective study. *Chronobiology International*, *27*(5), 987–996.

American Academy of Sleep Medicine. (2007, June 13). Sleep disorders highly prevalent among police officers. *Science Daily.* http://www.sciencedaily.com/releases/2007/06/070612075008.htm.

Anderson, A. (2011). Intimate partner violence within law enforcement families. *Journal of Interpersonal Violence*, *26*(6), 1176–1193.

Arendt, J. (2010). Shiftwork: Coping with the biological clock. *Occupational Medicine (London)*, *60*(1), 10–20. doi:10.1093/occmed/kqp162.

Brinkley, M. (2010). Effects on health for the night shift worker. http://www.livestrong.com/article/112321-effects-health-night-shift-worker.

Canadian Centre for Occupational Health and Safety (CCOHS). (2010). Rotational shiftwork. http://www.ccohs.ca/oshanswers/ergonomics/shiftwrk.html.

Choy, M., & Salbu, R.L. (2011). Jet lag: Current and potential therapies. *Pharmacy and Therapeutics*, *36*(4), 221–224, 231.

Dickinson, H., Campbell, F., Beyer, F., Nicolson, D.J., Cook, J., et al. (2008). Relaxation therapies for the management of primary hypertension in adults: A Cochrane review. *Journal of Human Hypertension*, *22*(12), 807–808.

Filipski, E. (2002). Host circadian clock as a control point in tumor progression. *Journal of the National Cancer Institute*, *94*(9), 690–697.

Gooneratne, N.S. (2008). Complementary and alternative medicine for sleep disturbances in older adults. *Clinical Geriatric Medicine*, *24*(1), 121–138.

Health Canada. (2012). *Eating well with Canada's Food Guide.* http://www.hc-sc.gc.ca/fn-an/food-guide-aliment/order-commander/index-eng.php.

International Association for Human Values. (2004). *Integra survey 2000.* http://www.niosh.com.

Janszky, I., & Ljung, R. (2008). Shifts to and from Daylight Saving Time and incidence of myocardial infarction. *New England Journal of Medicine*, *359*, 1966–1968.

National Institute for Occupational Safety and Health (NIOSH). (2004). Work-related roadway crashes. http://www.cdc.gov/niosh/docs/2004-137.

National Sleep Foundation. (2011a). Narcolepsy and sleep. http://www.sleepfoundation.org/article/sleep-related-problems/narcolepsy-and-sleep.

National Sleep Foundation. (2011b). RLS (restless legs syndrome) diagnosis. http://www.sleepfoundation.org/article/rls-restless-legs-syndrome-diagnosis.

National Sleep Foundation. (2011c). Sleep apnea and sleep. http://www.sleepfoundation.org/article/sleep-related-problems/obstructive-sleep-apnea-and-sleep.

National Sleep Foundation. (2012). http://www.sleepfoundation.org.

Nurmine, T. (1998). Shiftwork and reproductive health. *Scandinavian Journal of Work Environment*, *24* (Suppl. 3), 28–34.

Vila, B. (2000). *Tired cops: The importance of managing police fatigue.* Washington, DC: Police Executive Research Forum.

Violanti, J. (2011). Shift work may be hazardous to your health. *The Jimston Journal.* http://www.jimstonjournal.com/id136.html.

Violanti, J.M., Andrew, M., Burchfiel, C.M., Hartley, T.A., Charles, L.E., et al. (2007). Post-traumatic stress symptoms and cortisol patterns among police officers. *Policing: An International Journal of Police Strategies & Management*, *30*(2): 189–202.

Violanti, J.M., Burchfiel, C.M., Hartley, T.A., Mnatsakanova, A., Fekedulegn, D., et al. (2009). Atypical work hours and metabolic syndrome among police officers. *Archives of Environmental & Occupational Health*, *64*(3), 194–201.

Waters, J., & Ussery, W. (2007). Police stress: History, contributing factors, symptoms and interventions. *Policing: An International Journal of Police Strategies & Management*, *30*(2), 169–189.

Wedderburn, A.A.I., & King, C. (1996). *Shiftworkers' health: Evaluation of a self-help guidebook. The shiftworker's guide.* Edinburgh: Heriot-Watt University.

14

Common Injuries

LEARNING OBJECTIVES

After completing this chapter, you should be able to:

- Explain the causes, and the signs and symptoms, of common musculoskeletal injuries.
- Describe the treatments that are available for common musculoskeletal injuries.
- Describe delayed-onset muscle soreness (DOMS), its prevention, and its treatment.
- Explain the signs and symptoms of heat- and cold-related injuries.
- Understand the risks associated with heat- and cold-related injuries.
- Describe treatments for heat- and cold-related injuries.

OVERVIEW

Exercise-related injuries can be painful and frustrating. They always seem to happen when we're the most motivated to participate in an exercise program. It's no secret why this happens—people who have not exercised for a long time try to push their body past a safe level in an attempt to get back what they had. Many people try to achieve their training goals in too short a period of time. Some people leave training for the BFOR test to just weeks before it's scheduled to take place. Overtraining has resulted in many injuries. This chapter looks at various injuries, their causes, and treatments for them.

General Treatments for Musculoskeletal Injuries

Many sport injuries are the result of too much, too soon. By overdoing it, you increase your risk for sprained joints, strained muscles, and other minor musculoskeletal injuries. One important but simple way to decrease your risk of injury is to make sure that you warm up properly before exercising or doing sports and cool down after. A good warm-up consists of performing your regular activity at a lesser intensity. (Refer to the *Fit for Duty, Fit for Life Training Guide*, which accompanies this textbook, for more information.) Remember that there is a difference between feeling uncomfortable because you are out of shape and being in pain. Don't believe that "no pain, no gain" is true. Trying to exercise through pain will likely just cause an injury or make an existing injury worse.

General treatment for a musculoskeletal injury involves backing off. Proper care during the first day or two after the injury may reduce the time it takes to heal. Remember that even though something may hurt only slightly while you are exercising, it may get worse when you stop. Endorphins, a chemical released by the brain during exercise, tend to dull the sensation of pain. After an injury occurs, the damaged area may bleed (internally or externally) and become inflamed. Healing starts as collagen, the primary component of scar tissue, replaces the damaged tissue. In order for an individual to return to the activity, ideally, the scar tissue should be completely repaired. In the case of acute musculoskeletal injuries, follow the RICE principle.

The RICE Principle

The RICE principle (rest, ice, compression, and elevation) is immediate, simple treatment for a musculoskeletal injury. You can ease pain and assist the healing process if you act quickly. If you are unsure of the extent of your injury, keep the affected part of your body immobilized, follow the RICE principle, and seek medical help as soon as possible.

Rest

Reduce regular exercise or daily activities as needed. Rest is important to protect the injured muscle, tendon, ligament, or other tissue from further damage. Rest is also important in order to conserve the energy needed to heal the injury most effectively. Depending on the severity of the injury, do not put any weight on an injured area for 48 hours. If you cannot put weight on an ankle or knee, crutches may help.

Ice

To reduce swelling, apply an ice pack (a gel pack, a plastic bag of ice or snow, or a bag of frozen peas) wrapped in a towel to the injured area for 20 minutes at a time, four to eight times a day. Never put ice directly on the tissue, as it may damage your skin.

Compression

Compression of an injured ankle, knee, or wrist may help reduce swelling. You might use elastic wraps, compression bandages, special boots, air casts, or splints. Ask your doctor for advice on which one to use.

delayed-onset muscle soreness (DOMS)
soreness of muscles 12 hours or more after exercise

Elevation

If possible, keep the injured part elevated on a pillow, above the level of your heart, to help decrease swelling.

Sorting Out Muscle Soreness

Aside from the pain of muscle injuries such as strains, there are two common kinds of exercise-related muscle soreness: acute soreness, which occurs during or immediately after exercise, and **delayed-onset muscle soreness (DOMS)**, which develops 12 hours or more after exercise.

Acute muscle soreness during and immediately after exercise usually reflects simple fatigue caused by a buildup of chemical waste products (lactic acid and hydrogen ions). The discomfort will often subside after a minute or two of rest when the muscles can replace energy substrates and oxygen. Once the soreness goes away, you can usually continue exercising with no residual effects. If discomfort persists despite a rest period, stop your activity and rest the part of the body that is hurting. Don't proceed with your workout until you're able to exercise that area without pain.

DOMS after a workout is common, particularly if you aren't used to the activity. If, for example, you haven't exercised for six months, and then you suddenly jump on the treadmill for 5 kilometres and do some push-ups and sit-ups, you may feel soreness throughout much of your body the next morning. You may also notice muscle stiffness and weakness. Such symptoms are a normal response to unusual exertion and are part of an adaptation process that leads to greater strength once the muscles recover. The soreness is generally at its worst in the first two days following the activity and subsides over the next few days.

DOMS is thought to be a result of microscopic tearing of the muscle fibres. The amount of tearing depends on how hard and long you exercise and what type of exercise you do. For example, exercises in which muscles forcefully contract while they are lengthening tend to cause the most soreness. These eccentric contractions (explained in Chapter 6) provide a braking action. Examples include running

TOP TIPS ...

For Preventing and Treating DOMS

Try these tips to prevent and treat DOMS:

- Warm up and stretch the muscles that you will be using and do a few minutes of a light, low-impact aerobic activity such as walking or biking. This should help to increase blood flow to the affected muscles and help to reduce soreness.
- Build up slowly in terms of intensity, duration, and frequency of the exercise. In weight lifting, for example, start with lighter weights, fewer sets, and fewer repetitions.
- Avoid the weekend warrior approach, where you only play a pickup game of football or basketball without some type of aerobic activity during the week.
- Applying ice, gently stretching, and massaging the affected muscles can help.
- Non-steroidal anti-inflammatory medications may reduce the soreness temporarily, but they won't speed healing.
- Try yoga. There is some evidence that yoga may reduce DOMS (Boyle, Sayers, Jensen, Headley, & Manos, 2004).
- Rest. Let your muscles heal before you attempt to go back to the activity.

down stairs, running downhill, lowering weights, and performing the downward movements of squats, chin-ups, and push-ups.

In addition to microscopic tearing, swelling may take place in and around a muscle, which can contribute to delayed soreness. Such swelling increases pressure on the neighbouring structures, resulting in greater muscle pain and stiffness.

Common Sport-Related Musculoskeletal Injuries

Certain types of injuries plague sport participants. Although most are minor, knowing the early signs, symptoms, and what to do can help prevent them from becoming chronic conditions.

Sprain

sprain
a stretching or tearing injury to a ligament

A **sprain** is an injury to a ligament—a stretching or tearing. The severity of the injury depends on the extent of injury to a single ligament (whether the tear is partial or complete) and the number of ligaments involved. A sprain can result from a fall, a sudden twist, or a blow to the body that forces a joint out of its normal position. This results in overstretching or tearing of the ligament supporting that joint. Typically, sprains occur when people fall and land on an outstretched arm, slide into base, land on the side of their foot, or twist a knee with the foot planted firmly on the ground when involved in an altercation with a suspect. The three most common sites of sprains are ankles, knees, and wrists.

There are three levels of sprains:

- *Mild sprains* happen when ligaments are stretched excessively or torn slightly. They are somewhat painful, especially with movement. There is not a lot of swelling, and you can put weight on the joint.
- *Moderate sprains* occur when there is partial rupture of the fibres. The area is painful and tender. There is swelling and discolouration, and it is hard to move and bear weight on the joint.
- *Severe sprains* take place when one or more ligaments are torn. You can't put weight on the joint or move it easily. There is swelling, discolouration, and pain. It is hard to distinguish a severe sprain from a fracture or dislocation. You may need a brace to stabilize the joint, and surgery may be required to repair the ligaments.

Signs and Symptoms of a Sprain

The usual signs and symptoms of a sprain include the following:

- varying degrees of pain
- swelling
- bruising
- inability to move and use the joint

Sometimes people feel a pop or tear when the sprain happens. An X-ray may be needed to determine whether a fracture is causing the pain and swelling.

Strain

Twisting or pulling a muscle or tendon causes a **strain**. Strains can be acute or chronic. An acute strain is caused by trauma or an injury such as a blow to the body; improperly lifting heavy objects or overstressing the muscles can also cause it. Chronic strains are usually the result of overuse—prolonged, repetitive movement of the muscles and tendons.

strain
a twisting or pulling injury to a muscle or tendon

The two most common sites for a strain are the back and the hamstring muscle (located in the back of the thigh). Law enforcement officers risk injury when they go from prolonged sitting in a cruiser and then are faced with a physical confrontation or other demand on their body. Contact sports such as soccer, football, hockey, boxing, and wrestling put people at risk for strains. Gymnastics, tennis, rowing, golf, and other sports that require extensive gripping can increase the risk of hand and forearm strains. Elbow strains sometimes occur in people who participate in racquet sports, throwing, and contact sports.

Signs and Symptoms of a Strain

Signs and symptoms of a strain include the following:

- pain, muscle spasm, and muscle weakness
- localized swelling, cramping, or inflammation and, with a minor or moderate strain, usually some loss of muscle function
- pain in the injured area and general weakness of the muscle when you try to move it
- in the case of severe strains that partially or completely tear the muscle or tendon, extreme pain due to significant bleeding, swelling, and bruising around the muscle
- a complete lack of muscle function, if the muscle has been torn away completely from the bone

Treatment for Sprains and Strains

You should see a doctor about a sprain or strain if you have severe pain, you cannot move the joint, it is tender to touch, there are lumps and bumps (other than swelling), you are experiencing numbness, and you cannot put any weight on the injured joint. You may see redness or red streaks spreading out from the injury.

Treatment for sprains and strains is similar and can be thought of as having two stages. The goal during the first stage is to reduce swelling and pain. At this stage, doctors usually advise patients to follow the RICE formula (rest, ice, compression, and elevation) for the first 24–48 hours after the injury. A doctor may prescribe a non-steroidal anti-inflammatory drug, such as acetylsalicylic acid (Aspirin®, Entrophen®) or ibuprofen (Advil®, Motrin®), to help decrease pain and inflammation.

For people with a moderate or severe sprain, particularly of the ankle, a hard cast may be applied. Severe sprains and strains may require surgery to repair the torn ligaments, muscles, or tendons.

The second stage of treating a sprain or strain is rehabilitation, whose overall goal is to improve the condition of the injured part and restore its function. An exercise program designed to prevent stiffness, improve range of motion, and restore the joint's normal flexibility and strength is key. Some people may need physical therapy during this stage.

Tendinitis, Impingement Syndrome, and Bursitis of the Shoulder

These conditions are closely related and may occur alone or in combination. Repeated motion involving the arms, or the aging process, may irritate and wear down the tendons, muscles, and surrounding structures.

tendinitis
inflammation of a tendon

Tendinitis is inflammation (redness, soreness, and swelling) of a tendon. In tendinitis of the shoulder, the rotator cuff (the group of muscles that surround the shoulder) and/or biceps tendon become inflamed, usually as a result of being pinched by surrounding structures. The injury may vary from mild to severe inflammation.

When the rotator cuff tendon becomes inflamed and thickened, it may get trapped under the outer edge of the shoulder blade, where the collarbone is attached. Squeezing of the rotator cuff is called **impingement syndrome**. If left untreated, the muscle can actually tear in two, resulting in a rotator cuff tear.

impingement syndrome
squeezing of the rotator cuff (the group of muscles that surrounds the shoulder)

bursitis
inflammation of a bursa (a sac of fluid near a joint)

Tendinitis and impingement syndrome are often accompanied by inflammation of the bursa sacs (sacs of fluid near joints) that protect the shoulder. An inflamed bursa is called **bursitis**. Inflammation caused by a disease such as rheumatoid arthritis may cause rotator cuff tendinitis and bursitis. Sports that involve overuse of the shoulder and occupations that require frequent overhead reaching are other potential causes of irritation to the rotator cuff or bursae, and may lead to inflammation and impingement.

Signs and Symptoms

Signs and symptoms of tendinitis, impingement syndrome, and bursitis of the shoulder include the following:

- the slow onset of discomfort and pain in the upper shoulder or upper third of the arm
- difficulty sleeping on the shoulder
- pain when the arm is lifted away from the body or overhead (such as when trying to put on a coat)
- if tendinitis involves the biceps tendon (the tendon located in front of the shoulder that helps bend the elbow and turn the forearm), pain in the front or side of the shoulder that may travel down to the elbow and forearm (pain may also occur when the arm is forcefully pushed upward)
- when the rotator cuff tears, significant weakness, making it difficult for the person to elevate his or her arm

Treatment

These injuries are treated with rest, ice, and anti-inflammatory medicines. In some cases, the doctor or therapist will use ultrasound (gentle sound wave vibrations) to warm deep tissues and improve blood flow. Gentle stretching and strengthening exercises are added gradually, preceded or followed by use of an ice pack. If there is no improvement, the doctor may inject a corticosteroid medicine into the space under the acromion (these injections must be used with caution because they may lead to tendon rupture). Severe cases may need surgery to repair damage and relieve pressure on the tendons and bursae.

Dislocated Shoulder

As shown in Figure 14.1, the shoulder comprises a large number of muscles, tendons, and bones that work together to provide movement, structure, and strength. Fifteen muscles move and stabilize the scapula. Nine muscles stabilize the gleno-humeral joint, and six muscles support the scapula on the thorax. The rotator cuff is made up of a group of four muscles (supraspinatus, infraspinatus, teres minor, and subscapularis) that support the shoulder joint. The muscles attach to the skeletal elements by tendons. The rotator cuff stabilizes the gleno-humeral joint to provide rotation, elevation, depression, protraction, and retraction.

A dislocation of the shoulder joint happens when the ball of the joint (the end of the arm bone, or humerus) and the socket (part of your shoulder blade, or scapula) making up the shoulder move apart. When the ball part of the joint is dislocated in front of the socket, it is called an anterior dislocation, the most common type. When it is dislocated behind the socket, it is called a posterior dislocation. In severe cases, ligaments, tendons, and nerves also can be stretched and injured.

An anterior dislocation can be caused by a fall onto your outstretched hand or onto the shoulder itself. A posterior dislocation may occur as a result of a powerful direct blow to the front of your shoulder. A violent twisting of your upper arm, such as that caused by an electric shock or seizure, may also cause it. Dislocated shoulders are common in contact sports such as football, rugby, hockey, and lacrosse. Other sports that may cause the injury include downhill skiing, volleyball, and soccer. In law enforcement, officers sometimes deal with altercations where someone is pulling at their arms or aggressively pushing or punching.

Signs and Symptoms

Signs and symptoms of a dislocated shoulder include the following:

- pain in the shoulder and upper arm that is made worse by movement
- shoulder instability and deformation
- shoulder tenderness and weakness
- possible numbness in the shoulder area, arm, or hand

Treatment

Put ice on the shoulder immediately to reduce swelling caused by internal bleeding and the buildup of fluids in and around the injured area, and put the arm in a sling. See a doctor to reposition the head or ball of the joint back into the joint socket. The doctor may give you a prescription for pain, a muscle relaxant, and anti-inflammatory medication. If your shoulder joint becomes weak because of repeated dislocations, your doctor may recommend an operation to tighten the ligaments that hold the joint together. The healing process may take 4–12 weeks, depending

FIGURE 14.1 Shoulder Joint

The shoulder joint is the most frequently dislocated joint in the body. It occurs when an impact or force moves the shoulder outward (abduction) or forces extreme rotation of the head of the humerus, causing it to pop out of the socket.

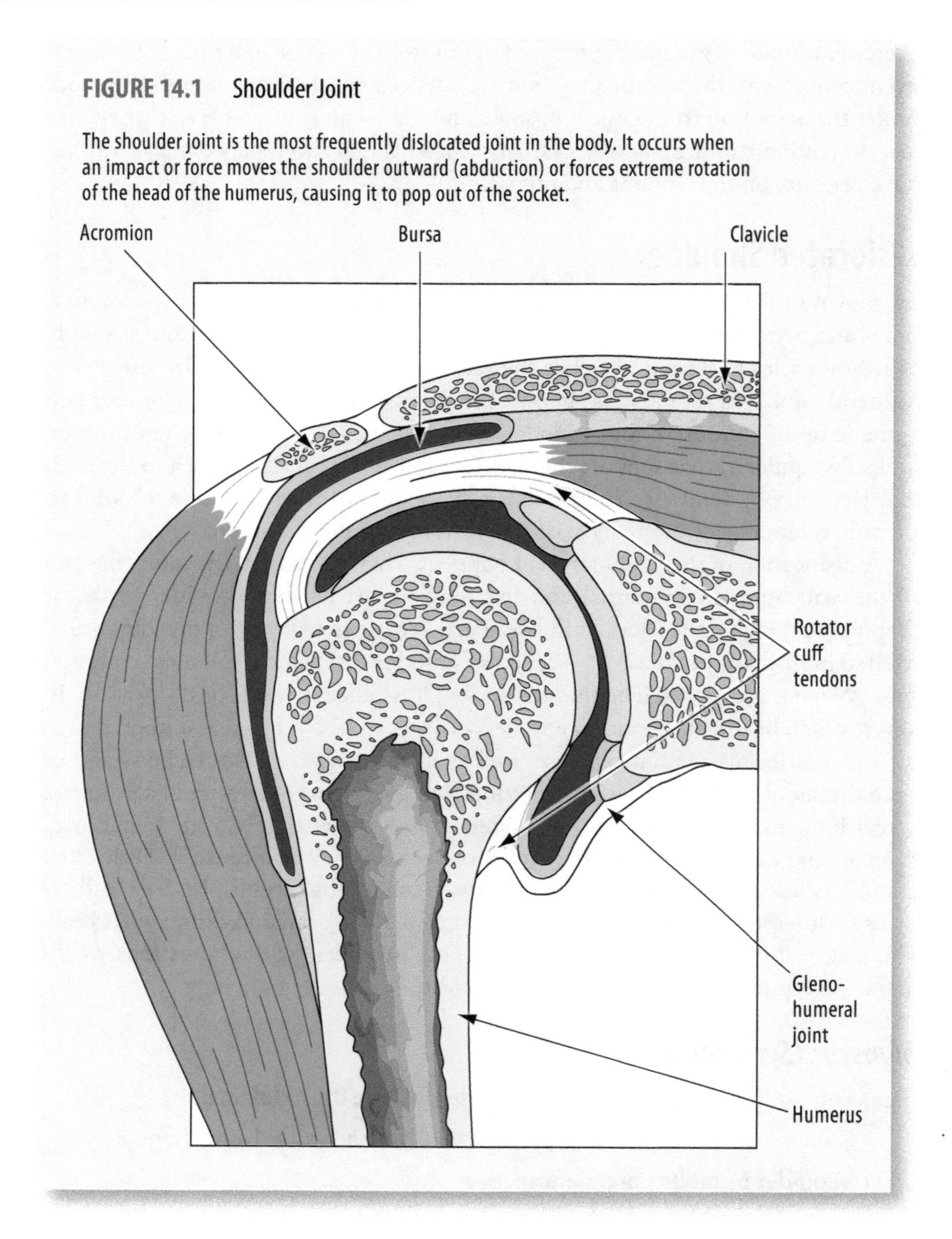

DID YOU KNOW?

In Ontario, common musculoskeletal injuries account for 42 percent of all lost-time claims, 42 percent of all lost-time claim costs, and 50 percent of all lost-time days on the job.

SOURCE: OHSCO, 2007.

on the extent of your injury. With proper healing and rehabilitation exercise, you should regain full movement of your shoulder.

Broken Ribs

A broken or fractured rib is a common injury when there is trauma to the chest, such as from a fall, a motor vehicle accident, or an impact during an altercation with a suspect. People who have weak bones (for example, from osteoporosis) have greater risk of ribs breaking when there is strain on the rib cage, such as during a strong coughing spell. The risk of injury also increases with age due to lessening elasticity of the ribs.

Signs and Symptoms

When ribs are broken, it is very difficult to take a deep breath. Pain is worse when you press on the injured area or when you bend, twist, or attempt physical exertion. Complications can include puncturing the lungs and surrounding tissue, which can cause blood (hemothorax) or air (pneumothorax) to accumulate between the lungs and the walls of the chest. Depending on the amount of blood or air in the pleural cavity (the closed space that surrounds the lungs), a collapsed lung can result, leading to respiratory and hemodynamic failure (tension pneumothorax), which can be life-threatening. Treatment involves stopping the bleeding, removing the blood or air in the pleural space, and re-expanding the lung.

Treatment

It is very important to rest broken ribs, and to use ice for pain and swelling. Over-the-counter pain medication, including acetaminophen (Tylenol®) and non-steroidal anti-inflammatory drugs such as ibuprofen (Advil®, Motrin®), can help relieve discomfort while ribs heal. Doctors usually do not recommend compression wraps, as they increase the likelihood of respiratory complications (such as pneumonia). It can take upward of two months for ribs to heal.

Patello-Femoral Syndrome (Chondromalacia Patella)

Patello-femoral syndrome, or chondromalacia (KON-dro-mah-LAY-she-ah, the old term), refers to softening of the kneecap cartilage. This disorder occurs most often in young adults, especially females, and can be caused by injury, overuse, parts out of alignment, or muscle weakness in the inner thigh. Instead of gliding smoothly across the lower end of the thigh bone, the kneecap rubs against it, roughening the cartilage underneath the kneecap (Figure 14.2). The damage may range from a slightly abnormal surface of the cartilage to a surface that has been worn away to the bone. It is the result of muscle tightness in the calf, hamstring, or other muscles. The disorder is common in runners and is also seen in skiers, cyclists, and soccer players.

Signs and Symptoms

Signs and symptoms of patello-femoral syndrome include the following:

- dull pain around or under the kneecap that worsens when walking down stairs or hills
- pain when climbing stairs or when the knee bears weight as it straightens
- grinding and clicking in the knee

Treatment

Apply the RICE formula (rest, ice, compression, and elevation). Perform low-impact exercises that strengthen muscles, particularly the muscles in the inner part of the quadriceps, without injuring joints and as long as the knee doesn't bend more than 90 degrees. Tape the knee to keep the kneecap in line. Electrical stimulation may also be used to strengthen the muscles. Arthroscopic surgery may be used to smooth the surface of the cartilage and "wash out" the cartilage fragments that

FIGURE 14.2 Patello-Femoral Syndrome

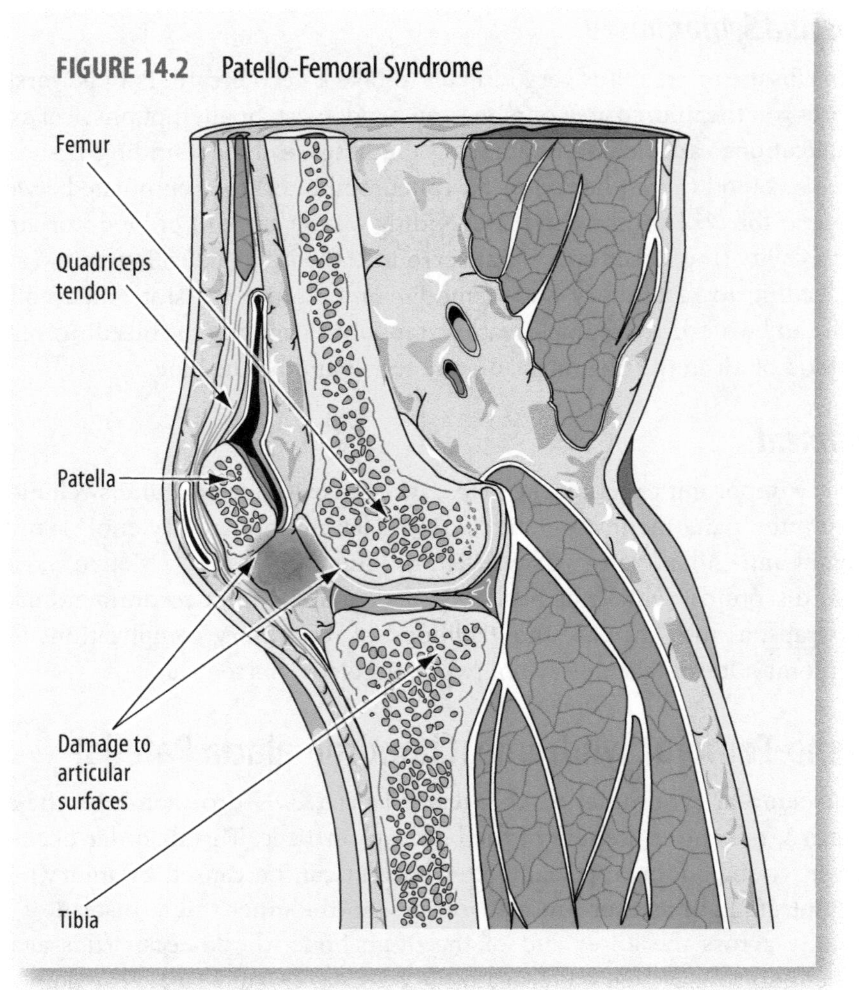

cause the joint to catch during bending and straightening. In more severe cases, more invasive surgery may be necessary to correct the angle of the kneecap and relieve friction with the cartilage or to reposition parts that are out of alignment.

Shin Splints (Tibial Stress Syndrome)

Shin splints are pain along the shin (tibia) and are commonly seen as an overuse injury in runners (Figure 14.3). They usually develop gradually over a period of weeks to months, but may occur after a single excessive bout of exercise.

Shin splints can be caused by running on the insides of your feet. They often occur in both legs. This usually happens when someone is beginning a running program, doing excessive downhill running, or engaging in sports that require rapid starts and stops which cause damage to the muscle, resulting in pain.

Signs and Symptoms

Signs and symptoms of shin splints include the following:

- pain on the side of the shin and the back of the calf (often experienced by runners)
- noticeable pain when exercise starts, which then decreases or goes away as exercise continues; worse after exercise stops or the following morning

Treatment

Rest. This means dramatically decreasing both the frequency and the duration of exercise and increasing (doubling or tripling) the time between workouts. Put ice directly on the sore area. Massage the muscles that are affected. A doctor may prescribe anti-inflammatory medications. If the shin splints are caused by the way your feet turn in when you walk or run (overpronation or flat feet), you may need a good arch support in the form of an orthotic (a shoe insert that corrects the alignment of the foot). Changing your running shoes every 800 kilometres is another good idea.

FIGURE 14.3 Shin Splints

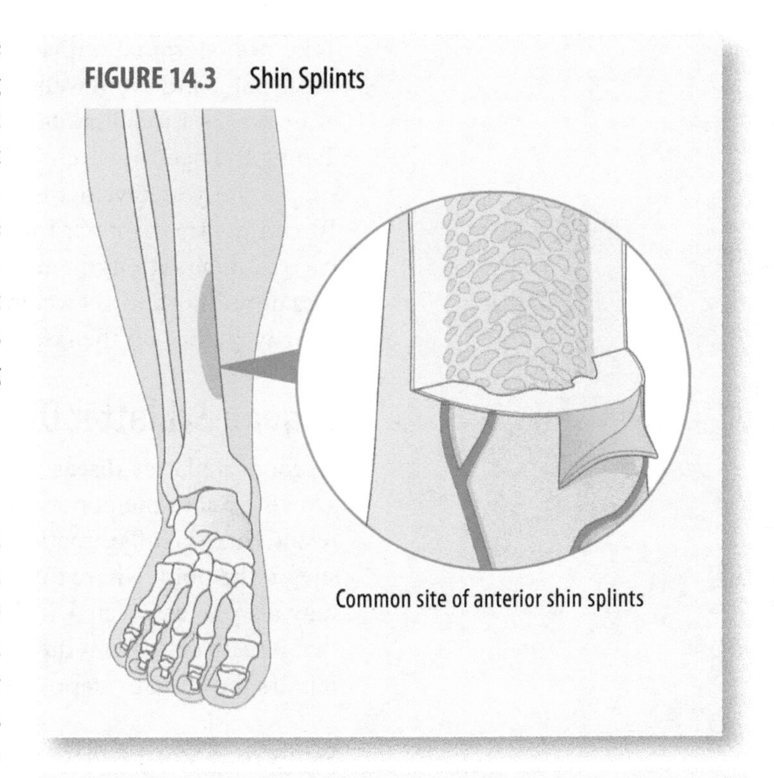

Plantar Fasciitis

Plantar fasciitis is the most common cause of pain on the bottom of the heel (Figure 14.4). The fascia, a thin strip of tissue at the bottom of the foot, stretches to the point of developing small tears. Pain occurs with the onset of activity such as walking and running, or even the first few morning steps. The pain subsides as the activity progresses, and usually returns after resting and then resuming activity.

Plantar fasciitis is considered a chronic inflammatory response. It is common in runners, who repetitively flex their feet and toes. It is also common in people who experience sudden weight gain. Shoes with poor cushioning can contribute to the tearing of the fascia. People who work in occupations that require prolonged standing or weight-bearing activities may strain the fascia. The leather boots that law enforcement officers used to wear had no cushioning or arch support, which led to frequent occurences of this injury. Directing traffic or walking the beat for extended periods of time can contribute to this condition.

FIGURE 16.4 Plantar Fasciitis

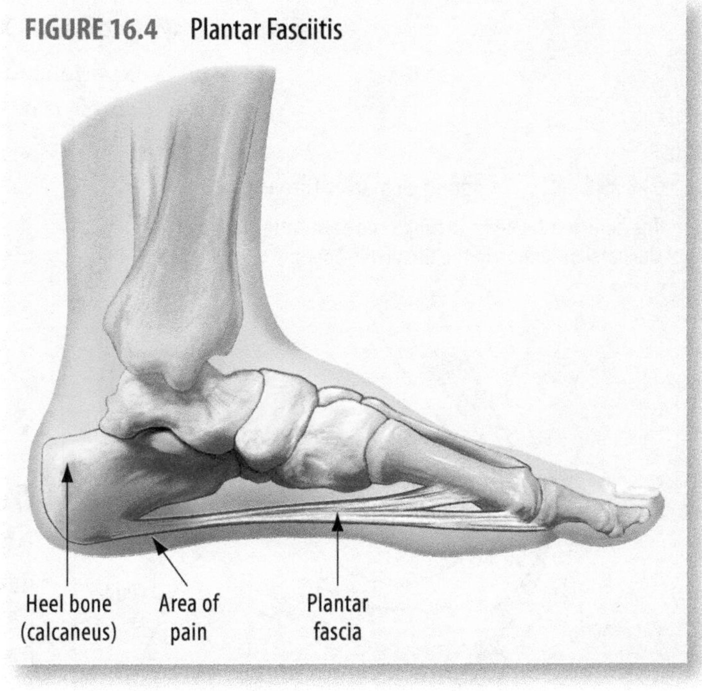

Signs and Symptoms

Signs and symptoms of plantar fasciitis include the following:

- heel pain that is at its worst during the first steps of the morning
- pain at the start of exercise and when exercise is resumed after resting
- tight Achilles tendon
- sometimes a heel spur (a calcium deposit on the bottom of the heel), but it is typically not a cause

Treatment

Take non-steroidal anti-inflammatory drugs (ask a doctor). Avoid activities that cause pain, and avoid walking barefoot on hard surfaces. Lose weight if your weight is a cause of the injury. Stretch the heel cord (Achilles tendon) and plantar fascia. Taping the heel and arch may also help to reduce pain. You may need to wear arch supports if you have flat feet. Massaging the fascia by rolling your foot over a 7- to 10-centimetre diameter tube, such as a rolling pin or soup can, has been an effective treatment. Strengthening exercises include scrunching up a hand towel with the toes or pulling a towel weighted with a soup can across the floor. After any physical activity, put ice on the fascia. Buy proper footwear with arch support.

Osgood-Schlatter Disease

Osgood-Schlatter disease is caused by repetitive stress or tension on part of the growth area of the upper tibia (the leg bone between the knee and the ankle). As a result, there is inflammation of the tendon in the kneecap and surrounding soft tissues at the point where the tendon is attached to the tibia (Figure 14.5). The disease may also be associated with an injury in which the tendon is stretched so much that it tears away from the tibia and takes a fragment of bone with it. The body then repairs the bone by depositing calcium, which results in a buildup of bone.

Signs and Symptoms

Signs and symptoms of Osgood-Schlatter disease include the following:

- Pain is experienced just below the knee joint; the pain usually worsens with activity and is relieved by rest.
- A bony bump that is particularly painful when pressed may appear on the upper edge of the tibia, below the kneecap. Although knee motion is usually not affected, it can be very difficult to kneel or sit on your knees.
- Pain may last a few months and may recur until the individual's growth is completed. Teens are especially prone to the pain, which can carry on into their 20s.
- X-rays show that the growth area is in fragments.

FIGURE 14.5 Osgood-Schlatter Disease

The bone is inflamed and broken up at the attachment of the patellar tendon to the tibia (shin bone).

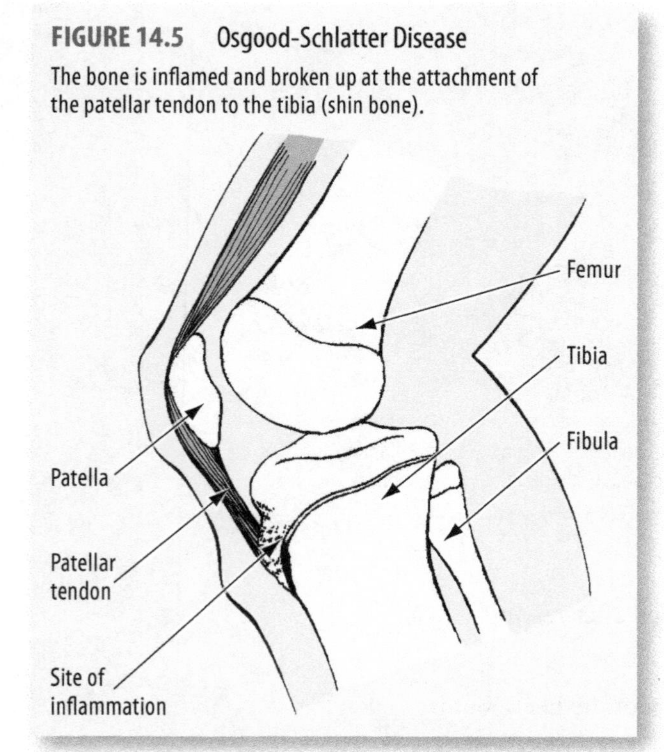

Treatment

When pain begins, apply ice to the knee to help relieve inflammation. Do stretching and strengthening exercises, and limit your participation in vigorous sports. Wear knee pads for protection when you are taking part in sports, and apply ice to the knee afterward.

Iliotibial Band Syndrome

Iliotibial band (ITB) syndrome is an overuse condition in which inflammation results when a band of a tendon rubs over the outer bone of the knee (Figure 14.6). Although ITB syndrome may be caused by direct injury to the knee, it is most often caused by the stress of long-term overuse, such as sometimes occurs in sports training.

FIGURE 14.6
Iliotibial Band Syndrome (side view)
The iliotibial band runs down the thigh, stabilizing the knee, but continual rubbing of the band over the lateral femoral epicondyle causes inflammation.

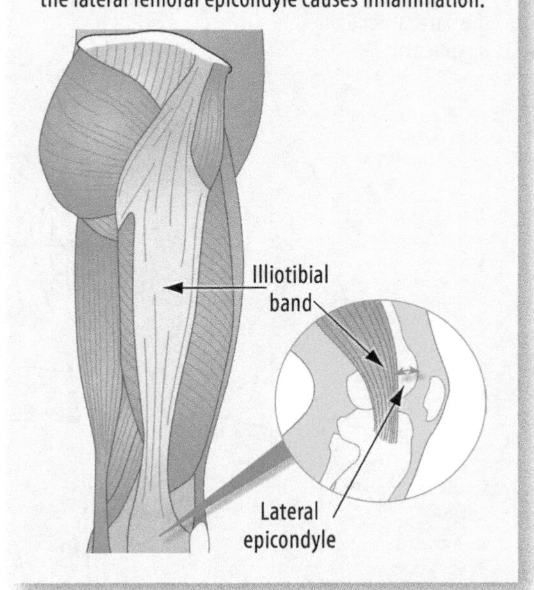

Signs and Symptoms

Signs and symptoms of iliotibial band syndrome include the following:

- ache or burning sensation at the outer side of the knee during activity
- pain at the side of the knee or radiating up the side of the thigh
- a snap felt when the knee is bent and then straightened

Note that there is usually no swelling and knee motion is normal.

Treatment

Reduce activity and do stretching exercises followed by muscle-strengthening exercises. In rare cases, when the syndrome doesn't disappear, surgery may be necessary to split the tendon so that it isn't stretched too tightly over the bone.

Ligament Injuries of the Knee

Four ligaments connect the leg bones and give the knee joint strength and stability (Figure 14.7):

1. the medial collateral ligament (MCL), which provides stability to the inner (medial) part of the knee
2. the lateral collateral ligament (LCL), which provides stability to the outer (lateral) part of the knee
3. the anterior cruciate ligament (ACL), in the centre of the knee, which limits rotation and the forward movement of the tibia (the shin bone)
4. the posterior cruciate ligament (PCL), also in the centre of the knee, which limits backward movement of the tibia

The ACL is most often stretched, torn, or both (that is, sprained) by a sudden twisting motion (for example, when the feet are planted one way and the knees are turned another). This can happen when you stretch your upper torso while keeping your legs planted, such as when an officer must drag someone out of a car. The PCL is most often injured by a direct impact, such as in an automobile accident (trying to brake) or a football tackle. The MCL is more easily injured than the LCL. The cause is most often a blow to the outer side of the knee that stretches and tears the ligament on the inner side of the knee. Such blows frequently occur in contact sports like football or hockey. In law enforcement, they can occur during altercations or when performing self-defence manoeuvres.

FIGURE 14.7 Ligaments of the Knee

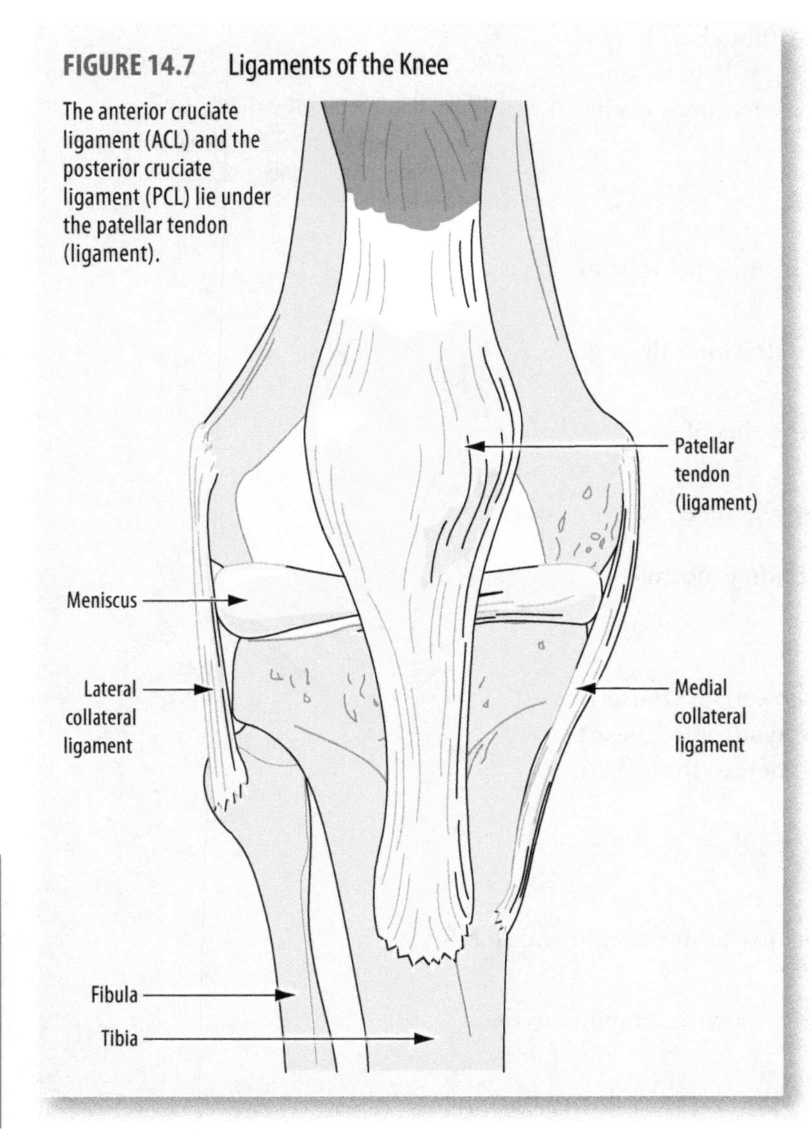

Signs and Symptoms

Signs and symptoms of ligament injuries of the knee include the following:

- a popping sound
- swelling
- leg buckling when you try to stand
- top part of leg moves while lower leg remains stationary

Note that there may or may not be pain, depending on which ligament is injured.

Treatment

Immediate treatment includes the RICE approach. If there is an incomplete tear, an exercise program can strengthen the surrounding muscles. You may need to wear a brace to protect the knee during activity. You may also need surgery to reattach or reconstruct a ligament that is completely torn.

Injuries to the Meniscus

Separating the bones of the knee are pads of connective tissue called the menisci (muh-NISS-sky), or meniscus (muh-NISS-kus) in the singular. The menisci are divided into two crescent-shaped discs positioned between the leg bones on the outer and inner sides of each knee. They act like shock absorbers, cushioning the lower part of the leg from the weight of the rest of the body, as well as enhancing stability. (The removal of all four of former hockey player Bobby Orr's menisci, one at a time, left his knees unstable, which eventually led to his retirement from hockey.)

Through degeneration over time or too much concentrated force, the meniscus can be torn, as shown in Figure 14.8. The entire rim of the medial meniscus can be torn. Symptoms include pain along the joint line and locking of the leg as it is extended and pulled back. In essence, the knee locks so that it cannot be straightened or fully bent. Swelling occurs as synovial fluid (fluid the body sends as part of an immune response) rushes to the area in response to the deterioration on the surface.

Signs and Symptoms

Signs and symptoms of injuries to the meniscus include the following:

- There may be some pain, particularly when the knee is straightened. If the pain is mild, the person may continue moving. Severe pain may occur if a fragment of the meniscus catches between the leg bones.

- Swelling may occur soon after injury if blood vessels are disrupted, or swelling may occur several hours later if the joint fills with fluid produced by the joint lining as a result of inflammation.
- The knee may click, lock, or feel weak, and pain is persistent.
- On examination, when the leg is rotated outward and inward while extended, there is pain and audible clicking, suggesting a tear. An MRI scan can confirm this.

FIGURE 14.8 Injuries to the Meniscus

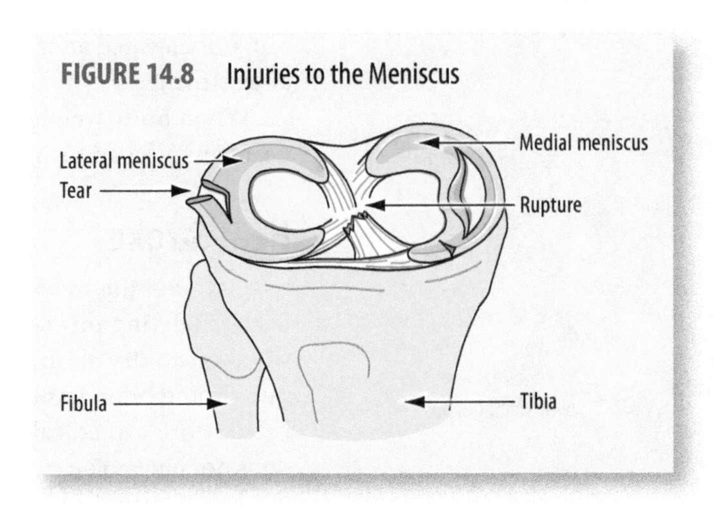

Treatment

Immediate treatment includes the RICE approach for sprains. Muscle-strengthening programs for the knee (quadriceps and hamstrings) can help. Surgery may be needed to repair the tear if there is good blood supply to the area. If the blood supply is poor, parts of the meniscus, or the entire meniscus, may need to be removed. Artificial meniscus replacement has met with limited success to date.

Heat-Related Injuries and Illnesses

Heat-related injuries have become a huge issue in athletics. In recent summers, a number of athletes have died due to heat-related injuries. You need to be aware of the symptoms. If you do volunteer work with children's sports teams, be especially vigilant, because children's body temperatures easily fluctuate and they can quickly suffer from heat-related injuries.

Heat Cramps

Heat cramps are caused by a deficiency of water and sodium and feel like severe muscle pulls. They occur in worked muscles after exertion, often after profuse sweating and drinking water without adequate electrolyte replacement. Heat cramps cause painful muscle contractions (for example, in the hamstring area). They are usually not life-threatening, but ignoring them can lead to more serious heat-related illnesses. Treatment for heat cramps includes water, cool air, and rest.

heat cramps
illness caused by a water and sodium deficiency; heat cramps feel like severe muscle pulls

Heat Exhaustion

Heat exhaustion is caused by extreme body heat. Excessive heat (a hot environment) and dehydration can cause the body to overreact, thus raising your body temperature to 38–40 °C (102–104 °F). Sweating still occurs. Symptoms of heat exhaustion include paleness, nausea, extreme fatigue, dizziness, light-headedness, vomiting, fainting, and cool, clammy skin. Heat exhaustion is a serious illness and should be carefully monitored.

heat exhaustion
illness caused by extreme body heat; excessive heat and dehydration can raise body temperature to 38–40 °C (100–104 °F)

Treatment includes a cool, shady environment; liquids; cool rags or ice packs placed on various areas of the body; and replacement of electrolytes (such as those found in sports drinks). Make sure there is good ventilation. If body temperature remains elevated after treatment or the person is continually vomiting, seek medical treatment.

When body weight drops 1–2 percent (0.7–1.4 kg in a 70-kg person), exercise performance can be impaired and heat exhaustion becomes a possibility.

Heat Stroke

heat stroke
illness caused by failure of the body's heat-regulating mechanism; may lead to permanent disability or death

Heat stroke, the most severe form of heat-related illness, occurs when the body's heat-regulating mechanism fails. Body temperature may be above 40 °C (104 °F), with warm, dry skin. The very high body temperature damages tissues, including muscle and brain tissue. Heat stroke may lead to permanent disability or death, and is therefore a medical emergency. Unlike other forms of heat illness, heat stroke does not have to be caused by exercise or exertion. High temperatures, lack of body fluids, and overexposure to the elements can all bring about heat stroke. Very young and very old people are particularly susceptible to the hazards of this illness, especially those playing sports. Symptoms include a red, flushed face; a body temperature of 40 °C (104 °F) or higher; headache; rapid pulse; and unconsciousness.

Anyone exhibiting the signs and symptoms of heat stroke should be rushed to the nearest hospital or clinic. Treat the person with water, cool down his or her body by ventilating the area (fan or windows down in car), and remove any tight clothing and head covering from the person en route to medical treatment. The person may need fluids pumped into his or her body for rehydration.

Preventing Heat-Related Injuries

Sweating is your body's main system for getting rid of extra heat. When you sweat, water evaporates from your skin. The heat that evaporates the sweat comes mainly from your skin.

As long as blood is flowing properly to your skin, extra heat from the core of your body is "pumped" to the surface and removed by sweat evaporation. If you do not have good blood flow or do not sweat enough, you cannot get rid of extra heat well. If you are dehydrated, you won't sweat as much, and your body will try to keep blood away from the skin to keep your blood pressure at the right level in the core of your body (your other organs get the needed fluid first). Because you lose water when you sweat, you must make up that water to keep from becoming dehydrated. If the air is humid, it's harder for your sweat to evaporate. This means that your body cannot get rid of extra heat as well when the weather is muggy, compared to when the air is dry. This factor is an issue in southern Ontario, where the summers are very humid. Here are some ways to prevent heat injuries and illnesses:

- Drink. Staying hydrated is key. Sport drinks are a good choice, but water works fine. As you become heat-acclimatized, you will sweat more, so you will need more fluids. Two to three hours before exercising, you should drink 500–600 millilitres of fluid, with another 200–300 millilitres 10–20 minutes before the event. You should be drinking 200–300 millilitres every 10–15 minutes during the event. Post-exercise hydration, or rehydration, should aim to correct any fluid loss accumulated during the practice or event. Ideally completed within two hours, rehydration should contain water to restore hydration status, carbohydrates to replenish glycogen stores, and electrolytes to speed rehydration. The primary goal is the immediate return of physiologic function. When rehydration must be quick, you need to replace sweat and urine losses by drinking 25–50 percent more than what was lost to sweat. That means upward of 500 millilitres for every half-kilogram of weight loss within two hours of finishing training or competition to be at optimal hydration four to six hours after the event (Casa, Armstrong, & Hillman, 2000).

- Keep ventilation going (fan, air conditioner).
- Wear light-coloured, loose-fitting clothing (an issue with sports like football).
- Wear a hat outdoors.
- Limit your activity in hot, humid conditions.

Under Ontario's *Occupational Health and Safety Act*, employers and employees are required to take every precaution reasonable in the circumstances for the protection of workers. For example, law enforcement officers are issued baseball caps and sunscreen to help reduce the effects of heat. For more information, see Ministry of Labour (2011) (in References).

FYI

Recognizing Dehydration in Individuals

There are signs and symptoms of dehydration that you can watch for. If you identify the condition early enough, you can limit the degree of heat-related illness.

- Early signs and symptoms include thirst, general discomfort, and irritability, followed by flushed skin, weariness, cramps, and apathy.
- Greater water deficits result in dizziness, headaches, vomiting, nausea, heat sensations on the head or neck, and decreased performance.
- Dyspnea (difficult or laboured breathing) may also be present.

SOURCE: American College of Sports Medicine, 1996; Armstrong & Maresh, 1993.

Cold-Related Injuries and Illnesses

Under most conditions, your body is able to maintain a healthy temperature. But when you are exposed to a cold environment, if you are not dressed appropriately, more heat can escape from your body than you can produce. When the body's control mechanism can no longer maintain normal body temperature, **hypothermia** can set in. Prolonged exposure in cases such as directing traffic in January, overseeing an accident on the highway, or tracking a lost skier may lead to deadly results. Hypothermia can also happen on cool days when it is wet and windy, because evaporation from your skin helps to lower your core temperature.

hypothermia
condition occurring when the body's control mechanism can no longer maintain a normal body temperature, and the body's temperature drops to an abnormally low level

Who Is at Risk?

Hypothermia usually comes on gradually. At first, your body shivers (muscles contract) in an attempt to generate heat. Then, as your nervous system is affected, you begin to mumble, fumble, grumble, and stumble. You may lose consciousness and experience loss of fine motor coordination. Additional signs and symptoms include slurred speech, slowed breathing, cold, pale skin, and fatigue that is accompanied by lethargy or apathy. If not dealt with, severe hypothermia can lead to cardiac and respiratory failure and, ultimately, death.

In addition, people who have spent prolonged periods of time in cold environments or cool, wet, and windy environments; who are very young or very old; or who are substance abusers, have impaired mental status, or have been immersed in cold water, are at increased risk for hypothermia.

One-sixth of Ontario's terrain is covered with lakes, rivers, and streams (Encyclopedia of Canadian Provinces, 2007). Many officers are called upon to assist and rescue individuals who have fallen into the water. Immersion in cold water numbs the extremities quickly to the point that the individual cannot grasp rescue lines, fasten lifejacket straps, or hang on to an object such as a boat. Shivering and the sensation of cold begin when the body temperature decreases from the normal temperature of 37 °C (98.6 °F) to approximately 35.8 °C (96.5 °F). Amnesia can start at approximately 35 °C (95 °F), unconsciousness at 30 °C (86 °F), and death at approximately 26.1 °C (79 °F) (US Search and Rescue Task Force, n.d.). Although it is imperative to get out of the water as soon as possible, physical exertion causes the body to lose heat at a fast rate, because blood is being sent to the extremities and quickly cooled. Survival time can be shortened by more than 50 percent (US Search and Rescue Task Force, n.d.). See Table 14.1 for expected survival times for prolonged exposure to cold water.

DID YOU KNOW?

Cold water robs the body of its heat 32 times faster than cold air.

TABLE 14.1 Expected Survival Time in Cold Water

WATER TEMPERATURE	EXHAUSTION OR UNCONSCIOUSNESS	EXPECTED SURVIVAL TIME
21–27 °C (70–80 °F)	3–12 hours	3 hours to indefinitely
16–21 °C (60–70 °F)	2–7 hours	2–40 hours
10–16 °C (50–60 °F)	1–2 hours	1–6 hours
4–10 °C (40–50 °F)	30–60 minutes	1–3 hours
0–4 °C (32.5–40 °F)	15–30 minutes	30–90 minutes
<0 °C (<32 °F)	under 15 minutes	under 15–45 minutes

SOURCE: US Search and Rescue Task Force, n.d.

Signs and Symptoms of a Cold-Water Drowning Victim

Typical symptoms include the following:

- cyanotic (blue) skin colouration
- pupils fully dilated (opened)
- no detectable breathing
- no apparent pulse or heartbeat

In spite of these symptoms, remember that heart rates can go down to as little as six to eight beats per minute (diving reflex). So it is important to try resuscitation efforts in accordance with your CPR training.

First Aid Considerations for Cold-Water Victims

It is important to treat hypothermia as quickly as possible. Some treatments include the following:

- Remove wet clothes and replace with dry clothes or blankets.
- Use the rescuer's body heat if nothing else is available.
- Avoid massaging the extremities.
- Lay the semi-conscious person face up with his or her head slightly lowered to get oxygen to the brain.
- Rewarm the body in a bath of 40.5–43.3 °C (105–110 °F), but keep the arms and legs out to prevent cold blood from limbs cooling the core temperature any further. If a tub is not available, use hot, wet towels or blankets on the victim's head, neck, chest, groin, and abdomen, avoiding warming the arms or legs.
- Begin CPR if there is no discernible pulse or breathing.

Exercising in Cold Temperatures

As long as we maintain core temperature, it is rarely too cold to exercise. In cold conditions, although we can wear scarves to warm inhaled air, most times the air will naturally warm up to a safe temperature by the time it reaches the lungs. Aerobic exercise helps to maintain core temperature by producing three-quarters of the energy in the form of heat. Aerobic capacity is not adversely affected as long as core temperature is maintained. If we stand around for long periods of time, or stop exercising but stay outside, the cold air begins to affect our body.

As core temperature drops, muscles set off a greater anaerobic metabolism, producing more lactic acid and associated muscle burn in an attempt to maintain core temperature. This results in an overall reduction in the strength and power that can be produced by the muscle tissue in severely cold weather. Combined with cold water in the form of rain, hail, or snow, along with fatigue, these factors can make police officers easy targets for hypothermia.

Frostnip is a mild form of frostbite, where only the top layer of skin freezes. There may be a painful tingling or burning sensation; skin appears yellowish or white, but feels soft to the touch. **Frostbite** is a more severe condition, where both the skin and the underlying tissue (fat, muscle, bone) are frozen. The area is numb. Skin appears white and waxy, and is hard to the touch. At this point, medical attention is necessary.

frostnip
a mild form of frostbite, where only the top layer of skin freezes

frostbite
severe condition where both the skin and the underlying tissue (fat, muscle, and bone) are frozen

wind chill index (WCI)
measure representing how the temperature would feel on your skin if the wind were reduced to a walking pace of 4.8 km/h

When headed outdoors, you need to be aware of the **wind chill index (WCI)** instead of just consulting outside air temperatures. The wind chill represents how the temperature would feel on your skin if the wind were reduced to a walking pace of 4.8 kilometres per hour. Wind increases the rate at which insulating air surrounding the body is whisked away; the warmer air is then replaced by the colder outside air. When the wind chill index is −27 °C (−18 °F) or warmer, the risk of frostbite is low. At a wind chill factor between −28 °C (−20 °F) and −39 °C (−39 °F), the risk of frostbite rapidly increases. When the wind chill reaches a factor of −40 °C (−40 °F), frostbite will occur in less than 10 minutes on exposed skin for most people. At a wind chill factor of −55 °C (−68 °F), frostbite will occur in two minutes or less on exposed skin for most people. As a general rule, if the WCI is less than −28 °C (−20 °F), caution must be taken when participating in outdoor activities. See Table 14.2 for wind chill and frostbite risk levels, health concerns, and their remedies.

Proper apparel and common sense are key to preventing hypothermia. You can wear up to four layers of clothing, with a ventilation layer next to the skin. It is important to wear gloves and a hat, as large amounts of heat are lost through your head. Keep your neck and throat area covered. Change your socks if your feet get wet.

Biological and Chemical Hazards in Policing

Emergency response teams encounter hazardous products on a daily basis. Sources of biological hazards include bacteria, viruses, insects, plants, birds, animals, and humans. Methamphetamine laboratories in homes, hepatitis, tuberculosis, anthrax, Lyme disease (bacterial infection acquired from the bite of an infected tick), and HIV/AIDS are just a few hazards that officers may face when they respond to a call. Their health can be affected in ways ranging from skin irritation, allergies, and res-

TABLE 14.2 Wind Chill Hazards and What to Do

WIND CHILL (°C)	RISK OF FROSTBITE	OTHER HEALTH CONCERNS	WHAT TO DO
0 to −9	Low	• Slight increase in discomfort	• Dress warmly • Stay dry
−10 to −27	Low	• Uncomfortable • Risk of hypothermia if outside for long periods without adequate protection	• Dress in layers of warm clothing, with an outer layer that is wind-resistant • Wear a hat, mittens or insulated gloves, a scarf, and insulated, waterproof footwear • Stay dry • Keep active
−28 to −39	Risk: Exposed skin can freeze in 10–30 minutes	• Risk of frostnip or frostbite: Check face and extremities for numbness or whiteness • Risk of hypothermia if outside for long periods without adequate clothing or shelter from wind and cold	• Dress in layers of warm clothing, with an outer layer that is wind-resistant • Cover exposed skin • Wear a hat, mittens or insulated gloves, a scarf, neck tube or face mask, and insulated, waterproof footwear • Stay dry • Keep active
−40 to −47	High risk: Exposed skin can freeze in 5–10 minutes*	• High risk of frostbite: Check face and extremities for numbness or whiteness • Risk of hypothermia if outside for long periods without adequate clothing or shelter from wind and cold	• Dress in layers of warm clothing, with an outer layer that is wind-resistant • Cover all exposed skin • Wear a hat, mittens or insulated gloves, a scarf, neck tube or face mask, and insulated, waterproof footwear • Stay dry • Keep active
−48 to −54	Very high risk: Exposed skin can freeze in 2–5 minutes*	• Very high risk of frostbite: Check face and extremities frequently for numbness or whiteness • Serious risk of hypothermia if outside for long periods without adequate clothing or shelter from wind and cold	• Be careful—dress very warmly in layers of clothing, with an outer layer that is wind-resistant • Cover all exposed skin • Wear a hat, mittens or insulated gloves, a scarf, neck tube or face mask, and insulated, waterproof footwear • Be ready to cut short or cancel outdoor activities • Stay dry • Keep active
−55 and colder	Extremely high risk: Exposed skin can freeze in less than 2 minutes*	• DANGER! Outdoor conditions are hazardous	• Stay indoors

* In sustained winds over 50 km/h, frostbite can occur faster than indicated.

SOURCE: Environment Canada, 2012.

piratory infections to contraction of diseases, including HIV/AIDS and various cancers.

Chemical hazards include individual chemicals, mixtures like petroleum solvents, and synthetic polymers (plastics). In 1988, the national **Workplace Hazardous Materials Information System (WHMIS)** was developed to familiarize workers with safety information about potentially hazardous products in the workplace (CCOHS, 2007). Workers are required to learn the WHMIS symbols and their meanings, the labels on products, and how to read and understand material safety data sheets. These sheets provide information about the physical, chemical, and environmental characteristics of a material, along with information regarding toxicity and potential hazards (such as whether it is reactive, flammable, combustible, or toxic). Data sheets will also include preparation and production information about the substance, as well as the appropriate first aid measures that should be taken upon exposure.

Workplace Hazardous Materials Information System (WHMIS)
a system that familiarizes workers with safety information about potentially hazardous products in their workplace

The aim of the program is to provide basic health and safety measures to protect individuals, and to prevent workplace injuries and illness. WHMIS provides information on supplier and workplace labels, material safety data sheets, fundamentals of chemical safety and emergency first aid, and other helpful resources. The State of New Jersey Department of Health (2012) (see References) provides a database of approximately 1,700 fact sheets on important hazardous substances found in workplaces and the environment.

The Canadian Centre for Occupational Health and Safety (CCOHS) provides information on biological and chemical hazards. Each police service and community is required to develop an emergency response plan based on risk assessment (what is in a community that could expose its members to hazardous materials). Each community must develop a comprehensive emergency preparedness policy and response program to deal with each emergency in the safest and most efficient manner possible. For more information, see CCOHS (2012) (in References).

KEY TERMS

bursitis, 322
delayed-onset muscle soreness (DOMS), 319
frostbite, 335
frostnip, 335
heat cramps, 331
heat exhaustion, 331
heat stroke, 332
hypothermia, 333
impingement syndrome, 322
sprain, 320
strain, 321
tendinitis, 322
wind chill index (WCI), 335
Workplace Hazardous Materials Information System (WHMIS), 337

EXERCISES

True or False?

1. Overuse problems are more common when someone is beginning a fitness program, and account for the majority of injuries.
2. Alternating a high-impact activity with a low-impact activity may prevent overuse of specific muscle groups.
3. Being fatigued during a workout will not make you more susceptible to developing an injury.
4. Mild muscle soreness that develops at the beginning of a new exercise program will usually disappear in one to three days.

Multiple Choice

1. The most common preventable cause of exercise injury is
   - **a.** overuse
   - **b.** poor nutrition
   - **c.** sudden trauma
   - **d.** dehydration
   - **e.** muscular endurance
2. To help prevent overuse of muscles, you should
   - **a.** work through the soreness
   - **b.** increase the length of your workout each day to toughen your muscles
   - **c.** exercise seven days a week to toughen your muscles
   - **d.** alternate days spent on aerobic and strength conditioning
   - **e.** do two-a-day workouts to toughen your muscles
3. According to the RICE principle, for a mild ankle sprain you should
   - **a.** rest the injured area for 12 hours
   - **b.** apply ice for 20 minutes after 24 hours
   - **c.** apply tape and leave it wrapped for 12 hours
   - **d.** keep exercising unless there is extreme pain
   - **e.** raise the ankle up and apply ice
4. Injury to a ligament caused by a sudden force is called a
   - **a.** cramp
   - **b.** bursitis
   - **c.** sprain
   - **d.** strain
   - **e.** plantar fasciitis
5. Injury to a tendon caused by a sudden force is called a(n)
   - **a.** pull
   - **b.** sprain
   - **c.** strain
   - **d.** inversion
   - **e.** eversion
6. Heat cramps may be treated by
   - **a.** increased salt intake
   - **b.** water, cool air, and rest
   - **c.** alternating heat with ice on the affected area
   - **d.** wrapping the affected muscle
   - **e.** applying more clothes to keep the muscle warm

Short Answer

1. What is the RICE principle?

2. Why do people suffer from delayed-onset muscle soreness?

3. Differentiate between a sprain and a strain.

4. How do you treat a sprain or a strain?

5. What are shin splints? How do you prevent shin splints?

6. Name and briefly explain the three heat-related illnesses.

7. How do you treat heat-related illnesses?

8. What is hypothermia? What are some of its signs and symptoms?

9. How do you treat someone who has developed hypothermia?

10. What are some of the biological or chemical hazards that an officer may face while working?

REFERENCES

American College of Sports Medicine. (1996). Position stand: Heat and cold illnesses during distance running. *Medicine & Science in Sports & Exercise, 28*(12), i–x.

Armstrong, L.E., & Maresh, C.M. (1993). The exertional heat illness: A risk of athletic participation. *Medicine, Exercise, Nutrition and Health, 2*, 125–134.

Boyle, C.A., Sayers, S.P., Jensen, B.E., Headley, S.A., & Manos, T.M. (2004). The effects of yoga training and a single bout of yoga on delayed onset muscle soreness in the lower extremity. *Journal of Strength and Conditioning Research, 18*(4), 723–729.

Canadian Centre for Occupational Health and Safety (CCOHS). (2007). What is WHMIS? http://www.ccohs.ca/headlines/text51.html.

Canadian Centre for Occupational Health and Safety (CCOHS). (2012). http://www.ccohs.ca.

Casa, D.J., Armstrong, L.E., & Hillman, S.K. (2000). National Athletic Trainer's Association position statement: Fluid replacement for athletes. *Journal of Athletic Training, 35*(2), 212–224.

Encyclopedia of Canadian Provinces. (2007). Ontario. http://www.nationsencyclopedia.com/canada/Nunavut-to-Yukon/Ontario.html.

Environment Canada. (2012). Canada's wind chill hazards and what to do. http://www.ec.gc.ca/meteo-weather/default.asp?lang=en&n=5FBF816A-1#table1.

Ministry of Labour. (2011). A guide to the *Occupational Health and Safety Act*. http://www.labour.gov.on.ca/english/hs/pdf/ohsa_g.pdf.

Occupational Health and Safety Council of Ontario (OHSCO). (2007, February). *Resource manual for the MSD prevention guideline for Ontario. Part 2.* http://www.osach.ca/misc_pdf/MSDResource.pdf.

State of New Jersey Department of Health. (2012). http://www.state.nj.us/health.

United States (US) Search and Rescue Task Force. (n.d.). Cold water survival. http://www.ussartf.org/cold_water_survival.htm.

PART 5

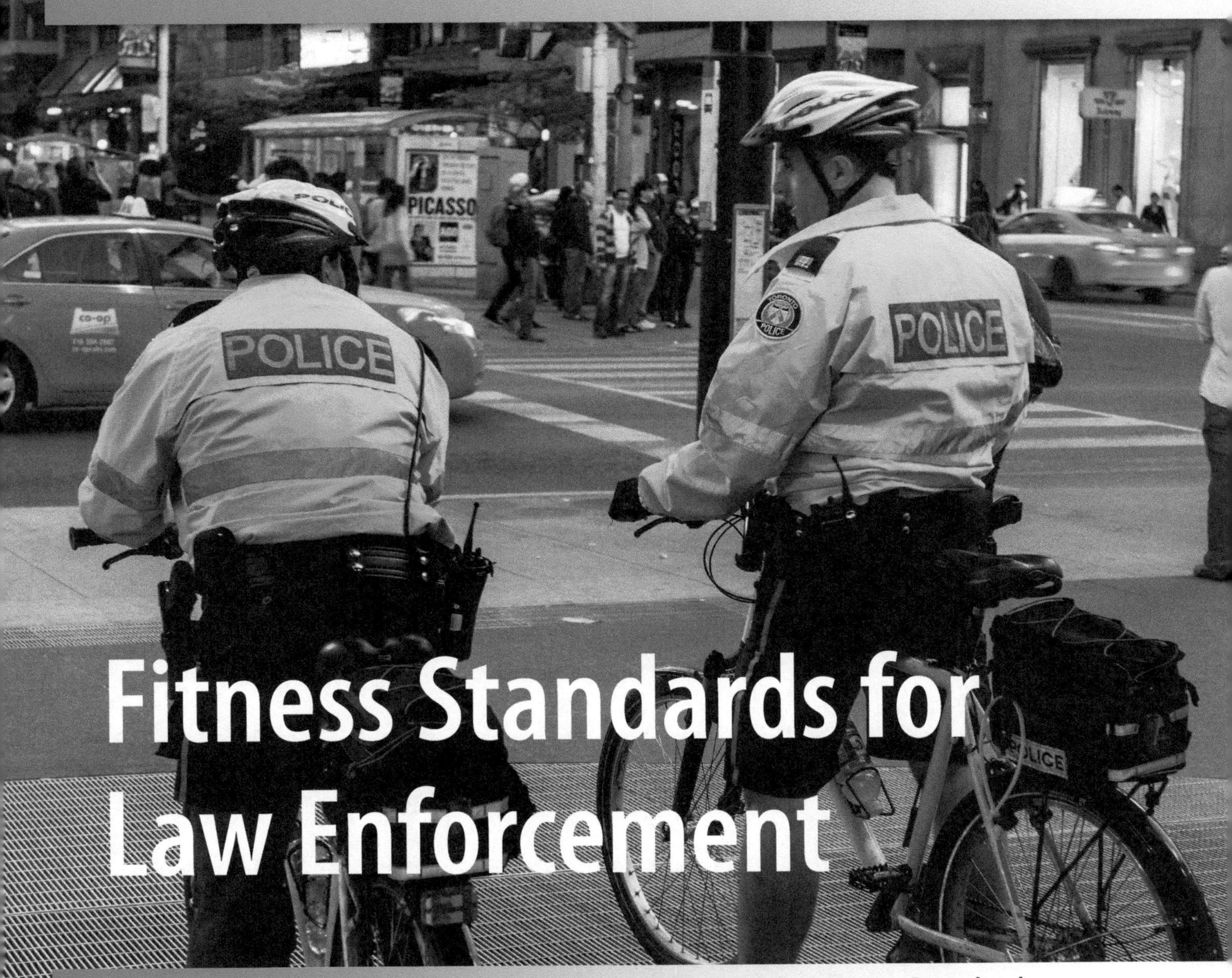

Fitness Standards for Law Enforcement

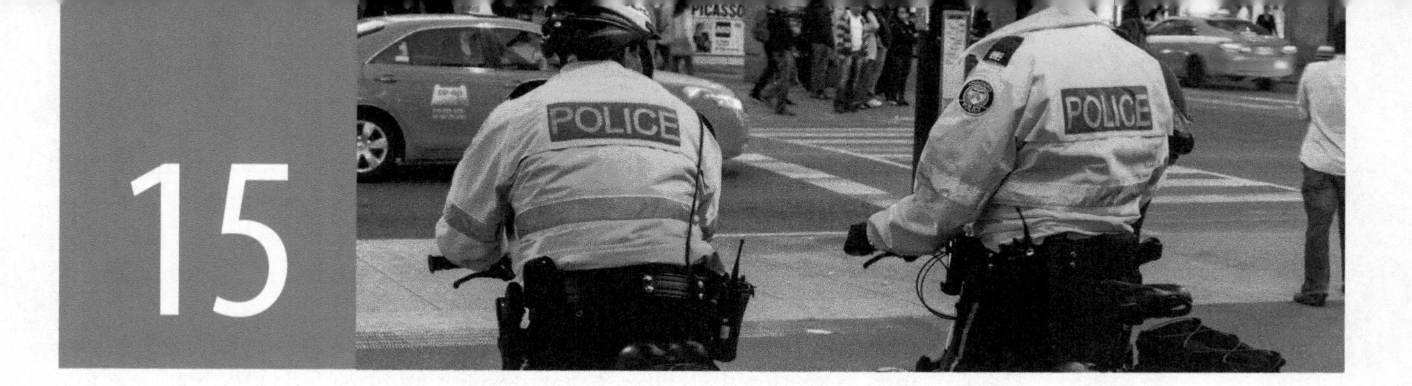

Preparing to Meet Law Enforcement Fitness Standards

LEARNING OBJECTIVES

After completing this chapter, you should be able to:

- Briefly describe the purposes of the Physical Readiness Evaluation for Police (PREP) test, the Physical Abilities Requirement Evaluation (PARE) test, the Ontario Police Fitness Award (OPFA) Standards, and the Peel Regional Police Service Fitness Standards.
- Briefly describe the main features of the PREP test, the PARE test, and the OPFA Standards.
- Identify exercises that can help you prepare for the PREP test, the PARE test, and the OPFA Standards.

OVERVIEW

The Ontario Police College first developed physical fitness standards in the 1970s based on the fitness levels of the general Canadian population. Until the late 1970s, minimal height requirements and weight standards were used as part of police service selection criteria. The tests typically had the effect of excluding many women and some minority groups.

In the late 1980s, the RCMP, and in 1992, the Ontario Ministry of the Solicitor General and Correctional Services, began developing Bona Fide Occupational Requirements (BFOR) for assessing recruits' job readiness in Ontario. They looked at the specific demands of policing and corrections, respectively, to determine what physical components were essential to perform jobs in these areas. These BFOR standards were implemented to address human rights issues so that one standard is applied to all applicants, regardless of age, sex, or race. It was critical to eliminate the adverse impact of entry-level physical assessment, so it included all successful candidates without excluding qualified visible minorities.

The RCMP and Ontario Ministry of the Attorney General and Correctional Services documented the physical activities that are essential for policing (content validity) and predicted successful job performance (criterion-related validity). After looking at other BFOR protocols in Canada and around the world, the ministry's policing and fitness experts spent two years developing the Physical Readiness Evaluation for Police (PREP) test. In January 1999, the PREP test became the required standard in Ontario for police applicant physical fitness testing.

In 2013, over a two-year process, the PREP was re-evaluated

> to confirm and/or expand on the tasks that were identified in the original PREP report as important, physically demanding and frequently occurring tasks that are encountered by front-line police constables in emergency conditions and not skill dependent or learned behaviours with particular attention to possible changes over the past 15 years. (Gledhill & Jamnik, 2015)

As a result, based on importance, physical demands, and frequency of occurrence for each of the identified on-the-job emergency police constable tasks, tests were added for wearing a weighted vest, scaling a 1.8-metre (6-ft) wall, and crawling under a barrier, and changes were made to the push/pull component, dragging a victim farther with different coefficients, and the requirement to demonstrate greater aerobic fitness.

In the 1980s, the Justice Institute of British Columbia developed the Police Officer's Physical Abilities Test (POPAT) for use in British Columbia. The RCMP's Physical Abilities Requirement Evaluation (PARE) test is a modified version of the POPAT. The PARE is used for applicant and recruit testing, and as a motivational tool for RCMP staff. Currently, incumbents with the RCMP are required to run through the protocol, with specialized units being required to meet certain standards.

The Ontario Police Fitness Award (OPFA) is a provincial incentive program developed to motivate Ontario police officers and police service employees to remain physically fit throughout their entire careers. The OPFA program is sanctioned by the policing services division of the Ministry of the Solicitor General and the Ontario Association of Chiefs of Police. As of 2012, the testing includes push-ups, core endurance (modified back extension), trunk flexion (sit and reach), and the 1.5-mile (2.4-km) run or the shuttle run. The OPFA program is designed and implemented by the Police Fitness Personnel of Ontario (PFPO) executive and delivered through its membership throughout Ontario.

The OPFA Standards, developed in the early 1980s, are used to assess the fitness level of police officers. The standard of comparison is the general population of Canada. Whereas BFOR standards assess physical readiness for the job, the OPFA fitness standards assess general fitness level. Those individuals who achieve a 75 percent grade are awarded the OPFA pin.

Over a three-year period (March 1996 to March 1999), Mr. Peter Shipley, Physiological Health Science Coordinator at the Provincial Police Academy, conducted a cost–benefit analysis within the Ontario Provincial Police (Shipley, 2000). His research indicated that OPP officers who had earned their five-year OPFA pin used, on average, 4.24 fewer sick days per year than the average OPP officer. With all these benefits in mind, it is felt that police services should be concerned about their officers' physical fitness levels, not just during the initial hiring phase but throughout their careers. The OPFA program was designed to assist police services in monitoring and motivating their officers' physical health.

This chapter reproduces the testing protocols for the OPFA Standards, as well as standards for the PREP and PARE (BFOR) tests. Many forces still use the OPFA Standards as benchmarks in hiring cadets and special constables, and in recruit training and promotions. Since the inception of the fitness pin award, Correctional Services, private police services (for example, Bruce Nuclear, Ontario Power/Pickering Station), and various emergency response teams have adopted the pin standards as their own.

Physical Readiness Evaluation for Police (PREP) Test

Fit to Serve: Preparing for the PREP (Ministry of Community Safety and Correctional Services, 2015) will be available electronically through police services sites and the Ministry website. This is the standard that must be achieved to graduate from the Ontario Police College. It outlines the components of the PREP:

1. pre-exercise clearance, which includes the 2015 PAR-Q+ and, if required, the directive from the online ePARmed–X+ at www.eparmedx.com (Warburton et al., 2015) and your "Informed Consent for PREP Testing/ Consent for Release of Information" form; blood pressure, heart rate, a demonstration, and a period of time to get acquainted with the various equipment used in the test
2. pursuit/restraint circuit
3. aerobic fitness test (Léger 20-metre shuttle run)

Pursuit/Restraint Circuit

The pursuit/restraint circuit (Figure 15.1) simulates a police foot chase that includes obstacles, the control of a person who resists arrest, and the dragging of an incapacitated person. This test assesses your physical and occupational readiness to perform the duties of a police officer in the province of Ontario.

Throughout the pursuit/restraint circuit, you must wear a 9-pound (4.1-kg) soft belt around your waist and a 9-pound (4.1-kg) vest, which together simulate the weight of standard police equipment. Performing this circuit simulates an emergency

FIGURE 15.1 PREP Test: Pursuit/Restraint Circuit

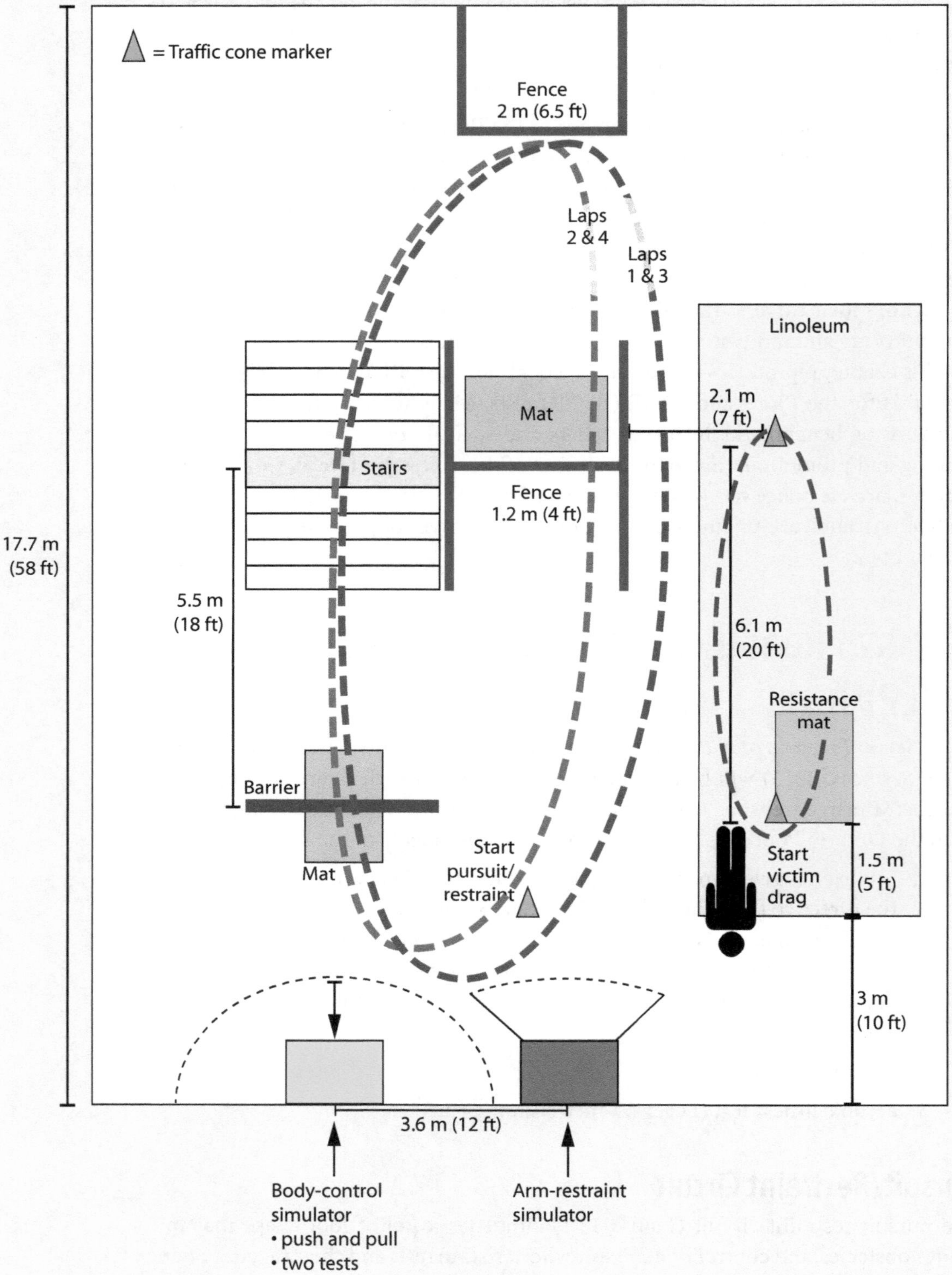

= Traffic cone marker
Fence
2 m (6.5 ft)
Laps
2 & 4
Laps
1 & 3
Linoleum
Mat
2.1 m
(7 ft)
Stairs
Fence
1.2 m (4 ft)
17.7 m
(58 ft)
5.5 m
(18 ft)
6.1 m
(20 ft)
Resistance
mat
Barrier
Start
pursuit/
restraint
Mat
Start
victim
drag
1.5 m
(5 ft)
3 m
(10 ft)
3.6 m (12 ft)
Body-control
simulator
• push and pull
• two tests
Arm-restraint
simulator

SOURCE: Ministry of Community Safety and Correctional Services, 2015.

response in which a police constable pursues an offender a total distance of 100 metres (332 ft) while climbing up and down a set of stairs four times, scaling a 1.2-metre (4-ft) fence twice, pulling one's own body weight up to look over a 2-metre (6.5-ft) fence twice, crawling under a low barrier four times, engaging in a physical altercation to accomplish the control and restraint of a resisting offender twice, and pulling an accident victim from a car, then dragging the victim to a triage area (Gledhill & Jamnik, 2015).

The following is the sequence of the pursuit/restraint circuit:

1. During the first and third laps of the circuit, you will pull yourself up to look over the far 2-metre (6.5-ft) fence with a toehold and to indicate to the appraiser whether the light is on or off, climb up and down a set of stairs, drop to the floor, and crawl under a barrier of 61 centimetres (24 in).
2. During the second and fourth laps, you will scale the near 1.2-metre (4-ft) fence with no toehold, climb up and down a set of stairs, then drop to the floor and crawl under a barrier of 61 centimetres (24 in).

   After completing the second and fourth laps, you will be directed to go to the body-control simulator (force = 35.5 kg/78 lb). "Push" or "pull" commands will indicate the action you are required to perform; "right," "centre," and "left" commands will indicate the direction in which you should move. Next, you will proceed to the arm-restraint simulator (grip = 14.5 kg/32 lb; retraction = 16 kg/35 lb). Depress the grips and force the arms together, then return them to their starting position.
3. After the fourth lap, you will be directed over to the Victim Drag. Using the handle attached to the back of the mannequin's neck, you will drag it over a resistive mat that requires the same force needed to pull a body out of a car. You will continue to pull the mannequin around the pylon and back until the heels pass the Start pylon (mannequin weight = 77 kg/170 lb; force required over resistive mat = 55 kg/121 lb; force required over rest of floor = 35 kg/77 lb).

A time of 157 seconds or less is required for the successful completion of the pursuit/restraint circuit.

Note: Participants are allowed a 15-minute rest following the pursuit/restraint circuit before beginning the aerobic fitness test.

Aerobic Fitness Test: Léger 20-Metre Shuttle Run

The aerobic fitness test consists of a 20-metre (67-ft) shuttle run to evaluate your aerobic fitness and work capability during physically demanding policing tasks as well as everyday policing activities (Léger & Lambert, 1982). In this test, you run back and forth between two marked lines over a 20-metre course in time with a recorded audio signal. The time permitted to cover the 20 metres decreases progressively until you are unable to maintain the pace. The time permitted to cover the 20 metres initially requires a slow jog. In each leg of the run, warning lines, placed 2 metres (7 ft) from each of the 20-metre lines, must be reached before the permitted time elapses. You will be cautioned when you miss a warning line. The test is terminated when two consecutive warning lines are missed. To successfully complete the minimum requirement of the aerobic fitness test for the PREP, you must achieve stage 7 in the 20-metre shuttle run.

Instructions for the shuttle run are given prior to the test and are as follows:

Test Description: The Léger 20-Metre Shuttle Run provides an evaluation of aerobic fitness which is relied on by Correctional Officers during everyday activities and in particular while performing physically demanding tasks. In this test, the participant runs back and forth over a 20-metre (66-ft.) course in time with audio signals recorded on a CD. The time permitted to cover the 20-metres initially requires a very slow jog, then the time is made progressively shorter so that the participant runs faster until he or she completes stage 7 or is no longer able to maintain the required pace.

In each leg of the Shuttle Run, at least one foot *must touch the end line* and the warning lines (situated 2 metres (6.6 ft.) from each of the 20 metre end lines) *must be reached before* the permitted time elapses.

The participant is warned when he or she misses a warning line. However, he or she must still reach the end line. The test is terminated and the participant receives a rating of "DOES NOT MEET STANDARD" when two *consecutive* warning lines are missed and the participant is instructed to exit out the end of his or her lane and not to cut across lanes.

If the participant fails to reach an *end* line, he or she will be cautioned. If, after two cautions, at any time during the test the participant's foot does not touch on or over the end line, on a third occasion the test will be terminated and his or her performance will be rated "DOES NOT MEET STANDARD".

Scoring the Aerobic Shuttle Run: Candidates who complete stage 7 in the Léger 20-Metre Shuttle Run receive a "*Meets Standard*" rating.

SOURCE: Ministry of Community Safety and Correctional Services, 2015.

Physical Abilities Requirement Evaluation (PARE) Test

The PARE is a police occupational abilities test of skills-related fitness components (Thompson, Gordon, & Pescatello, 2010, p. 3) for speed, power, balance, agility, and mobility. As such, it has nine essential gross-motor tasks that simulate a scenario in which a police officer must get to the scene of a problem or occurrence (the obstacle course), physically solve the problem (body-control push/pull activity), and remove objects or persons from the scene (the torso bag carry) (RCMP, 2005, updated 2011). This type of job simulation is termed a content-valid test for policing because the exact skills are tested in the job simulation (Eid, 2001). The RCMP PARE tests nine essential gross-motor skills: running, jumping, climbing and descending stairs, vaulting small- (18-in/45.7-cm) and medium-height (3-ft/0.9-m) barriers, dynamic pushing and pulling (80 lb/36 kg), controlled falls to the floor and back up, and walking and carrying 100 pounds (45 kg) of dead weight at waist level.

The standard reflects a level of ability that is designed to demonstrate a safe and efficient performance of police work for the public, yourself, and your partner (Trottier & Brown, 1994) at a satisfactory level. On the basis of police task analysis, the RCMP developed the PARE from the original police abilities test, called the Police Officer's Physical Abilities Test (POPAT) (Farenholtz & Rhodes, 1986). Small changes to the POPAT included placing the vaulting in the six-circuit run versus repeating it 12 times after the circuit, to get maximal intensity. PARE already solicited near or maximum levels of metabolic activation (max heart rate) after just two laps, in some cases. Another small change was shortening the jump mat from 6 feet to 5 feet (Shephard & Bonneau, 2002) to avoid adverse impact for smaller-statured persons. Thus, the PARE is represented as a Bona Fide Occupational Requirement (BFOR) test that legally discriminates for adequate levels of skill-related fitness without contravening protected human rights areas such as age and gender. Every item of the PARE circuit has been recently validated by serving officers and subject matter experts through a discrete item analysis completed by a large cross-section of RCMP officers across Canada (Anderson & Plecas, 2008).

The PARE is a BFOR that assesses whether you can perform the basic physical skills necessary to do the job, based on your level of skill-related fitness, safely. It is a content-valid, job-specific evaluation of physical ability, designed to assess a person's capacity to meet the minimal critical physical demands of police work (RCMP, 2005, updated 2011). The PARE test sections are quoted below and are illustrated in Figure 15.2.

FIGURE 15.2 PARE Test Stations

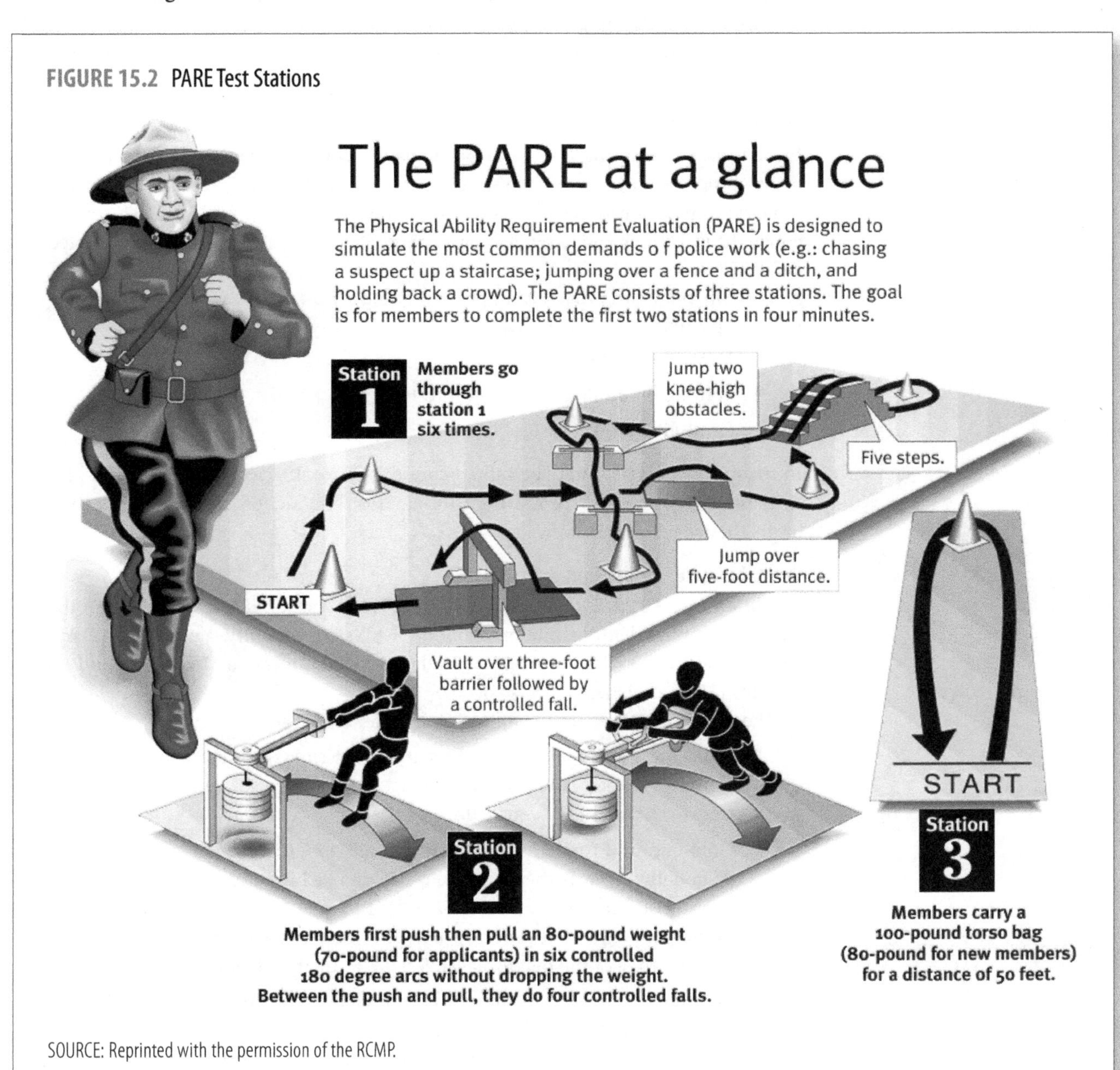

SOURCE: Reprinted with the permission of the RCMP.

PARE is divided into three sections:

1. Obstacle Course
2. Push/Pull Station
3. Torso Bag Carry

The first two stations (1. Obstacle Course and 2. Push/Pull) are timed and must be completed in less than/equal to 4 minutes 45 seconds for applicants, and less than/equal to 4 minutes for members applying for specialized duties and cadets before graduating from Depot. [For example, as of spring 2002, air marshals in the Canadian Air Career Protective Service must be fit for duty at the PARE standard of 4 minutes; as of 2007, VIP bodyguards must also pass the standard (R. Séguin, division fitness lifestyle adviser, RCMP, Central Region, London, ON; personal communication, 2007).] The last section (the torso bag carry) is a pass or fail activity and is not timed. [Note: Penalties are handed out to those who commit an error in performance (such as knocking down a stick, throwing a bag over the shoulders, or walking with the bag resting on the knees). Participants may be required to re-perform a manoeuvre or may be given a time penalty.]

Screening

Prior to attempting the PARE, all participants, both applicants and incumbents, must complete an informed consent, pass a same-day pre-screening called the Physical Activity Readiness Questionnaire ["PAR-Q and You"; CSEP, 2002] for adequate health status and provide a current medical clearance prior to being tested at a PARE test site.

Participants failing the resting pre-screening with any of the following indices may not participate in PARE that day:

a. Heart Rate > 99 bpm
b. Systolic Blood Pressure > 144 mm Hg
c. Diastolic Blood Pressure > 94 mm Hg

In many cases, anxiety may be influencing the above. If attempts to relax the participant, after 5 minutes' rest, bring the values on the second screening under the limits they may participate.

Pursuit Course: Agility Run

The first part of PARE consists of a 1,148 ft. (350 metre) obstacle run where the participant must demonstrate gross motor [skills] of mobility, agility, power and general endurance. The course is typically performed in about 2 minutes and 30 seconds (25 seconds/lap per 6 laps).

The course is laid out in the following manner [see Figure 15.3]:

1. From the start marker (#1), the participant runs diagonally to the left, towards #2 marker placed 20 ft. (6.1 metres) out from #1, and 10 ft. (3.05 metres) to the left of the centre line.
2. Going around the left side of this marker (#2), the participant runs inside diagonally towards the #3 marker. Before reaching marker #3, the participant must jump over and clear a 5 ft. (1.52 metre) mat. Upon landing, the participant turns left around marker #3 and proceeds towards the stairs. The last edge of the mat is placed 5 ft. (1.52 metres) from marker #3.
3. The stairs are placed in the centre of the course in such a manner that the centre of the top platform is exactly 60 ft. (18.29 metres) from the start marker (#1), 20 ft. (6.1 metres) from marker #4 and directly in line with the centre. The participant must run up and down the stairs, stepping on at

FIGURE 15.3 PARE Test Obstacle Course

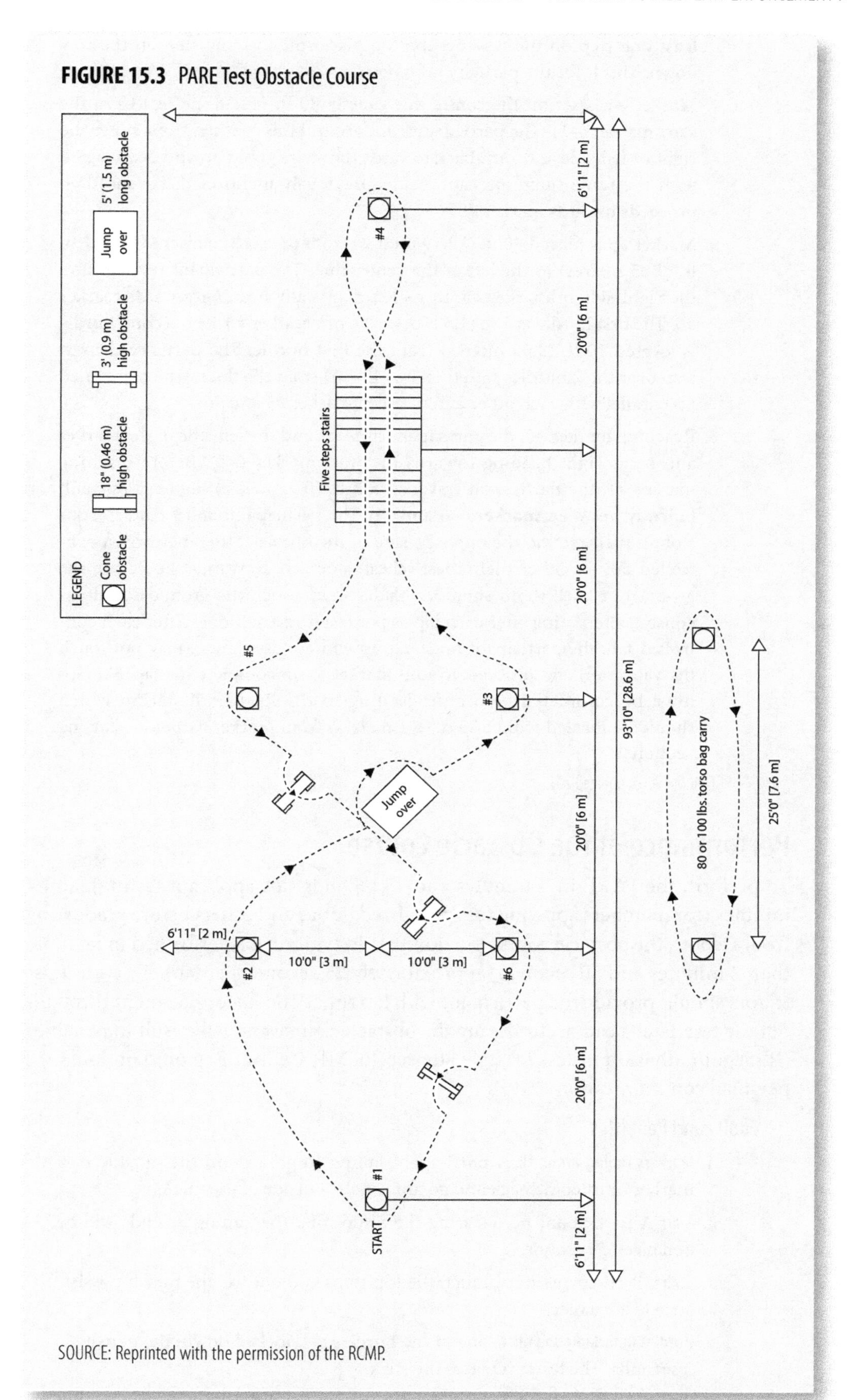

SOURCE: Reprinted with the permission of the RCMP.

least one step on the way up, the top platform, and one step on the way down. This is for the participant's safety.

4. Marker #4 is set on the centre line exactly 80 ft. (24.38 metres) from the start marker (#1). The participant runs around this marker, from either the right or left side and runs back towards the stairs going up and down again with the same safety precautions as previously mentioned. He/she then proceeds towards marker #5.
5. Marker #5 is placed 40 ft. (12.19 metres) from the start marker (#1) and 10 ft. (3.05 metres) to the left of the centre line. The participant runs around the right side of marker #5, turns left diagonally heading towards marker #6. The first hurdle is 5 ft. (1.52 metres) from marker #5. The second hurdle is located 10 ft. (3.05 metres) from the first hurdle. The participant must leap over the 2 hurdles raised 18 in. (45 cm) from the floor, which are lined up parallel with each other and between marker #5 and #6.
6. Reaching marker #6, the participant runs around the left side of the marker and turns right heading towards the start marker (#1). Before reaching marker #1, the participant traverses a 3 ft. (0.91 metre) high railing vault **halfway between markers #6 and #1**. The participants must land in control on their feet on the opposite side of the obstacle, then perform a controlled fall on either their chest (chest, stomach, hips must be flat on the ground) or back (both shoulder blades must touch the ground simultaneously), alternating after each lap as per tester instructions. After each controlled fall, the participant must get up without assistance (may not touch the vault rail) and proceed around marker #1 to complete the lap. Six laps must be completed before proceeding to the Push/Pull station which should be located within 20 ft. (6.1 metres) from marker #1 before starting Section 2.

SOURCE: RCMP, 2005, updated 2011.

Performance of the Obstacle Course

To perform the PARE in 4 minutes and 45 seconds (for applicant testing), and 4 minutes (for members applying for specialized duties and cadets before graduating from Depot), the obstacle course portion should typically be performed in no more than 2 minutes and 30 seconds (approximately 25 seconds per lap). Test administrators should provide the participant with lap times and encouragement throughout the test. Faults can occur during the obstacle course and will result in penalties (R. Séguin, division fitness lifestyle adviser, RCMP, Central Region, London, ON; personal communication, 2013):

Faults and Penalties

i. **Markers (going around):** A participant failing to go around the outside of a marker must come back and go around the outside of the marker.

ii. **Mat:** A participant not clearing the 5 foot mat (beginning or end) will be penalized 5 seconds.

iii. **Stairs:** Participants must touch the top steps and not use the rails for assistance just balance.

iv. **Hurdles (knocking down):** If one of the hurdles is knocked down, the penalty is 2 seconds. The tester replaces the stick.

v. **Hurdles (going outside):** A participant jumping over the hurdle with his/her trail leg outside the cone will be assessed a 2 second penalty.

vi. **Vault (traversing):** If a participant is unable to traverse the vault, the test is terminated. The way a participant traverses the vault is not specifically directed; however, it must be in a controlled manner. The participant may touch the vault with any parts of his/her body but must remain in control at all times.

vii. **Vault (landing):** A participant not landing in a controlled manner after traversing the vault is required to go back and traverse the vault again, landing in control on both feet.

viii. **Controlled falls (getting up):** Using the vault or mat to pull oneself to a standing position will require the participant to repeat the controlled fall.

ix. **Controlled falls (proper form):** A participant who does not land touching his/her chest, stomach, hips or both shoulder blades during the front and back falls, must repeat the controlled fall.

Once the sixth lap is completed [the pursuit section is typically performed in about 2 minutes and 30 seconds], the participant proceeds to the body control simulator, to begin Section 2. Please note that the body control simulator should be within 20 ft. (6.1 metres) from the start marker.

Apprehension Section

Upon finishing the obstacle run, the participant moves immediately to the body control simulator, mounted on a high traction surface (carpet or rubber). The maximum allowed distance between the end of the obstacle course (marker #1) and the push/pull apparatus is 20 ft. (6 metres).

The participant may perform this activity in the order he/she chooses (i.e., push first, then pull, or vice versa). Since the push is more difficult to perform, it is recommended to do this activity first. [This second part of the test is typically performed in 65 to 70 seconds.]

Push Activity

Upon reaching the body control simulator, the participant grasps the handles and pushes the weight, 70 lb. (32 kg) for applicants or 80 lb. (36 kg) for members, *off the base of the machine*, then proceeds to complete six controlled 180° arcs. In order to complete an arc, the participant's body must face the machine along the arm of the machine.

The participant's chest stays well away from the machine, with at least 90° or more extension of the arms. The arms must remain bent at the elbow throughout the performance of the activity. The elbows or hands must not be touching the chest or shoulders.

This activity should typically last no longer than 30 seconds. It is important to watch that the abdominal muscles are co-contracted with back extensors and the back maintains a neutral spine position. If after one reminder the participants fail to correct their technique and form, the specific arc must be repeated.

Controlled Falls

After six arcs are completed, the weight is lowered with control. The participant then moves away from the unit about 3 feet (1 metre) and faces the wheel or wall (marked at wheel height). The participant must perform a controlled fall on their front with chest, stomach and hips on the ground and get up executing a push-up like movement. The chest must completely touch the floor with legs out behind. The participant must then come to a standing ready position, touch the wheel or wall with two hands and execute a second fall, this time on their back with both shoulder blades on the ground. A sit-up like manoeuvre is required to come back up to the standing ready position. This sequence—front and back falls returning to a ready position between each—is repeated until the participant has completed two front falls and two back falls. This procedure should be demonstrated by the tester and practised by the participant before the test. The participant **must not use the wheel or wall for assistance to get up** from the falls. This activity should typically last no longer than 30 seconds.

The participant must always face the wall or the machine. Turning the back to the machine or wall is considered a fault and the participant is asked to repeat the fall. This activity typically lasts 20 seconds.

Pull Activity

Once the sequence of falls is completed, the participant grasps the tricep rope (on any portions of the rope) using both hands and pulls so the weight plates lift off the base of the body control simulator machine. The participant then proceeds to completing six 180° arcs.

In order to complete an arc, the participant's body (head and trunk) must face the push/pull machine at all times during this activity (i.e., shoulders not turning away from the machine). The participant must remain in control throughout the arcs while keeping his/her elbows, hips and knees bent and his/her shoulders facing the machine. The participant may not lean back during the pull activity as it would demonstrate a lack of control. The shoulders should be in front of above the hips at all times. The pull activity should typically last no longer than 30 seconds.

The administrator should advise the participant to "sit down" in a squat position, keeping the back in a neutral posture (not flexed at waist—flexed at hip with knees bent. If proper technique is not maintained, the participant is provided a warning. Failing to comply will result in repeating the arc).

The tester stops the clock once the sixth arc is completed when the participant puts the weight down in a controlled fashion and touches the wheel.

The timed section of PARE is finished when the participant completes the Apprehension Section.

SOURCE: RCMP, 2005, updated 2011.

Performance of the Push/Pull Section of the PARE

To perform the PARE in 4 minutes or less, the push/pull section should typically be performed in no more than 1 minute and 30 seconds. Test administrators should provide direction and encouragement to the participant throughout this section. Faults can occur during the push/pull section and will result in penalties (R. Séguin, division fitness lifestyle adviser, RCMP, Central Region, London, ON; personal communication, 2013):

Faults and Penalties

Arcs

i. **Dropping weights:** A participant failing to maintain the weight off the base of the machine during a controlled arc will be asked to perform an additional correct arc.

ii. **Straight elbows:** A participant failing to maintain elbows bent in the push or pull activity (participant is allowed one warning) will be asked to perform an additional arc.

iii. **Leaning back or leaning forward on handles:** A participant leaning back during the pull activity (or forward on handles during push) is allowed one warning or failing to keep the elbows, hips and knees bent at 90°, participant is allowed one warning, and will be asked in either or both cases to perform an additional arc.

iv. **Incomplete arc:** A participant failing to complete an entire 180° arc will be asked to perform an additional arc.

Falls

When a fault of the following nature occurs, the participant must repeat the controlled fall.

v. **Proper position:** Participant failing to come to a controlled, ready position between falls will be required to redo the controlled fall.

vi. **Touching the wheel/wall:** Participant not touching the pad or wall with both hands between the falls will be required to redo the controlled fall.

vii. **Not facing the wheel:** Participant falling and turning away from the pad or wall will be required to redo the controlled fall.

viii. **Getting up:** Participant using the body control simulator to assist with getting up will be required to redo the controlled fall.

ix. **Proper technique:** Participant not touching their chest, stomach, hips or both shoulder blades during the front and back falls, will be required to redo the controlled fall.

Torso Bag Carry Section

The Torso Bag Carry section of PARE is a pass/fail untimed activity. The participant must be able to pick up a weight, 80 lb. (36 kg) for applicants or 100 lb. (45 kg) for members, and carry it using arms only, over a distance of 50 ft. (15 metres). This activity should begin 60 to 120 seconds after completion of the timed part of the test.

The resistance is placed within a bag made of waterproof material. On either side of the bag, enough material is provided to allow the participant a secure grip. Being able to lift the bag demonstrates good muscular strength in the forearms, wrists and fingers. Participants are allowed to wrap their arms around the bag and lift. The lift must be with the legs, and not the back, to avoid injury. The bag must be carried in front of the participant, NOT over the shoulders (fireman carry) *and not resting on the knees while walking.*

Once the torso bag is lifted, the participant must carry it to a cone placed 25 ft. (7.6 metres) from the start cone, go around it and come back to the start cone where the bag is lowered to the floor, **in a controlled manner.**

SOURCE: RCMP, 2005, updated 2011.

Performance of the Torso Bag Carry

The participant must demonstrate sufficient strength and endurance to manipulate, lift, and carry heavy objects. The participant will have a maximum of three trials to complete the torso bag carry in the proper manner over a distance of 50 feet (15 metres) (see Figure 15.3). Faults can occur during the weight-carry activity and will trigger penalties (R. Séguin, division fitness lifestyle adviser, RCMP, Central Region, London, ON; personal communication, 2013):

Faults and Penalties

i. **Unable to lift the bag:** Participant failing to pick up the bag will be given a maximum of three trials to complete the weight carry.

ii. **Dropping the bag:** Participant picking up the bag but dropping it before completing the task must redo the entire weight carry section.

iii. **Improper carry:** Participant throwing the bag over the shoulder or walking with the bag resting on the thighs will be asked to redo the entire weight carry section.

iv. **Lowering the bag:** Participant failing to lower the bag in a controlled manner at the end of the activity will be asked to redo the entire weight carry section.

An unsuccessful carry *after three failed attempts* will constitute a PARE failure.

SOURCE: RCMP, 2005, updated 2011.

Ontario Police Fitness Award (OPFA) Standards

The OPFA Standards, developed in the early 1980s, are used to assess the fitness level of police officers. The standard of comparison is the general population of Canada. Whereas BFOR standards are for assessing your physical readiness for the job, the OPFA Standards are for assessing your general fitness level.

The tables on the following pages are adapted from the OPFA Standards. They cover five fitness assessments—push-ups, core endurance (modified back extension), trunk forward flexion, and aerobic assessments consisting of the 1.5-mile (2.4-km) run and maximal shuttle run—that can help you prepare for the PREP and similar tests. Each table provides benchmarks that allow you to score your performance and gauge your improvement as you work toward your goal of meeting law enforcement fitness standards. Descriptions of push-ups, core endurance, trunk forward flexion, and the 1.5-mile run precede each set of tables. Officers who meet 75 percent of the OPFA Standards receive a fitness pin that they wear on their uniform, sponsored by the Police Fitness Personnel of Ontario (PFPO) and the Ontario Association of Chiefs of Police. Some services require recruits to meet this fitness level in order to attend recruit training at the Ontario Police College (OPC). Some services require cadets to meet the 75-percent standard in order to be hired. However, the PREP is the graduation standard for the OPC.

Push-ups

Push-ups are a test of muscular endurance, which is defined as the ability of a muscle to perform repeated contractions over a period of time.

Procedure

It is imperative that the participant is well instructed in the correct performance of the push-up prior to beginning the test. The push-ups are to be performed consecutively and without a time limit. The test is terminated when the participant has completed as many push-ups as possible, the form deviates too much from the procedure, or there is more than a two-second pause between repetitions. If the upper body does not stay in a straight line, or the individual does not go to full extension, or the individual is forcibly straining over two consecutive repetitions, the test is terminated.

Males

The participant lies on his stomach, legs together. His hands, *pointing forward*, are positioned under the shoulders. To begin, the participant pushes up from the mat by fully straightening the elbows, using the toes as the pivotal point. The upper body must be kept in a straight line (Figure 15.4). The participant returns to the starting

FIGURE 15.4 Push-up, Males: (a) Start Position, (b) Full Extension

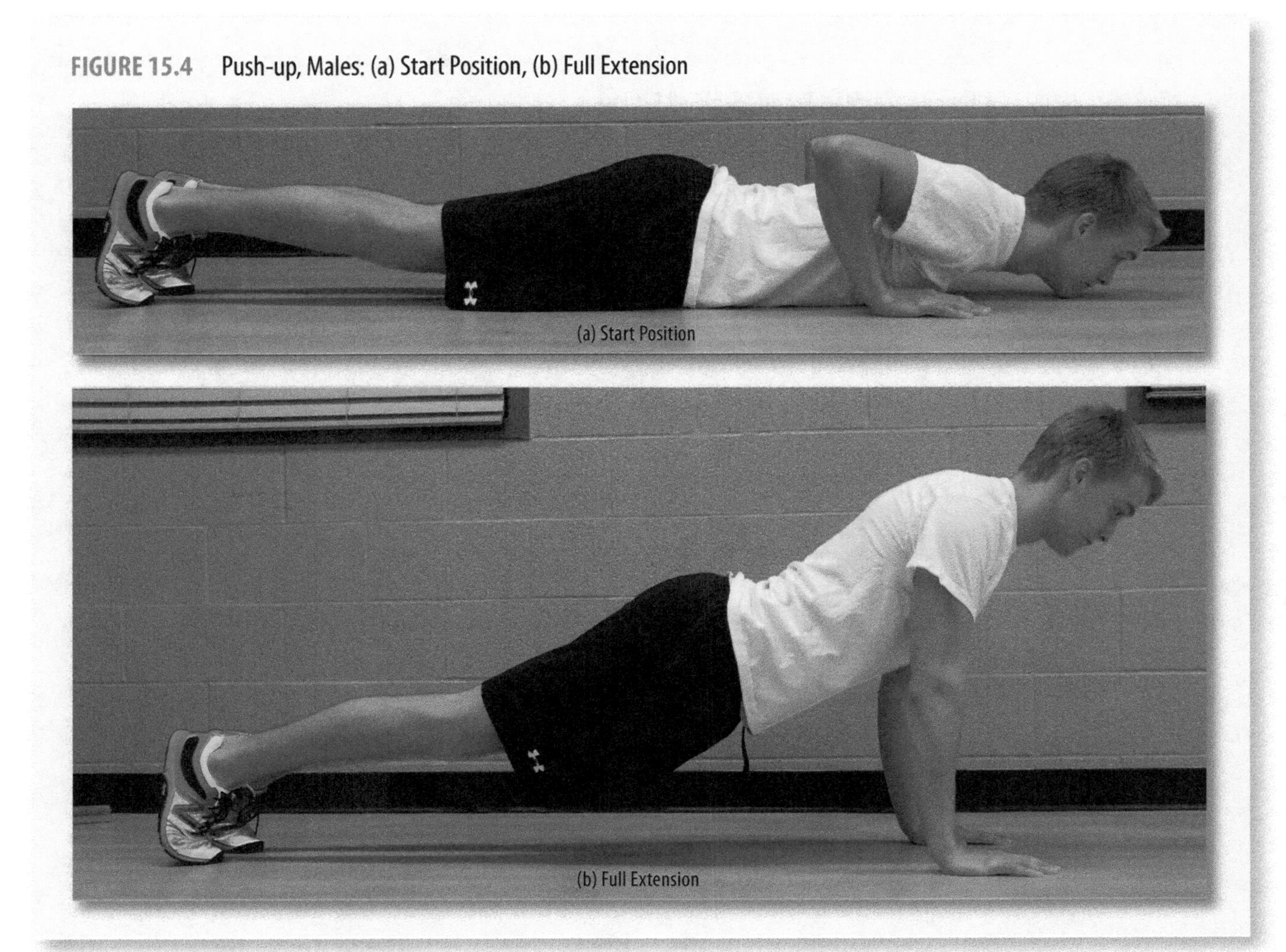

FYI

OPFA Protocol: Push-ups

In many cases, lack of compliance with the OPFA protocol (that is, arching the back on a push-up, not going down far enough, moving hands farther apart, failing to keep the upper body in a straight line, not going to full extension, or forcibly straining) terminates the test. If the person corrects the technique, the inappropriate push-up is not counted, and the participant can continue until he or she deviates in two consecutive repetitions.

It is not acceptable for either females or males to have their feet against a wall or for an additional mat to be placed under the chin.

position, chin to the mat. Neither the stomach nor the thighs should touch the mat.

Females

The participant lies on her stomach with legs together. Her hands, *pointing forward*, are positioned under the shoulders. She then pushes up from the mat by fully straightening the elbows, using the knees as the pivot point. Flexing at the elbows, she lowers the body, maintaining a neutral spine (body held in a straight line). The elbow must be flexed to 90 degrees at the bottom of the movement (Figure 15.5). The participant returns to the starting position with only the chin to the mat. The stomach and hips *cannot* touch the mat. The participant *must* have the lower leg remain in contact with the mat, ankles plantar-flexed. The participant may not flex the hip, strain forcibly, or hold her breath.

Table 15.1 shows standard results and scores for males and females.

FIGURE 15.5 Push-up, Females: (a) Start Position, (b) Full Extension

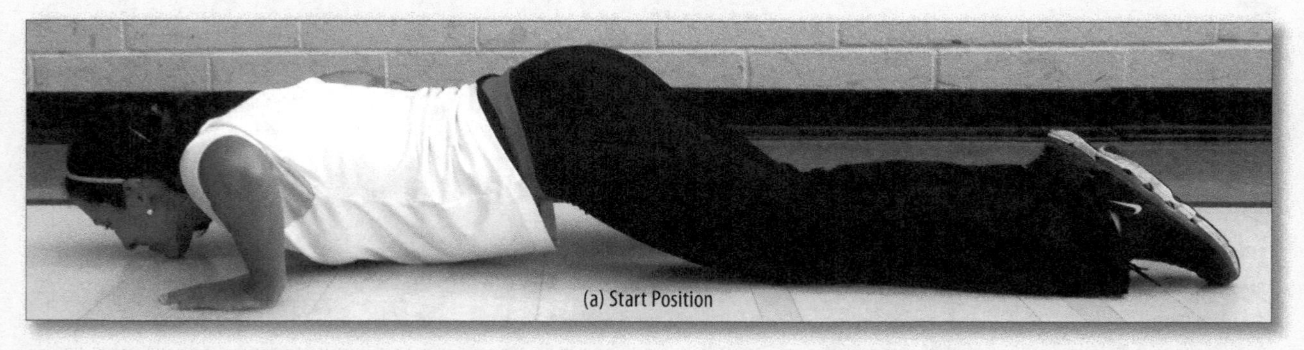

(a) Start Position

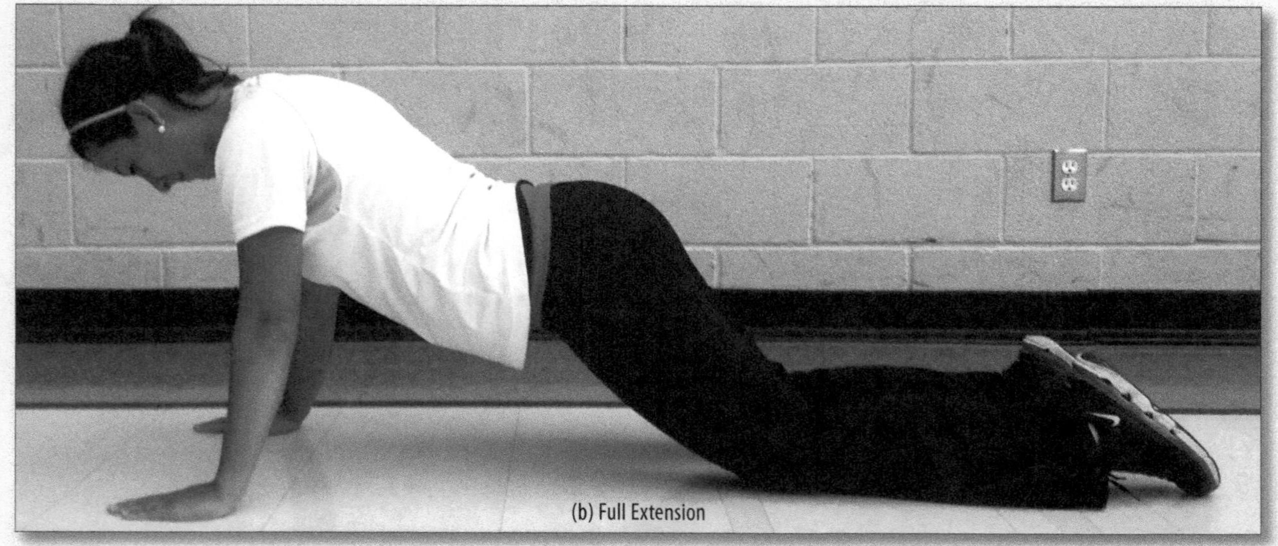

(b) Full Extension

TABLE 15.1 Push-ups Results and Scores, Male and Female

SCORE	AGE									
	20–29		30–39		40–49		50–59		60+	
	Male	*Female*	*Male*	*Female*	*Male*	*Female*	*Male*	*Female*	*Male*	*Female*
20	49+	38+	37+	37+	31+	33+	29+	31+	28+	31+
19	48	37	36	36	30	32	28	30	25–27	30
18	36–47	30–36	30–35	27–35	22–29	24–31	21–27	21–29	18–24	17–29
17	32–35	24–29	25–29	22–26	20–21	20–23	15–20	15–20	13–17	13–16
16	29–31	21–23	22–24	20–21	17–19	15–19	13–14	12–14	11–12	12
15	27–28	20	21	17–19	16	14	12	11	10	10–11
14	25–26	18–19	20	16	15	13	11	10	10	9
12	24	16–17	19	14–15	13–14	12	10	9	9	6–8
10	21–23	14–15	16–18	12–13	12	10–11	9	5–8	7–8	4–5
8	18–20	11–13	14–15	10–11	10–11	7–9	7–8	3–4	6	2–3
6	16–17	9–10	11–13	7–9	8–9	4–6	5–6	1–2	4–5	1
4	11–15	5–8	8–10	4–6	5–7	2–3	4	—	2–3	—
2	10	4	7	3	4	1	3	—	1	—
0	≤9	≤3	≤6	≤2	≤3	0	≤2	0	0	0

SOURCE: Adapted with permission of the PFPO (2012).

FIGURE 15.6 Pre-screening for Back Extension, (a) Leg Lift Only, (b) Leg Lift with Opposite Arm

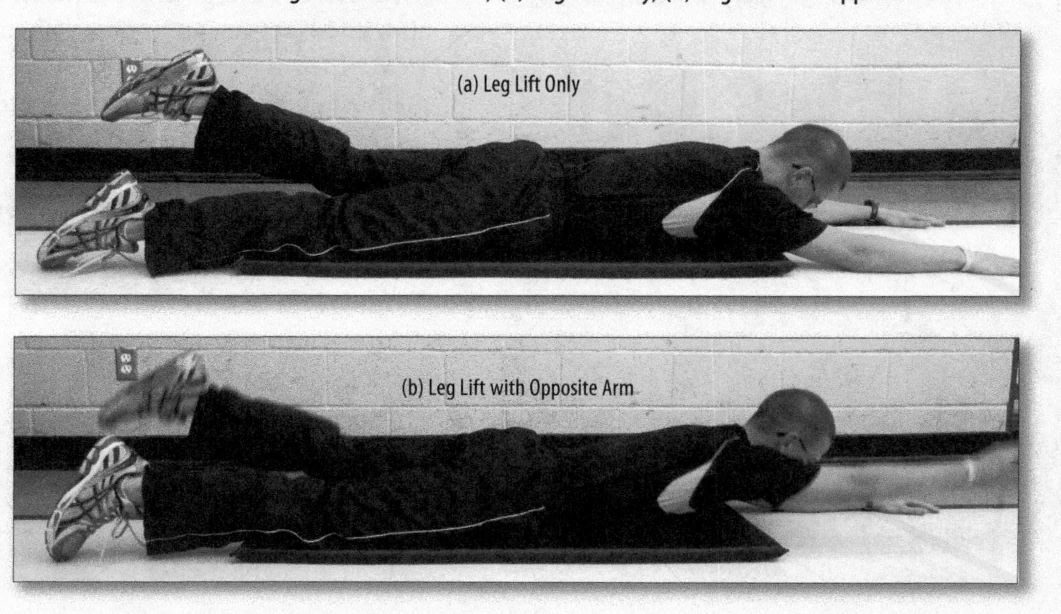

FIGURE 15.7 Biering-Sorensen Back Assessment: (a) Correct Body Position, (b) Incorrect Body Position (one warning, then test terminated)

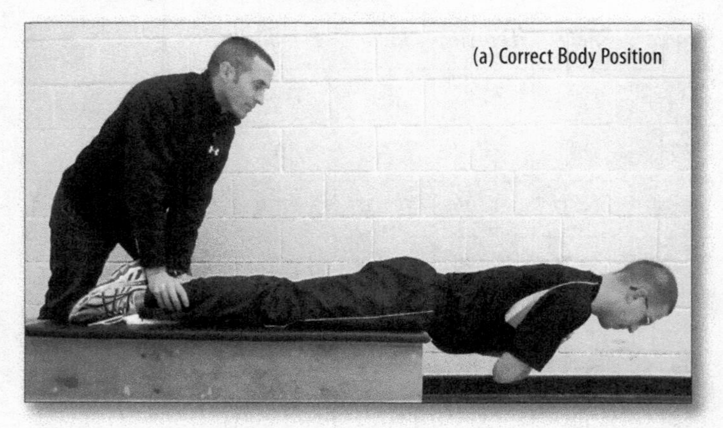

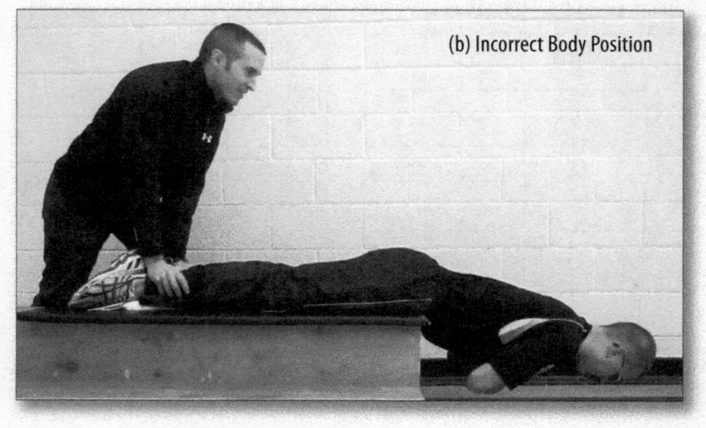

FIGURE 15.8 Biering-Sorensen Back Assessment: Body Position Using Straps

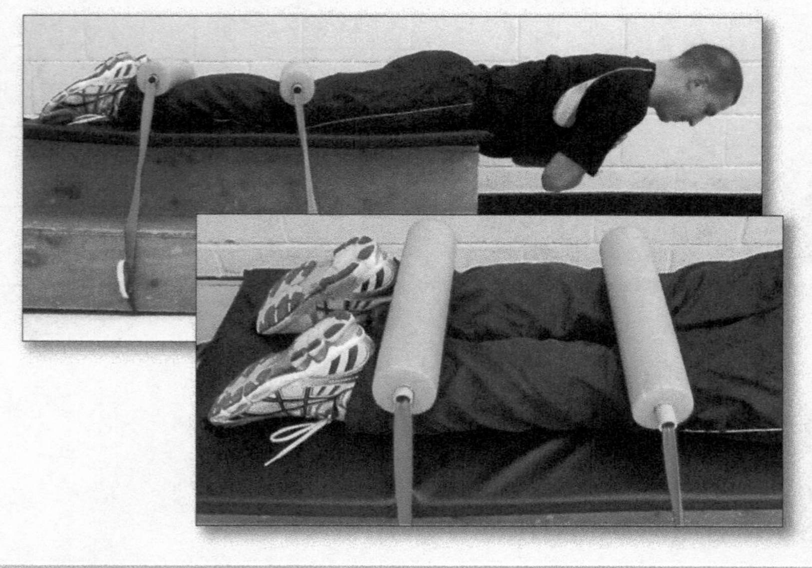

Core Endurance Test

(Note: Standards are based on the modified Sorenson back extension).

As of spring 2012, the OPFA test replaces the curl-up with a back assessment to evaluate core endurance. Back injury is one of the most common reasons for law enforcement officers to take time off work. Officers are subject to back injury whether they are on the road sitting long hours in a vehicle, sitting at a computer writing reports, or making rounds at an institution or on an employer's property while wearing their duty belt. For that reason, the modified Biering-Sorenson back assessment was chosen. It is endorsed by the Canadian Society for Exercise Physiology and used in the *Canadian Physical Activity, Fitness and Lifestyle Approach* (CSEP, 2003).

The assessment is for those participants who are asymptomatic and pass the prescreening for having no back problems. The participant must have filled out his or her PAR-Q and must have no restrictions.

Pre-screening

The participant lies face down on a mat and performs a straight leg extension with the right leg and then the left, with arms outstretched in front. If there is no pain, then he or she is told to repeat the same movements with the opposing arm outstretched and lifted at the same time (Figure 15.6). Then the participant returns to the starting position. If no pain is indicated, he or she proceeds to the test.

Biering-Sorensen Back Assessment

The equipment required for the back assessment is as follows:

1. Stopwatch or clock with a second hand
2. Padded bench or flat surface that is at least 40 centimetres off the floor (with a mat on top of it, or a step with four risers on each side can be used)

3. Securing straps or a partner to hold the participant
4. Towel (to be placed under ankles to maintain flexion)

The participant lies face down on top of the bench with the lower body on the bench. The iliac crest is positioned at the edge of the bench. The client needs to be secured by either straps or a partner while supporting his or her upper body with the arms outstretched until the test begins (Figures 15.7 and 15.8). Before starting the test, the participant is told to use the abdominal muscles throughout the test. A towel may be placed under the ankles to add support. This may allow the calves to stay in a relaxed state.

Once the participant is secured, he or she is instructed to raise the upper body until it is parallel with the lower body. The entire body forms one straight line, with no rotation or lateral shifting. The participant stays in this position for as long as possible to a maximum of 180 seconds. Participants are allowed one warning to re-position themselves if they drop below parallel.

The score is based on the number of seconds that the test is performed.

Cautions:

1. Do not raise your head. It should be parallel with the floor.
2. Keep neck straight and neutral.
3. Do not arch your back.
4. Breathe normally.

Table 15.2 shows standard results and scores for males and females.

TABLE 15.2 Biering-Sorensen Back Assessment: Core Endurance Test Results and Scores, Male and Female

SCORE	AGE									
	20–29		30–39		40–49		50–59		60+	
	Male	*Female*	*Male*	*Female*	*Male*	*Female*	*Male*	*Female*	*Male*	*Female*
20	3:00	3:00	3:00	3:00	2:45–3:00	3:00	2:41–3:00	2:36–3:00	2:00–3:00	2:29–3:00
19	2:57–2:59	2:40–2:59	2:41–2:59	2:50–2:59	2:30–2:44	2:40–2:59	2:21–2:40	2:13–2:35	1:53–1:59	2:00–2:28
18	2:49–2:56	2:30–2:39	2:27–2:40	2:40–2:49	2:10–2:29	2:20–2:39	2:00–2:20	1:50–2:12	1:44–1:52	1:31–1:59
17	2:36–2:48	2:20–2:29	2:16–2:26	2:30–2:39	2:00–2:09	2:00–2:19	1:50–1:59	1:38–1:49	1:35–1:43	1:14–1:30
16	2:23–2:35	2:10–2:19	2:05–2:15	2:20–2:29	1:50–1:59	1:40–1:59	1:40–1:49	1:26–1:37	1:26–1:34	0:57–1:13
15	2:12–2:22	2:00–2:09	1:48–2:04	2:10–2:19	1:40–1:49	1:30–1:39	1:27–1:39	1:14–1:25	1:17–1:25	0:39–0:56
14	2:00–2:11	1:50–1:59	1:40–1:47	2:00–2:09	1:30–1:39	1:20–1:29	1:17–1:26	1:06–1:13	1:09–1:16	0:33–0:38
12	1:50–1:59	1:40–1:49	1:35–1:39	1:50–1:59	1:20–1:29	1:10–1:19	1:06–1:16	0:56–1:05	1:01–1:08	0:26–0:32
10	1:39–1:49	1:30–1:39	1:20–1:34	1:40–1:49	1:10–1:19	1:00–1:09	0:54–1:05	0:47–0:55	0:52–1:00	0:19–0:25
8	1:35–1:38	1:20–1:29	1:10–1:19	1:30–1:39	1:00–1:09	0:54–0:59	0:43–0:53	0:37–0:46	0:42–0:51	0:15–0:18
6	1:30–1:34	1:10–1:19	1:00–1:09	1:20–1:29	0:50–0:59	0:50–0:53	0:31–0:42	0:26–0:36	0:30–0:41	0:11–0:14
4	1:26–1:29	1:06–1:09	0:56–0:59	1:01–1:19	0:32–0:49	0:42–0:49	0:20–0:30	0:15–0:25	0:20–0:29	0:06–0:10
2	≤1:25	≤1:05	≤0:55	≤1:00	≤0:31	≤0:41	≤0:19	≤0:14	≤0:19	≤0:05
0	DID NOT ATTEMPT									

SOURCE: Adapted with permission of the PFPO, 2012.

Trunk Forward Flexion (Sit and Reach)

The trunk forward flexion test measures the flexibility of the hamstring and lower back muscles (Figure 15.9). Flexibility depends upon the elasticity of the muscles, tendons, and ligaments, and is the ability to bend without injury.

FIGURE 15.9 Trunk Forward Flexion

Procedure

Participants warm up for this test by performing slow stretching movements before the actual measurements are taken. Participants, without shoes, sit with legs fully extended and the soles of the feet placed flat against the flexometer. Keeping the knees fully extended, arms evenly stretched, and palms down, participants bend and reach forward (without jerking). The position of maximum flexion must be held for approximately two seconds. Participants are advised to lower their head during the motion to maximize the distance reached. Each participant takes a turn and then the procedure is repeated. Both results are recorded, with the higher result scored.

The trial does not count if:

- The knees are bent.
- The participant attempts to do a bouncing or jerking motion to reach the board.
- The participant is unable to hold the position for two seconds.

Table 15.3 shows standard results and scores for males and females.

TABLE 15.3 Trunk Forward Flexion Results and Scores, Male and Female

SCORE	AGE									
	20–29		30–39		40–49		50–59		60+	
	Male	*Female*	*Male*	*Female*	*Male*	*Female*	*Male*	*Female*	*Male*	*Female*
10	45+	46+	44+	46+	41+	44+	42+	44+	45+	41+
9.5	44	45	43	45	39–40	42–43	40–41	42–43	40–44	39–40
9	40–43	41–44	38–42	41–44	37–38	40–41	37–39	40–41	36–39	37–38
8.5	37–39	39–40	35–37	38–40	35–36	38–39	35–36	38–39	32–35	35–36
8	34–36	37–38	33–34	36–37	32–34	36–37	33–34	36–37	29–31	33–34
7.5	33	36	32	35	29–31	34–35	30–32	34–35	26–28	31–32
7	32	35	31	34	27–28	32–33	27–29	32–33	24–25	29–30
6	31	34	29–30	33	25–26	29–31	25–26	30–31	22–23	27–28
5	29–30	32–33	27–28	31–32	23–24	26–28	22–24	28–29	18–21	25–26
4	26–28	29–31	24–26	28–30	20–22	24–25	18–21	25–27	16–17	23–24
3	23–25	26–28	21–23	25–27	16–19	22–23	15–17	22–24	14–15	21–22
2	18–22	22–25	17–20	21–24	12–15	19–21	12–14	19–21	11–13	18–20
1	17	21	16	20	11	18	11	18	10	17

SOURCE: Adapted with permission of the PFPO, 2012.

TABLE 15.4 1.5-Mile Run Results and Scores, Male and Female

SCORE	AGE									
	20–29		30–34		35–39		40–59		50+	
	Male	*Female*	*Male*	*Female*	*Male*	*Female*	*Male*	*Female*	*Male*	*Female*
50	≤9:00	≤10:35	≤9:20	≤11:00	≤10:06	≤11:53	≤10:54	≤13:04	≤11:59	≤14:22
47.5	9:01–9:30	10:36–11:10	9:21–9:50	11:01–11:35	10:07–10:37	11:54–12:31	10:55–11:41	13:05–13:46	12:00–12:51	14:23–15:08
45	9:31–10:00	11:11–11:52	9:51–10:20	11:36–12:10	10:38–11:10	12:32–13:08	11:42–12:17	13:47–14:27	12:52–13:31	15:09–15:53
42.5	10:01–10:30	11:53–12:34	10:21–10:50	12:11–12:45	11:11–11:42	13:09–13:46	12:18–12:52	14:28–15:08	13:32–14:07	15:54–16:38
40	10:31–10:56	12:35–13:00	10:51–11:20	12:46–13:20	11:43–12:14	13:47–14:24	12:53–13:28	15:09–15:50	14:08–14:49	16:39–17:25
37.5	10:57–11:22	13:01–13:26	11:21–11:50	13:21–13:55	12:15–12:47	14:25–15:02	13:29–14:04	15:51–16:32	14:50–15:28	17:26–18:11
35	11:23–11:46	13:27–13:42	11:51–12:20	13:56–14:30	12:48–13:19	15:03–15:40	14:05–14:39	16:33–17:14	15:29–16:07	18:12–18:57
30	11:47–12:10	13:43–13:57	12:21–12:50	1431–15:05	13:20–13:52	15:41–16:17	14:40–15:15	17:15–17:55	16:08–16:47	18:58–19:42
25	12:11–12:35	13:58–14:12	12:51–13:20	15:06–15:40	13:53–14:24	16:18–16:55	15:16–15:50	17:56–18:21	16:48–17:25	19:43–20:11
20	12:36–12:59	14:13–14:27	13:21–13:50	15:41–16:15	14:25–14:56	16:56–17:33	15:51–16:26	18:22–19:18	17:26–18:05	20:12–21:14
15	13:00–13:30	14:28–14:42	13:51–14:20	16:16–16:50	14:57–15:29	17:34–18:11	16:27–17:02	19:19–20:06	18:06–18:44	21:15–22:00
10	13:31–14:00	14:43–14:57	14:21–14:50	16:51–17:25	15:30–16:01	18:12–18:29	17:03–17:37	20:07–20:41	18:45–19:23	22:01–22:45
5	14:01–14:30	14:58–15:12	14:51–15:20	17:26–18:00	16:02–16:34	18:50–19:26	17:38–18:13	20:42–21:22	19:24–20:02	22:46–23:30
0	DID NOT ATTEMPT OR FAILED TO MEET MINIMUM STANDARD TIME									

SOURCE: Adapted with permission of the PFPO, 2012.

1.5-Mile (2.4-Km) Run

The 1.5-mile (2.4-km) run is a test of aerobic fitness or cardiovascular endurance. It tests the combined efficiency of the lungs, heart, bloodstream, and local muscles in getting oxygen to the muscles and putting them to work.

Procedure

Participants are required to cover an accurately measured 1.5-mile distance in as short a time as possible.

Table 15.4 shows the standard results and scores for males and females.

Maximal 20-Metre Shuttle Run

The OPFA established a number of options for the aerobic component, including the maximal shuttle run, a bike test, and the Canadian Physical Activity, Fitness and Lifestyle Appraisal (CPAFLA) step test in place of the 1.5-mile (2.4-km) run. Because of obvious time constraints, the bike and CPAFLA step test are not practical.

Following the PREP shuttle run protocol, Table 15.5 shows the gradings that can be used in place of the scores obtained from the 1.5-mile run.

TABLE 15.5 OPFA Results Scores for Shuttle Run, Male and Female

SCORE	AGE									
	20–29		30–34		35–39		40–49		50+	
	Male	*Female*	*Male*	*Female*	*Male*	*Female*	*Male*	*Female*	*Male*	*Female*
50	≥12	≥9.5	≥11.5	≥9	≥10.5	≥8	≥9	≥6.5	≥7.5	≥5.5
47.5	11.5	9	11	8–8.5	10	7.5	8.5	6	7	5
45	11	8–8.5	10.5	7.5	9–9.5	7	7.5–8	5–5.5	6.5	4.5
42.5	10–10.5	7.5	9.5–10	7	8–8.5	6–6.5	7	4.5	5.5–6	4
40	9–9.5	7	8.5–9	6.5	7.5	5.5	6–6.5	4	5	3.5
37.5	8.5	6.5	8	6	7	5	5.5	3.5	4.5	2.5
35	8	6.0	7.5	5	6.5	4.5	5	3	4	2
30	7.5	5.5	7	4.5	6	4	4.5	2.5	3.5	1.5
25	7	5	6.5	4	5.5	3.5	4	2	3	1
20	6.5	4.5	5.5	3.5	5	3	3.5	1.5	2.5	0.5
15	6	4.5	5	3	4.5	2.5	3	1	2	—
10	5.5	4.5	4.5	2.5	4	2	2.5	0.5	1.5	—
5	5	4	4.5	2.5	3	1.5	2.5	—	1	—

NOTE: Age 35- to 39-year-old females, age 40- to 49-year old-females, and age 50+ males and females must complete a minimum of level 2 to be scored.

SOURCE: Adapted with permission of the PFPO, 2012.

Additional Fitness Standards

Additional fitness standards for the bench press, chin-ups, and 100-yard (91-m) sprint can be used to supplement the standards given above. The bench press tests upper body strength, the chin-ups test muscular endurance, and the 100-yard sprint tests anaerobic capacity (the body's ability to use energy stored in the muscles without having to draw on inhaled oxygen).

Standards for these additional tests appear in the *Fit for Duty, Fit for Life Training Guide* that accompanies this textbook.

Physical Fitness Log

As part of your physical fitness training goals, you should chart your progress throughout the course of your study. At the end of your first semester, you may have to change those goals that you have not been able to meet. Ultimately, it is your responsibility to know where you stand with your grades. Depending on the college and semester you are in, you will have certain standards to meet. By charting your results, you will know where you stand and the areas that you will have to address each semester.

To record the results of your running and workouts over time, see the running and daily workout logs in the *Fit for Duty, Fit for Life Training Guide* that accompanies this textbook.

REFERENCES

Anderson, G.S., & Plecas, D.B. (2008). Physical abilities requirement evaluation (PARE) phase 2: Discrete item analysis. http://www.ufv.ca/Assets/CCJR/Reports+and+Publications/PARE_Phase_2.pdf.

Canadian Society for Exercise Physiology (CSEP). (2002). Par-Q and you. http://www.csep.ca/cmfiles/publications/parq/par-q.pdf.

Canadian Society for Exercise Physiology (CSEP). (2003). *The Canadian physical activity, fitness & lifestyle approach (CPAFLA): CSEP-health & fitness program's health-related appraisal and counselling strategy* (3rd ed.). http://www.csep.ca/english/view.asp?x=609.

Eid, E. (2001). Challenges posed by the Supreme Court of Canada in the *Meoirin* decision to employers in physically demanding occupations. In N. Gledhill, J. Bonneau, & A. Salmon (Eds.), *Proceedings of the National Forum on Bona Fide Occupational Requirements*. Toronto: York University.

Farenholtz, D.W., & Rhodes, E.C. (1986). "Development of physical abilities test for municipal police officers in British Columbia." *Canadian Journal of Applied Sport Sciences, 11*(33).

Gledhill, N., & Jamnik, R. (2015). *PREP Technical Guide*. Toronto: Ontario Ministry of Community Safety and Correctional Services.

Léger, L.A., & Lambert, J. (1982). A maximal multistage 20-m shuttle run test to predict VO_{2max}. *European Journal of Applied Physiology, 49*, 1–5.

Ministry of Community Safety and Correctional Services. (2015). *Fit to serve: Preparing for the PREP—The physical readiness evaluation for police*. Toronto: Queen's Printer for Ontario.

Police Fitness Personnel of Ontario (PFPO). (1998). *The Ontario police fitness award program*. Toronto: Police Services Division of the Ministry of the Solicitor General and Correctional Services and the Ontario Association of Chiefs of Police.

Police Fitness Personnel of Ontario (PFPO). (2012). *Ontario police fitness standards*. Toronto: Queen's Printer for Ontario.

RCMP. (2005, updated 2011). *The Royal Canadian Mounted Police Physical Abilities Requirement Evaluation (PARE) protocol*. Ottawa: Author.

Shephard, R.J., & Bonneau, J. (2002). Assuring gender equity in recruitment standards for police officers. *Canadian Journal of Applied Physiology, 27*(3), 263–295. http://www.ncbi.nlm.nih.gov/pubmed/12180318.

Shipley, P.D. (2000, November). Cost–benefit analysis of Ontario Provincial Police, OPFA. Toronto: Queen's Printer for Ontario.

Thompson, W.R., Gordon, N.F., & Pescatello, L.S. (Eds.). (2010). *ACSM's guidelines for exercise testing and prescription*. Baltimore: Lippincott Williams & Wilkins.

Trottier, A., & Brown, J. (1994). *Police health: A physician's guide for the assessment of police officers*. Ottawa: Canada Communications Group.

Warburton, D.E.R., Jamnik, V.K., Bredin, S.S.D., & Gledhill, N. (2014). "The 2014 Physical Activity Readiness Questionnaire for Everyone (PAR-Q+) and Electronic Physical Activity Readiness Medical Examination (ePARmed-X+)." *Health & Fitness Journal of Canada*, 7(1): 80–83.

Appendix: Assignments

ASSIGNMENT 1.1 Wellness

Complete the following questionnaires to determine how ready you are to make healthier choices concerning habits, nutrition, stress management, and physical activity.

F•A•N•T•A•S•T•I•C LIFESTYLE CHECKLIST

INSTRUCTIONS:

Unless otherwise specified, place a ✓ beside the box which best describes your behavior or situation in the past month.

*See back for instructions

FAMILY **F**RIENDS	I have someone to talk to about things that are important to me	almost always	fairly often	some of the time	seldom	almost never
	I give and I receive affection	almost always	fairly often	some of the time	seldom	almost never
ACTIVITY	I am physically active (gardening, climbingstairs, walking, housework)	almost always	fairly often	some of the time	seldom	almost never
	I actively exercise for at least 20 min. eg. running, cycling, fast walk	5 or more times/week	4 times/week	3 times/week	1-2 times /week	less than once/week
NUTRITION	*I eat a balanced diet (See over)	almost always	fairly often	some of the time	seldom	almost never
	I often eat excess sugar or salt or animal fats or junk foods	none of these	one of these	two of these	three of these	four of these
	I am within ____ lbs. of my ideal weight	5 lbs (2 kg)	10 lbs (4 kg)	15 lbs (6 kg)	20 lbs (8 kg)	not within 20 lbs
TOBACCO **T**OXICS	I smoke tobacco	never smoked	quit over 5 yrs. ago	quit over a year ago	quit in past year	currently smoke
	I usually smoke ____ cigarets per day	none	5 or less	6-20	21-40	more than 40
	I use drugs such as marijuana, cocaine	never	almost never	only occasionally	fairly often	almost daily
	I overuse prescribed or "over the counter" drugs	never	almost never	only occasionally	fairly often	almost daily
	I drink caffeine-containing coffee, tea, or cola	never	1-2/day	3-6/day	7-10/day	more than 10/day
ALCOHOL	*My average alcohol intake per week is (See over)	0 - 7 drinks	8 - 10 drinks	11 - 13 drinks	14 - 20 drinks	more than 20 drinks
	I drink more than four drinks on an occasion	never	almost never	only occasionally	fairly often	almost daily
	I drive after drinking	never	almost never	only occasionally	once a month	often
SLEEP **S**EATBELTS **S**TRESS	I sleep well and feel rested	almost always	fairly often	some of the time	seldom	almost never
	I use seatbelts	always	most of the time	some of the time	seldom	never
	I am able to cope with the stresses in my life	almost always	fairly often	some of the time	seldom	almost never
	I relax and enjoy leisure time	almost always	fairly often	some of the time	seldom	almost never
TYPE OF **P**ERSON **A**LITY	I seem to be in a hurry	almost never	seldom	some of the time	fairly often	almost always
	I feel angry or hostile	almost never	seldom	some of the time	fairly often	almost always
INSIGHT	I am a positive or optimistic thinker	almost always	fairly often	some of the time	seldom	almost never
	I feel tense or uptight	almost never	seldom	some of the time	fairly often	almost always
	I feel sad or depressed	almost never	seldom	some of the time	fairly often	almost always
CAREER	I am satisfied with my job or role	almost always	fairly often	some of the time	seldom	never

STEP 1 Total the ✓s in each column ☐ ☐ ☐ ☐ ☐

STEP 2 Multiply the totals by the numbers indicated (Write in box below) X4 X3 X2 X1 0

STEP 3 Add your scores across the bottom for your grand total ☐ + ☐ + ☐ + ☐ = ☐ %

GRAND TOTAL

Name________________ Age________ Sex M☐ F☐

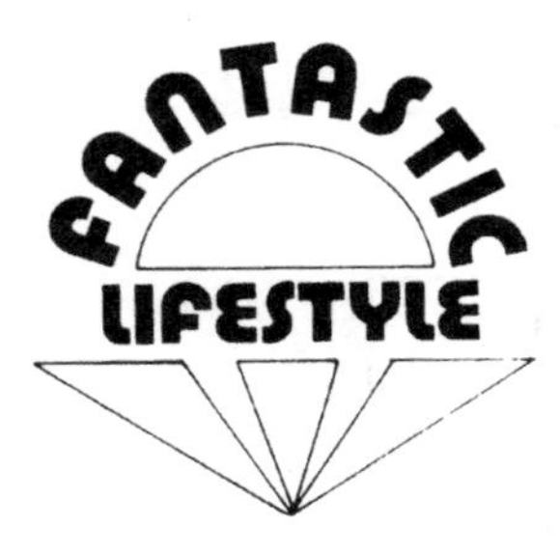

***A balanced diet each day consists of:**

Milk and Milk Products

Children up to 11 years 2-3 servings
Adolescents 3-4 servings
Pregnant and nursing women 3-4 servings
Adults 2 servings

Meat, Fish, Poultry and Alternates 2 servings

Breads and Cereals 3-5 servings whole grain or enriched

Fruits and Vegetables 4-5 servings Include at least two vegetables

***1 DRINK =**

		CANADIAN	METRIC	U.S.
1 bottle beer	5% alcohol	12 oz.	340.8 ml	10 oz.
1 glass wine	12% alcohol	5 oz.	142 ml	4.5 oz.
1 shot spirits	40% alcohol	1.5 oz.	42.6 ml	1.25 oz.

What does your score mean?

If you score:

85-100%—Congratulations—You are in control.

70- 84%—Good work—You are on the right track.

60- 69%—Fair

40- 59%—Somewhat low—you could take more control.

0- 19%—You are in the danger zone (but honesty is your real strength).

Note: The total score does not mean that you have failed. There is always the chance to change your lifestyle—starting now. Look at the areas where you scored a **0** or **1** and decide which areas you want to work on first.

Tips:

1. Don't try to change all the areas at once. This will be too overwhelming for you.
2. Writing down your proposed changes and your overall goal will help you to succeed.
3. Make changes in small steps towards the overall goal.
4. Enlist the help of a friend to make similar changes and/or to support you in your attempts.
5. Congratulate yourself for achieving each step. Give yourself appropriate rewards.
6. Ask your family physician, nurse or health department for more information on any of these areas.

Physical Activity Readiness Questionnaire - PAR-Q (revised 2002)

PAR-Q & YOU

(A Questionnaire for People Aged 15 to 69)

Regular physical activity is fun and healthy, and increasingly more people are starting to become more active every day. Being more active is very safe for most people. However, some people should check with their doctor before they start becoming much more physically active.

If you are planning to become much more physically active than you are now, start by answering the seven questions in the box below. If you are between the ages of 15 and 69, the PAR-Q will tell you if you should check with your doctor before you start. If you are over 69 years of age, and you are not used to being very active, check with your doctor.

Common sense is your best guide when you answer these questions. Please read the questions carefully and answer each one honestly: check YES or NO.

YES	NO		
☐	☐	1.	**Has your doctor ever said that you have a heart condition and that you should only do physical activity recommended by a doctor?**
☐	☐	2.	**Do you feel pain in your chest when you do physical activity?**
☐	☐	3.	**In the past month, have you had chest pain when you were not doing physical activity?**
☐	☐	4.	**Do you lose your balance because of dizziness or do you ever lose consciousness?**
☐	☐	5.	**Do you have a bone or joint problem (for example, back, knee or hip) that could be made worse by a change in your physical activity?**
☐	☐	6.	**Is your doctor currently prescribing drugs (for example, water pills) for your blood pressure or heart condition?**
☐	☐	7.	**Do you know of any other reason why you should not do physical activity?**

If you answered

YES to one or more questions

Talk with your doctor by phone or in person BEFORE you start becoming much more physically active or BEFORE you have a fitness appraisal. Tell your doctor about the PAR-Q and which questions you answered YES.

- You may be able to do any activity you want — as long as you start slowly and build up gradually. Or, you may need to restrict your activities to those which are safe for you. Talk with your doctor about the kinds of activities you wish to participate in and follow his/her advice.
- Find out which community programs are safe and helpful for you.

NO to all questions

If you answered NO honestly to all PAR-Q questions, you can be reasonably sure that you can:

- start becoming much more physically active – begin slowly and build up gradually. This is the safest and easiest way to go.
- take part in a fitness appraisal – this is an excellent way to determine your basic fitness so that you can plan the best way for you to live actively. It is also highly recommended that you have your blood pressure evaluated. If your reading is over 144/94, talk with your doctor before you start becoming much more physically active.

DELAY BECOMING MUCH MORE ACTIVE:

- if you are not feeling well because of a temporary illness such as a cold or a fever – wait until you feel better; or
- if you are or may be pregnant – talk to your doctor before you start becoming more active.

PLEASE NOTE: If your health changes so that you then answer YES to any of the above questions, tell your fitness or health professional. Ask whether you should change your physical activity plan.

Informed Use of the PAR-Q: The Canadian Society for Exercise Physiology, Health Canada, and their agents assume no liability for persons who undertake physical activity, and if in doubt after completing this questionnaire, consult your doctor prior to physical activity.

No changes permitted. You are encouraged to photocopy the PAR-Q but only if you use the entire form.

NOTE: If the PAR-Q is being given to a person before he or she participates in a physical activity program or a fitness appraisal, this section may be used for legal or administrative purposes.

"I have read, understood and completed this questionnaire. Any questions I had were answered to my full satisfaction."

NAME ______________________

SIGNATURE ______________________ DATE ______________________

SIGNATURE OF PARENT or GUARDIAN (for participants under the age of majority) ______________________ WITNESS ______________________

Note: This physical activity clearance is valid for a maximum of 12 months from the date it is completed and becomes invalid if your condition changes so that you would answer YES to any of the seven questions.

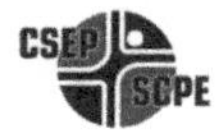

Supported by: 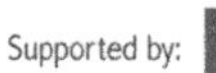 Health Canada Santé Canada

continued on other side...

...continued from other side

PAR-Q & YOU

Physical Activity Readiness
Questionnaire - PAR-Q
(revised 2002)

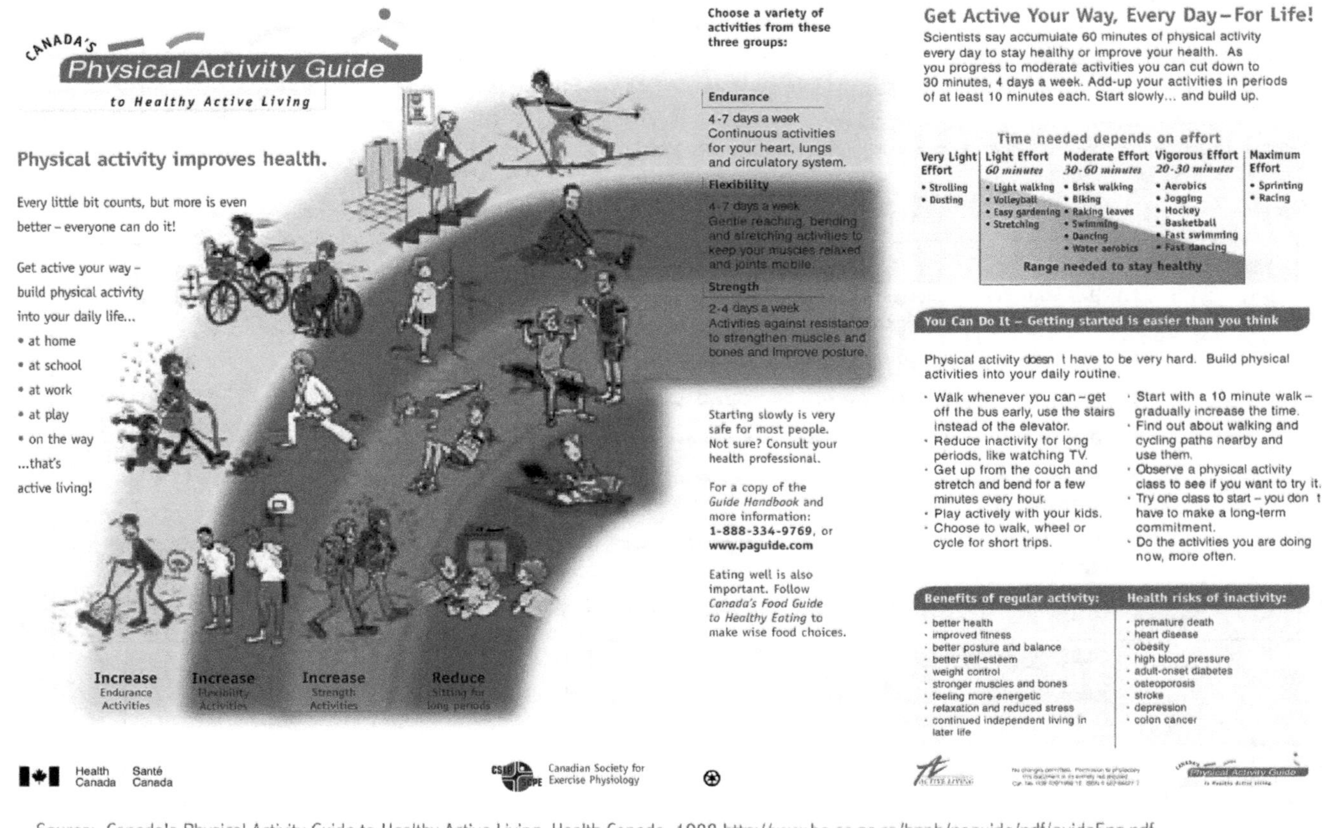

CANADA'S Physical Activity Guide
to Healthy Active Living

Physical activity improves health.

Every little bit counts, but more is even better – everyone can do it!

Get active your way – build physical activity into your daily life...
- at home
- at school
- at work
- at play
- on the way

...that's active living!

Choose a variety of activities from these three groups:

Endurance
4-7 days a week
Continuous activities for your heart, lungs and circulatory system.

Flexibility
4-7 days a week
Gentle reaching, bending and stretching activities to keep your muscles relaxed and joints mobile.

Strength
2-4 days a week
Activities against resistance to strengthen muscles and bones and improve posture.

Starting slowly is very safe for most people. Not sure? Consult your health professional.

For a copy of the *Guide Handbook* and more information: **1-888-334-9769**, or **www.paguide.com**

Eating well is also important. Follow *Canada's Food Guide to Healthy Eating* to make wise food choices.

Increase Endurance Activities | **Increase** Flexibility Activities | **Increase** Strength Activities | **Reduce** Sitting for long periods

Get Active Your Way, Every Day – For Life!

Scientists say accumulate 60 minutes of physical activity every day to stay healthy or improve your health. As you progress to moderate activities you can cut down to 30 minutes, 4 days a week. Add-up your activities in periods of at least 10 minutes each. Start slowly... and build up.

Time needed depends on effort

Very Light Effort	Light Effort *60 minutes*	Moderate Effort *30-60 minutes*	Vigorous Effort *20-30 minutes*	Maximum Effort
• Strolling • Dusting	• Light walking • Volleyball • Easy gardening • Stretching	• Brisk walking • Biking • Raking leaves • Swimming • Dancing • Water aerobics	• Aerobics • Jogging • Hockey • Basketball • Fast swimming • Fast dancing	• Sprinting • Racing

Range needed to stay healthy

You Can Do It – Getting started is easier than you think

Physical activity doesn t have to be very hard. Build physical activities into your daily routine.

- Walk whenever you can – get off the bus early, use the stairs instead of the elevator.
- Reduce inactivity for long periods, like watching TV.
- Get up from the couch and stretch and bend for a few minutes every hour.
- Play actively with your kids.
- Choose to walk, wheel or cycle for short trips.
- Start with a 10 minute walk – gradually increase the time.
- Find out about walking and cycling paths nearby and use them.
- Observe a physical activity class to see if you want to try it.
- Try one class to start – you don t have to make a long-term commitment.
- Do the activities you are doing now, more often.

Benefits of regular activity:
- better health
- improved fitness
- better posture and balance
- better self-esteem
- weight control
- stronger muscles and bones
- feeling more energetic
- relaxation and reduced stress
- continued independent living in later life

Health risks of inactivity:
- premature death
- heart disease
- obesity
- high blood pressure
- adult-onset diabetes
- osteoporosis
- stroke
- depression
- colon cancer

Health Canada Santé Canada

Canadian Society for Exercise Physiology

Source: Canada's Physical Activity Guide to Healthy Active Living, Health Canada, 1998 http://www.hc-sc.gc.ca/hppb/paguide/pdf/guideEng.pdf

FITNESS AND HEALTH PROFESSIONALS MAY BE INTERESTED IN THE INFORMATION BELOW:

The following companion forms are available for doctors' use by contacting the Canadian Society for Exercise Physiology (address below):

The **Physical Activity Readiness Medical Examination (PARmed-X)** – to be used by doctors with people who answer YES to one or more questions on the PAR-Q.

The **Physical Activity Readiness Medical Examination for Pregnancy (PARmed-X for Pregnancy)** – to be used by doctors with pregnant patients who wish to become more active.

References:

Arraix, G.A., Wigle, D.T., Mao, Y. (1992). Risk Assessment of Physical Activity and Physical Fitness in the Canada Health Survey Follow-Up Study. **J. Clin. Epidemiol.** 45:4 419-428.

Mottola, M., Wolfe, L.A. (1994). Active Living and Pregnancy, In: A. Quinney, L. Gauvin, T. Wall (eds.), **Toward Active Living: Proceedings of the International Conference on Physical Activity, Fitness and Health**. Champaign, IL: Human Kinetics.

PAR-Q Validation Report, British Columbia Ministry of Health, 1978.

Thomas, S., Reading, J., Shephard, R.J. (1992). Revision of the Physical Activity Readiness Questionnaire (PAR-Q). **Can. J. Spt. Sci.** 17:4 338-345.

For more information, please contact the:

Canadian Society for Exercise Physiology
202-185 Somerset Street West
Ottawa, ON K2P 0J2
Tel. 1-877-651-3755 • FAX (613) 234-3565
Online: www.csep.ca

The original PAR-Q was developed by the British Columbia Ministry of Health. It has been revised by an Expert Advisory Committee of the Canadian Society for Exercise Physiology chaired by Dr. N. Gledhill (2002).

Disponible en français sous le titre «Questionnaire sur l'aptitude à l'activité physique - Q-AAP (revisé 2002)».

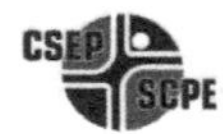

Supported by: 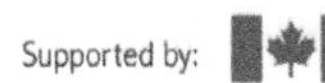 Health Canada Santé Canada

Physical Activity Readiness
Medical Examination
(revised 2002)

PARmed-X PHYSICAL ACTIVITY READINESS MEDICAL EXAMINATION

The PARmed-X is a physical activity-specific checklist to be used by a physician with patients who have had positive responses to the Physical Activity Readiness Questionnaire (PAR-Q). In addition, the Conveyance/Referral Form in the PARmed-X can be used to convey clearance for physical activity participation, or to make a referral to a medically-supervised exercise program.

Regular physical activity is fun and healthy, and increasingly more people are starting to become more active every day. Being more active is very safe for most people. The PAR-Q by itself provides adequate screening for the majority of people. However, some individuals may require a medical evaluation and specific advice (exercise prescription) due to one or more positive responses to the PAR-Q.

Following the participant's evaluation by a physician, a physical activity plan should be devised in consultation with a physical activity professional (CSEP-Professional Fitness & Lifestyle Consultant or CSEP-Exercise Therapist™). To assist in this, the following instructions are provided:

PAGE 1: • Sections A, B, C, and D should be completed by the participant BEFORE the examination by the physician. The bottom section is to be completed by the examining physician.

PAGES 2 & 3: • A checklist of medical conditions requiring special consideration and management.

PAGE 4: • Physical Activity & Lifestyle Advice for people who do not require specific instructions or prescribed exercise.

• Physical Activity Readiness Conveyance/Referral Form - an optional tear-off tab for the physician to convey clearance for physical activity participation, or to make a referral to a medically-supervised exercise program.

This section to be completed by the participant

A PERSONAL INFORMATION:

NAME ______________________

ADDRESS ______________________

____

TELEPHONE ______________________

BIRTHDATE ______________ GENDER ________

MEDICAL No. ______________________

B PAR-Q: Please indicate the PAR-Q questions to which you answered YES

- ❑ Q 1 Heart condition
- ❑ Q 2 Chest pain during activity
- ❑ Q 3 Chest pain at rest
- ❑ Q 4 Loss of balance, dizziness
- ❑ Q 5 Bone or joint problem
- ❑ Q 6 Blood pressure or heart drugs
- ❑ Q 7 Other reason: ______________________

C RISK FACTORS FOR CARDIOVASCULAR DISEASE:

Check all that apply

- ❑ Less than 30 minutes of moderate physical activity most days of the week.
- ❑ Currently smoker (tobacco smoking 1 or more times per week).
- ❑ High blood pressure reported by physician after repeated measurements.
- ❑ High cholesterol level reported by physician.
- ❑ Excessive accumulation of fat around waist.
- ❑ Family history of heart disease.

Please note: *Many of these risk factors are modifiable. Please refer to page 4 and discuss with your physician.*

D PHYSICAL ACTIVITY INTENTIONS:

What physical activity do you intend to do?

____

____

____

This section to be completed by the examining physician

Physical Exam:

Ht	Wt	BP i) /
		BP ii) /

Conditions limiting physical activity:

- ❑ Cardiovascular
- ❑ Respiratory
- ❑ Other
- ❑ Musculoskeletal
- ❑ Abdominal

Tests required:

- ❑ ECG
- ❑ Exercise Test
- ❑ X-Ray
- ❑ Blood
- ❑ Urinalysis
- ❑ Other

Physical Activity Readiness Conveyance/Referral:

Based upon a current review of health status, I recommend:

Further Information:
- ❑ Attached
- ❑ To be forwarded
- ❑ Available on request

- ❑ No physical activity
- ❑ Only a medically-supervised exercise program until further medical clearance
- ❑ Progressive physical activity:
  - ❑ with avoidance of: ______________________
  - ❑ with inclusion of: ______________________
  - ❑ under the supervision of a CSEP-Professional Fitness & Lifestyle Consultant or CSEP-Exercise Therapist™
- ❑ Unrestricted physical activity–start slowly and build up gradually

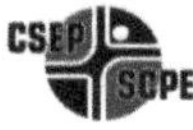

Supported by: 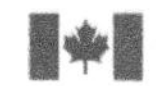 Health Canada Santé Canada

Physical Activity Readiness
Medical Examination
(revised 2002)

PARmed-X PHYSICAL ACTIVITY READINESS MEDICAL EXAMINATION

Following is a checklist of medical conditions for which a degree of precaution and/or special advice should be considered for those who answered "YES" to one or more questions on the PAR-Q, and people over the age of 69. Conditions are grouped by system. Three categories of precautions are provided. Comments under Advice are general, since details and alternatives require clinical judgement in each individual instance.

	Absolute Contraindications	Relative Contraindications	Special Prescriptive Conditions	ADVICE
	Permanent restriction or temporary restriction until condition is treated, stable, and/or past acute phase.	Highly variable. Value of exercise testing and/or program may exceed risk. Activity may be restricted. Desirable to maximize control of condition. Direct or indirect medical supervision of exercise program may be desirable.	Individualized prescriptive advice generally appropriate: • limitations imposed; and/or • special exercises prescribed. May require medical monitoring and/or initial supervision in exercise program.	
Cardiovascular	❑ aortic aneurysm (dissecting) ❑ aortic stenosis (severe) ❑ congestive heart failure ❑ crescendo angina ❑ myocardial infarction (acute) ❑ myocarditis (active or recent) ❑ pulmonary or systemic embolism—acute ❑ thrombophlebitis ❑ ventricular tachycardia and other dangerous dysrhythmias (e.g., multi-focal ventricular activity)	❑ aortic stenosis (moderate) ❑ subaortic stenosis (severe) ❑ marked cardiac enlargement ❑ supraventricular dysrhythmias (uncontrolled or high rate) ❑ ventricular ectopic activity (repetitive or frequent) ❑ ventricular aneurysm ❑ hypertension—untreated or uncontrolled severe (systemic or pulmonary) ❑ hypertrophic cardiomyopathy ❑ compensated congestive heart failure	❑ aortic (or pulmonary) stenosis—mild angina pectoris and other manifestations of coronary insufficiency (e.g., post-acute infarct) ❑ cyanotic heart disease ❑ shunts (intermittent or fixed) ❑ conduction disturbances • complete AV block • left BBB • Wolff-Parkinson-White syndrome ❑ dysrhythmias—controlled ❑ fixed rate pacemakers	• clinical exercise test may be warranted in selected cases, for specific determination of functional capacity and limitations and precautions (if any). • slow progression of exercise to levels based on test performance and individual tolerance. • consider individual need for initial conditioning program under medical supervision (indirect or direct).
			❑ intermittent claudication	progressive exercise to tolerance
			❑ hypertension: systolic 160-180; diastolic 105+	progressive exercise; care with medications (serum electrolytes; post-exercise syncope; etc.)
Infections	❑ acute infectious disease (regardless of etiology)	❑ subacute/chronic/recurrent infectious diseases (e.g., malaria, others)	❑ chronic infections ❑ HIV	variable as to condition
Metabolic		❑ uncontrolled metabolic disorders (diabetes mellitus, thyrotoxicosis, myxedema)	❑ renal, hepatic & other metabolic insufficiency	variable as to status
			❑ obesity ❑ single kidney	dietary moderation, and initial light exercises with slow progression (walking, swimming, cycling)
Pregnancy		❑ complicated pregnancy (e.g., toxemia, hemorrhage, incompetent cervix, etc.)	❑ advanced pregnancy (late 3rd trimester)	refer to the "PARmed-X for PREGNANCY"

References:

Arraix, G.A., Wigle, D.T., Mao, Y. (1992). Risk Assessment of Physical Activity and Physical Fitness in the Canada Health Survey Follow-Up Study. **J. Clin. Epidemiol.** 45:4 419-428.

Mottola, M., Wolfe, L.A. (1994). Active Living and Pregnancy, In: A. Quinney, L. Gauvin, T. Wall (eds.), **Toward Active Living: Proceedings of the International Conference on Physical Activity, Fitness and Health**. Champaign, IL: Human Kinetics.

PAR-Q Validation Report, British Columbia Ministry of Health, 1978.

Thomas, S., Reading, J., Shephard, R.J. (1992). Revision of the Physical Activity Readiness Questionnaire (PAR-Q). **Can. J. Spt. Sci.** 17: 4 338-345.

The PAR-Q and PARmed-X were developed by the British Columbia Ministry of Health. They have been revised by an Expert Advisory Committee of the Canadian Society for Exercise Physiology chaired by Dr. N. Gledhill (2002).

Disponible en français sous le titre
«Évaluation médicale de l'aptitude à l'activité physique (X-AAP)»

Continued on page 3...

Physical Activity Readiness
Medical Examination
(revised 2002)

	Special Prescriptive Conditions	ADVICE
Lung	❑ chronic pulmonary disorders	special relaxation and breathing exercises
	❑ obstructive lung disease ❑ asthma	breath control during endurance exercises to tolerance; avoid polluted air
	❑ exercise-induced bronchospasm	avoid hyperventilation during exercise; avoid extremely cold conditions; warm up adequately; utilize appropriate medication.
Musculoskeletal	❑ low back conditions (pathological, functional)	avoid or minimize exercise that precipitates or exasperates e.g., forced extreme flexion, extension, and violent twisting; correct posture, proper back exercises
	❑ arthritis—acute (infective, rheumatoid; gout)	treatment, plus judicious blend of rest, splinting and gentle movement
	❑ arthritis—subacute	progressive increase of active exercise therapy
	❑ arthritis—chronic (osteoarthritis and above conditions)	maintenance of mobility and strength; non-weightbearing exercises to minimize joint trauma (e.g., cycling, aquatic activity, etc.)
	❑ orthopaedic	highly variable and individualized
	❑ hernia	minimize straining and isometrics; stregthen abdominal muscles
	❑ osteoporosis or low bone density	avoid exercise with high risk for fracture such as push-ups, curl-ups, vertical jump and trunk forward flexion; engage in low-impact weight-bearing activities and resistance training
CNS	❑ convulsive disorder not completely controlled by medication	minimize or avoid exercise in hazardous environments and/or exercising alone (e.g., swimming, mountainclimbing, etc.)
	❑ recent concussion	thorough examination if history of two concussions; review for discontinuation of contact sport if three concussions, depending on duration of unconsciousness, retrograde amnesia, persistent headaches, and other objective evidence of cerebral damage
Blood	❑ anemia—severe (< 10 Gm/dl) ❑ electrolyte disturbances	control preferred; exercise as tolerated
Medications	❑ antianginal ❑ antiarrhythmic ❑ antihypertensive ❑ anticonvulsant ❑ beta-blockers ❑ digitalis preparations ❑ diuretics ❑ ganglionic blockers ❑ others	NOTE: consider underlying condition. Potential for: exertional syncope, electrolyte imbalance, bradycardia, dysrhythmias, impaired coordination and reaction time, heat intolerance. May alter resting and exercise ECG's and exercise test performance.
Other	❑ post-exercise syncope	moderate program
	❑ heat intolerance	prolong cool-down with light activities; avoid exercise in extreme heat
	❑ temporary minor illness	postpone until recovered
	❑ cancer	if potential metastases, test by cycle ergometry, consider non-weight bearing exercises; exercise at lower end of prescriptive range (40-65% of heart rate reserve), depending on condition and recent treatment (radiation, chemotherapy); monitor hemoglobin and lymphocyte counts; add dynamic lifting exercise to strengthen muscles, using machines rather than weights.

*Refer to special publications for elaboration as required

The following companion forms are available online: http://www.csep.ca/forms.asp

The **Physical Activity Readiness Questionnaire (PAR-Q)** - a questionnaire for people aged 15-69 to complete before becoming much more physically active.

The **Physical Activity Readiness Medical Examination for Pregnancy (PARmed-X for PREGNANCY)** - to be used by physicians with pregnant patients who wish to become more physically active.

For more information, please contact the:

Canadian Society for Exercise Physiology
202 - 185 Somerset St. West
Ottawa, ON K2P 0J2
Tel. 1-877-651-3755 • FAX (613) 234-3565 • Online: www.csep.ca

Note to physical activity professionals...

It is a prudent practice to retain the completed Physical Activity Readiness Conveyance/Referral Form in the participant's file.

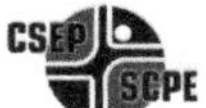

Supported by: 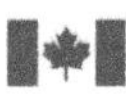 Health Canada Santé Canada

Continued on page 4...

Physical Activity Readiness
Medical Examination
(revised 2002)

PARmed-X PHYSICAL ACTIVITY READINESS MEDICAL EXAMINATION

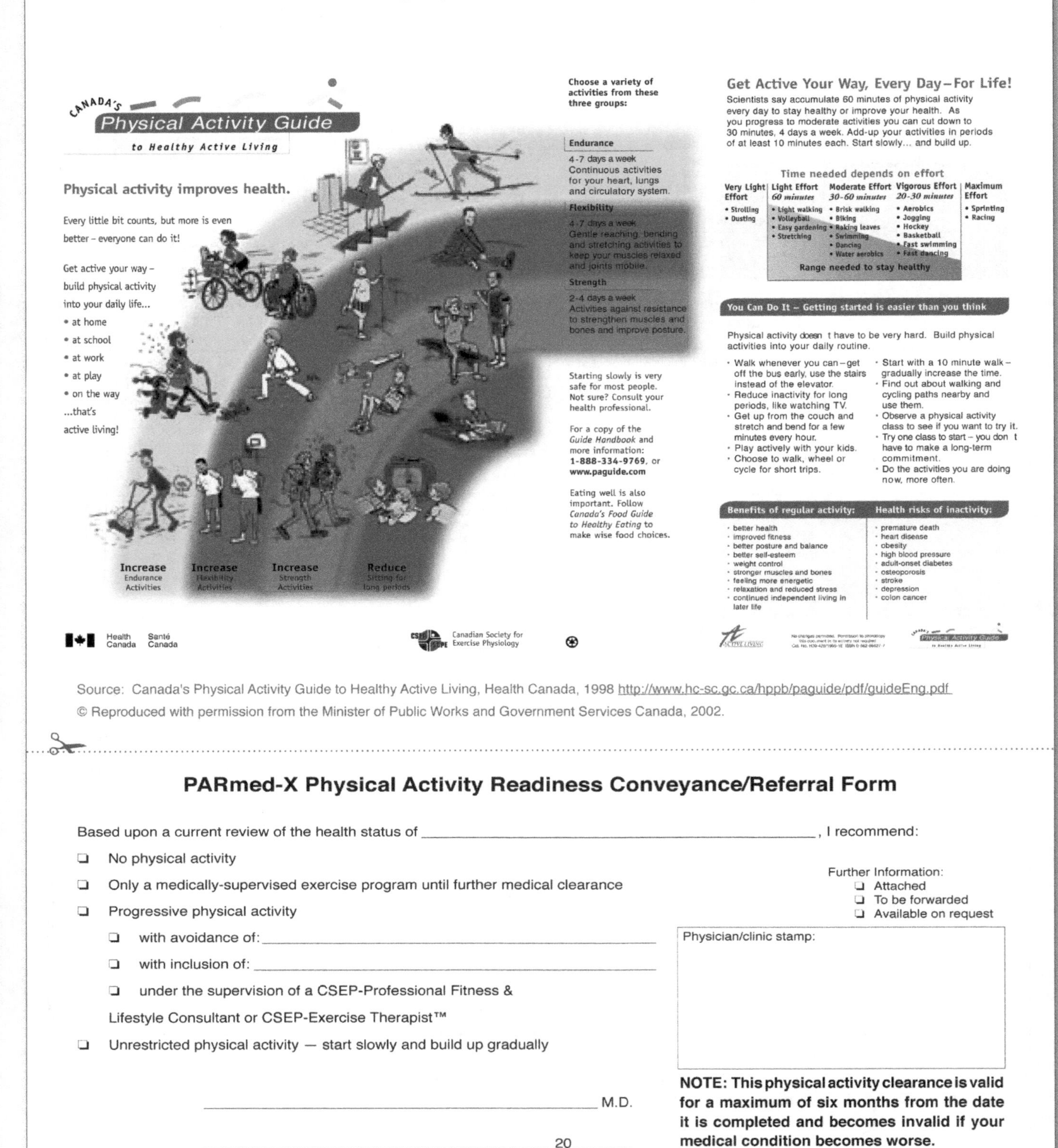

CANADA'S Physical Activity Guide to Healthy Active Living

Physical activity improves health.

Every little bit counts, but more is even better – everyone can do it!

Get active your way – build physical activity into your daily life...

- at home
- at school
- at work
- at play
- on the way

...that's active living!

Choose a variety of activities from these three groups:

Endurance
4-7 days a week
Continuous activities for your heart, lungs and circulatory system.

Flexibility
4-7 days a week
Gentle reaching, bending and stretching activities to keep your muscles relaxed and joints mobile.

Strength
2-4 days a week
Activities against resistance to strengthen muscles and bones and improve posture.

Increase Endurance Activities | **Increase** Flexibility Activities | **Increase** Strength Activities | **Reduce** Sitting for long periods

Starting slowly is very safe for most people. Not sure? Consult your health professional.

For a copy of the *Guide Handbook* and more information: **1-888-334-9769**, or **www.paguide.com**

Eating well is also important. Follow *Canada's Food Guide to Healthy Eating* to make wise food choices.

Get Active Your Way, Every Day–For Life!

Scientists say accumulate 60 minutes of physical activity every day to stay healthy or improve your health. As you progress to moderate activities you can cut down to 30 minutes, 4 days a week. Add-up your activities in periods of at least 10 minutes each. Start slowly... and build up.

Time needed depends on effort

Very Light Effort	Light Effort *60 minutes*	Moderate Effort *30-60 minutes*	Vigorous Effort *20-30 minutes*	Maximum Effort
• Strolling • Dusting	• Light walking • Volleyball • Easy gardening • Stretching	• Brisk walking • Biking • Raking leaves • Swimming • Dancing • Water aerobics	• Aerobics • Jogging • Hockey • Basketball • Fast swimming • Fast dancing	• Sprinting • Racing

Range needed to stay healthy

You Can Do It – Getting started is easier than you think

Physical activity doesn t have to be very hard. Build physical activities into your daily routine.

- Walk whenever you can – get off the bus early, use the stairs instead of the elevator.
- Reduce inactivity for long periods, like watching TV.
- Get up from the couch and stretch and bend for a few minutes every hour.
- Play actively with your kids.
- Choose to walk, wheel or cycle for short trips.
- Start with a 10 minute walk – gradually increase the time.
- Find out about walking and cycling paths nearby and use them.
- Observe a physical activity class to see if you want to try it.
- Try one class to start – you don t have to make a long-term commitment.
- Do the activities you are doing now, more often.

Benefits of regular activity:	Health risks of inactivity:
· better health · improved fitness · better posture and balance · better self-esteem · weight control · stronger muscles and bones · feeling more energetic · relaxation and reduced stress · continued independent living in later life	· premature death · heart disease · obesity · high blood pressure · adult-onset diabetes · osteoporosis · stroke · depression · colon cancer

Health Canada Santé Canada | Canadian Society for Exercise Physiology | Active Living | Canada's Physical Activity Guide to Healthy Active Living

Source: Canada's Physical Activity Guide to Healthy Active Living, Health Canada, 1998 http://www.hc-sc.gc.ca/hppb/paguide/pdf/guideEng.pdf

PARmed-X Physical Activity Readiness Conveyance/Referral Form

Based upon a current review of the health status of ______________________________, I recommend:

- ❑ No physical activity
- ❑ Only a medically-supervised exercise program until further medical clearance
- ❑ Progressive physical activity
  - ❑ with avoidance of: ______________________
  - ❑ with inclusion of: ______________________
  - ❑ under the supervision of a CSEP-Professional Fitness & Lifestyle Consultant or CSEP-Exercise Therapist™
- ❑ Unrestricted physical activity — start slowly and build up gradually

Further Information:
- ❑ Attached
- ❑ To be forwarded
- ❑ Available on request

Physician/clinic stamp:

______________________________ M.D.

______________________________ 20______
(date)

NOTE: This physical activity clearance is valid for a maximum of six months from the date it is completed and becomes invalid if your medical condition becomes worse.

4

ASSIGNMENT 1.2 Informed Consent for Training and BFOR Testing

After filling out the PAR-Q and prior to starting your fitness class, read and fill out this informed consent form. Make sure to ask your instructor if you have any questions. If you have answered yes to any of the questions in the PAR-Q, please see your instructor.

Informed Consent to Undertake Training to Be Fit for ____________ Course at ____________ College

I, ______________________________, understand that ______________________________ Fitness Class evaluates my physical capacity as it applies to police work. I understand that I will participate in training and testing of policing job simulation tests, metabolic assessments (shuttle run, timed 1.5-mile runs, sprints, stairs), and fitness assessments (e.g., back extension, push-ups, chin-ups, flexibility, bench press). The successful completion of this training and testing will show that I possess the minimal physical abilities deemed essential for the performance of police work.

Physical Demands

I understand that we will work at training and testing that is physically demanding. During training and testing my heart rate may reach its maximal level, and may remain there for several minutes, thus placing me under heavy physical stress. Training for and testing of various Bona Fide Occupational Requirements (BFOR) will also challenge my muscular strength, agility, and coordination skills. I will be required to run various distances, run stairs, carry heavy objects (36–45 kg), climb over a 1.2-m (4-ft) wall, run up and down stairs, drag a 68-kg (150-lb) victim, grasp a 15-kg (33-lb) mechanism and move the arms of the machine, and push/pull 32–36 kg (70–80 lb), jump hurdles, jump over a vault rail, and wear weighted vests.

I state that I have no known medical or physical problems that may place me at risk during or following my performance of the test. I have read and signed the PAR-Q. I have not taken any medication, supplements, or stimulants other than whole food prepared naturally today. (If I am taking any medication that is approved, it is indicated on my medical clearance in the PARmedX that was completed by my physician.) I have looked over the requirements for the career that I'm entering and have determined whether I can medically meet the requirements of that career. My health has not changed since my last medical examination. Prior to each class, I have followed the training/test preparation instructions, which include abstinence from alcohol and vigorous exercise for at least six hours prior to the test, abstinence from caffeinated products (including drinks that profess to provide you with energy and help keep you alert) for at least two hours prior to the test, avoidance of a *heavy* meal within three to four hours of the test, and abstinence from smoking for at least two hours prior to the test.

I understand the training/test as it has been explained and demonstrated to me, and I have had the opportunity to ask questions and practise on equipment. I will follow all safety procedures as outlined. Heart rate and blood pressure screening will be required, and I will remain at the testing session until successfully screened after the test. It is my obligation to immediately inform the appraiser of any pain, discomfort, fatigue, or other symptoms that I may suffer during or immediately following the test. My understanding is that there are potential risks associated with training and testing, such as light-headedness, fainting, chest discomfort, musculoskeletal injury, and nausea. I wilfully assume those risks.

No Compulsion

Any attempt of the BFOR or fitness training will be considered adherence to the college policy and will be recorded as such for my student file. I understand that UNDER NO CIRCUMSTANCES am I compelled to continue to complete a test should I decide to stop. I also will follow the instructions about safety, including slowing down or stopping immediately, IF INSTRUCTED TO DO SO by the test administrator and/or fitness instructor.

Full Effort

If I participate at full effort, I acknowledge that I have participated in physical activities such as sports or exercise requiring maximal exertion in the last two months and have a current medical clearance. If I am not used to maximal effort (last two months) then a maximal effort is NOT RECOMMENDED at this time.

Participant's Acknowledgment:

(Print Name) ______________________ (Signature) ______________________

Date: ____

Witness::

(Print Name) ______________________ (Signature) ______________________

Date: ____

Test Administrator/Fitness Instructor:

(Print Name) ______________________ (Signature) ______________________

College: ____

Date: ____

ASSIGNMENT 2.1 Assessing Your Values

1. Determine what values are important to you at this point in your life. Rank the following values on a scale of 1 (most important) to 5 (least important). Two or more values can share the same ranking. Space is provided at the end for adding values not mentioned in the list, if you wish. Knowing which values are most important to you will help you build short-term and long-term goals.

VALUE	RANK
Education	
Lifelong learning	
Keeping current on everyday legal issues	
Mental health	
Physical health	
Fitness and exercise	
Learning a new sport/skill	
Being employed in law enforcement	
Continuing education	
Being well paid	
Being financially stable	
Staying organized	
Volunteering your time	
Getting involved in student life	
Joining college sports teams	

VALUE	RANK
Serving on student council	
Time for yourself	
Time for family and friends	
Spiritual/religious life	
Creative/artistic endeavours	
A balanced lifestyle	
A healthy diet	
Free time/vacations	
Reading/studying	
Self-improvement	
Other values important to you:	

2. See if you can answer the following questions relating to personal values.
   a. What would you do with your life if you knew the world would end in the next year?

____

____

____

____

b. Think of someone who has influenced your life. What are the three top qualities that you admire in this person?

____

____

____

____

c. Who are you when you are at your absolute best?

____

____

____

____

d. Picture yourself the same age as your grandparents. What two or three lessons have you learned that are most important to you now?

____

____

____

____

e. What are your five most important values?

i) ____

ii) ____

iii) ____

iv) ____

v) ____

Return to "Short- and Long-Term Goals" in Chapter 2.

ASSIGNMENT 2.2 Determining What Success Means to You

Most people define "success" as fulfilling their goals in life. To set a path for success, it is important to set goals and work toward achieving them. Try to set goals that you would like to achieve in your life by using the values from **assignment 2.1** that you determined were important to you.

1. First, review the following questions to help you understand what your strengths, dreams, and desires are so that you can better define the goals you want to accomplish.
   a. What are you great at? (What does your biggest fan or parent think of you?)

   b. What do you love to do? What matters the most to you? What makes you the happiest? (Think in terms of values, beliefs, hobbies, and so on.)

   c. What would your dream life look like? (Think in terms of dream job, spouse, home, bank account, hobbies, and so on.)

   d. What skills do you want to master in your lifetime?

   e. What do you want to give back to the world?

2. Fill in five of your goals in each of the following sections.

GOAL SECTION	YOUR 5 GOALS
PERSONAL GOALS What are your personal goals? What commitment do you have to fitness? Do you have goals relating to your health? What courses do you want to take to improve yourself (for example, self-confidence, public speaking)? What type of fame—if any—do you want to achieve?	1. 2. 3. 4. 5.
FAMILY, FRIENDS, AND RELATIONSHIP GOALS What kinds of relationships do you want with your friends, parents, co-workers, and others? Do you want to be married, have children? How many close friends do you want?	1. 2. 3. 4. 5.
PROFESSIONAL GOALS What kind of work do you want to do? What skills do you need to prepare for a job interview? Do you have the basic skills that employers are looking for? Name specific career areas or occupations.	1. 2. 3. 4. 5.
FINANCIAL GOALS Are you choosing a career that will support your lifestyle? What types of material items do you want in life? Can you handle loans, credit cards, and other financial obligations? Do you have enough money to make it through the school year? Have you demonstrated a good credit rating (imperative for applying to a police agency)?	1. 2. 3. 4. 5.
LIFESTYLE GOALS What types of leisure activities do you want to pursue? What interests do you want to develop? What kinds of vacations do you want to take? What type of community involvement do you want? (Volunteer work is critical when you apply to a law enforcement agency.)	1. 2. 3. 4. 5.

3. Now try to rate and organize your goals by filling in the table below.
   a. In the "GOAL" column, write the 10 goals you consider most important, listing them in order of importance (the most important beside number 1, the second most important beside number 2, and so on).
   b. In the "DIFFICULTY" column, write the number that reflects how difficult it will be to achieve each of your 10 goals according to the following scale:
      3 — I will have to work very hard to reach this goal.
      2 — I can reach this goal if I work at it.
      1 — I can reach this goal fairly easily.
   c. In the "CONFLICTS WITH" column, write the number of each of the other goals with which your goal conflicts. If the goal does not conflict with any other goal, write "0."
   d. In the "HELPS" column, write the number of each of the other goals that is helped by achieving the goal. If the goal does not help any other goal, write "0."

   Remember: If goals are in conflict, you must either find ways for them to work together or decide which goal to achieve first before moving on to the next one.

	GOAL	DIFFICULTY	CONFLICTS WITH	HELPS
1.				
2.				
3.				
4.				
5.				
6.				
7.				
8.				
9.				
10.				

4. Based on all the goals that you have listed in this assignment, comment on what success means to you:

ASSIGNMENT 2.3

Developing Your Short-Term Goals to Achieve Long-Term Goals

1. Now that you have assessed your values, formulate one or two goals for each of the areas mentioned in **assignment 2.2** (personal, family and relationship, professional, financial, and lifestyle). These goals should be tied to the values you ranked the highest. Below are a number of questions you might want to ask yourself before writing down the goals and action plans to accomplish the ones you chose. Remember that you need to reassess at the end of each semester whether they are specific goals. Some of the questions that you may want to ask yourself include:

   - Have I prioritized my five most important goals for the next two years?
   - Do they reflect my most important values?
   - Do they follow the SMART principles?
   - Will my goals help me obtain the skills that law enforcement demands?
   - Am I physically fit to an acceptable level, and am I committed to maintaining fitness throughout my life?
   - Do I meet the academic, medical, and physical requirements for the career I am pursuing?

2. Now fill out the Smart Goal-Setting and Action Planner on the following page. After 4 weeks, using **assignment 2.4** (Summary of Goal-Setting Results: Successes, Barriers, and Strategies to Overcome Challenges chart), assess how you made out.

SMART Goal-Setting and Action Planner (4-Week Planner)

SMART: **S**pecific, **M**easurable, **A**ttainable, **R**elevant/Realistic, **T**imed

Start date: Completion date:

LONG-TERM GOAL AREAS	ACTION STEPS (Short-Term Goal Statements)	WEEKLY CHECK BOX (✓ or ✗ Depending on Achievement)				REWARDS
	Over the next 4 weeks, I will . . .	***Week 1***	***Week 2***	***Week 3***	***Week 4***	
Nutrition	1.					
	2.					
	3.					
Physical Activity	1.					
	2.					
	3.					
Time Management	1.					
	2.					
	3.					
Other	1.					
	2.					
	3.					

SUCCESS INDICATORS
1.
2.
3.
4.

THINGS TO RE-EVALUATE (FOR THE NEXT 4 WEEKS)
1.
2.
3.

SOURCE: Canadian Society for Exercise Physiology (CSEP). (2003). *The Canadian physical activity, fitness and lifestyle appraisal: CSEP's plan for healthy active living.* (3rd ed.). Adapted with permission from the Canadian Society for Exercise Physiology.

ASSIGNMENT 2.4 Summary of Goal-Setting Results: Successes, Barriers, and Strategies to Overcome Challenges

Two to three weeks before the end of the semester, assess how well you have done using the chart below.

Start date: ____________________ Completion date: ____________________

LONG-TERM GOAL AREAS	WHAT I FELT WENT WELL AND WHY	STRATEGIES FOR OVERCOMING FUTURE BARRIERS
Nutrition		
Physical Activity		
Time Management		
Other		

WHAT I LEARNED

WHERE I NEED TO GO FROM HERE

WHO/WHAT CAN HELP ME ACCOMPLISH MY GOALS

GOALS I WANT TO ADDRESS NEXT SEMESTER

INSTRUCTOR'S OBSERVATIONS/COMMENTS

ASSIGNMENT 2.5 Mission Statement

Prepare a mission statement that incorporates the goals you prioritized earlier.

FIVE TOP GOALS (FROM ASSIGNMENT 2.2)
1.
2.
3.
4.
5.

MISSION STATEMENT

ASSIGNMENT 3.1 Where Does All Your Time Go?

Think back over the past 7 days and estimate how much time you spent on each of the following activities:

ACTIVITY	HOURS
Classroom learning	
Homework	
Computer (games, Internet, word processing, etc.)	
Group work	
Time spent in the college cafeteria	
Library use	
Fitness training (outside of class)	
Recreational activities	
Meal preparation	
Meal consumption	
Grocery shopping	
Other shopping	
Laundry and other household chores	
Commuting	
Waiting in line	
Speaking on the telephone	
Text messaging (texting, tweeting, etc.)	
Searching the Internet, reading blogs, etc.	

ACTIVITY	HOURS
Chatting online (Facebook, etc.)	
Sleeping	
Grooming and personal hygiene	
Watching television	
Reading newspaper or books unrelated to academic work	
Time with family or significant other	
Time with friends	
Attending meetings of clubs and other organizations	
Volunteer work	
Paid work	
Other activities:	
TOTAL TIME	

Evaluating Your Time-Management Skills

1. A week has 168 hours. Was your total within 10 percent of this figure? If yes, can you explain why? What did you notice about where you used your time?

2. If your total was well below 168 hours, can you account for the lost time? Does the lost time indicate that there are issues and priorities in your life that are not being addressed? Are there areas where wasted time might be used more effectively? Do you think that your priorities relate to the goals you listed in Chapter 2? Be specific.

3. If your total was well above 168 hours, how do you account for this? Are you multitasking, or do you feel that you are not as productive with your time as you could be? How effective are you when you try to multitask? Be specific.

4. What have you learned about your time-management skills? What skills do you need to work on (procrastination, prioritizing your time, balancing work with personal choices, etc.)? What resources are available at your college to help balance your experience at school?

ASSIGNMENT 3.2 Tracking Your Time

1. For the next 7 days, use the time-management chart at the end of this assignment to track your activities. Colour-code the chart to analyze where you are spending your time. Try to confine yourself to the following categories:

BLACK	Time-wasters (wasting time between classes, standing in lines, etc.)
DARK BLUE	Duties, obligations (includes work hours)
LIGHT BLUE	School hours
DARK GREEN	Fitness and recreational activities
LIGHT GREEN	Physical needs, including grooming and personal hygiene (including the time it takes you to get ready for school, work, dates, etc.) and meal preparation and eating time
PINK	Transportation (getting to and from school, work, social activities)
ORANGE	Intellectual needs (reading, studying, doing research)
RED	Personal needs (time for yourself)
DARK PURPLE	Volunteer work
YELLOW	Fun activities, including social time (at school, and evenings and weekends)
LIGHT PURPLE	Time spent on the phone and Internet for personal reasons
GREY	Sleep

You may add additional colours to reflect additional responsibilities. Try to fill the chart out at least three times during the day—we all tend to forget the time we spend doing trivial things like checking email, sitting in the cafeteria talking to classmates, changing for gym class, making meals, doing dishes, tidying up, and talking on the phone. You may wish to include how you feel periodically during the day, whether you are alert, lethargic, tired, or energetic. This may help you assess whether your circadian rhythm (discussed in Chapter 13) affects your productivity or whether you need to look at your eating habits.

Some people who struggle with time management prefer to keep track of 15-minute increments so that they can see more clearly where their time is going. You may want to do this as well. Remember that this assignment takes only a few minutes a day if you do it during the day. You will not be as accurate if you record your activities only at the end of each day.

2. At the end of the 7 days, look over your chart and answer the following questions:
   a. Do you use your time effectively? Why or why not?

   b. Which time periods do you use most effectively?

   c. Which time periods do you use least effectively?

   d. Were you able to achieve all your goals for the week? Which goals did you achieve? Which goals did you not achieve? Can you explain why?

e. Did you spend most of your time on the activities/assignments that matter the most? Why or why not?

f. Does the time of day affect your productivity level (i.e., are there times during the day when you are more efficient, more alert, more energetic)? Be specific.

g. Do you have enough time to relax and unwind? Spend enough time with family and friends? Reward yourself for accomplishing tasks? Explain why or why not.

h. Does your time management for the week raise any issues that need to be addressed? What could you change to improve your time management? If there are no issues, what are you doing well?

Time-Management Chart

TIME	MONDAY	TUESDAY	WEDNESDAY	THURSDAY	FRIDAY	SATURDAY	SUNDAY
05:00							
05:30							
06:00							
06:30							
07:00							
07:30							
08:00							
08:30							
09:00							
09:30							
10:00							
10:30							
11:00							
11:30							
12:00							
12:30							
13:00							
13:30							
14:00							
14:30							
15:00							
15:30							
16:00							
16:30							
17:00							
17:30							
18:00							
18:30							
19:00							
19:30							
20:00							
20:30							
21:00							
21:30							
22:00							
22:30							
23:00							
23:30							
24:00							
00:30							
01:00							
01:30							
02:00							
02:30							
03:00							
03:30							
04:00							
04:30							

ASSIGNMENT 3.3 Your To-Do List for This Week

1. Using the activity headings below as a guideline, create a to-do list of essential, regular, and optional activities for this week. The list should include all of your formal job duties, special projects you want to complete, your daily/weekly routine responsibilities, and other tasks you would like to see accomplished.

ESSENTIAL ACTIVITIES	1.
	2.
	3.
	4.
REGULAR ACTIVITIES	1.
	2.
	3.
	4.
OPTIONAL ACTIVITIES	1.
	2.
	3.
	4.

2. Using the activity chart on the next page, consider these tasks and estimate the time each takes, their importance, priority, and whether the task could be delegated. Set dates for follow-up and deadlines for each task. This can be done on a weekly basis to assist you with developing an action plan for time management.

Activity chart for week of :

	ACTIVITY DESCRIPTION	ESTIMATED TIME	IMPORTANCE					POTENTIAL FOR DELEGATION	PERSON TO WHOM TASK IS DELEGATED	FOLLOW-UP DATE	PRIORITY					DEADLINE	COMPLETED
			1	2	3	4	5				1	2	3	4	5		
1.																	
2.																	
3.																	
4.																	
5.																	
6.																	
7.																	
8.																	
9.																	
10.																	
11.																	
12.																	

ASSIGNMENT 3.4 Assessing Your Level of Procrastination

Self-Assessment

1. What are your time-wasters? How do you, or how should you, deal with them (e.g., slow start/procrastination, disorganization, diversion, interruptions)?

TIME-WASTER	METHOD OF DEALING WITH TIME-WASTER

2. Everyone procrastinates at some point. How do you get yourself going on a project or completing a task? Be specific.

3. What techniques do you use to keep yourself going, especially on unpleasant or boring tasks? How do you motivate yourself to complete a task? Be specific.

4. How do you deal with or minimize interruptions? How should you deal with them?

5. Do you know how to delegate tasks? Why or why not?

6. Based on the answers above, do you need to work on procrastination skills? If so, what would be a good first step? If not, what can you do better?

Now, use the Project To-Do List sheet on the next page to help you accomplish a task over the next week.

Project To-Do List

Date:	Project due:
Project Overview:	

	STEP	TASKS	DEADLINE	DATE COMPLETED
1.		•		
		•		
		•		
2.		•		
		•		
		•		
3.		•		
		•		
		•		
4.		•		
		•		
		•		
5.		•		
		•		
		•		

ASSIGNMENT 4.1 Naming the Bones and Muscles of the Body

1. Identify the bones of the human skeleton that are numbered below.

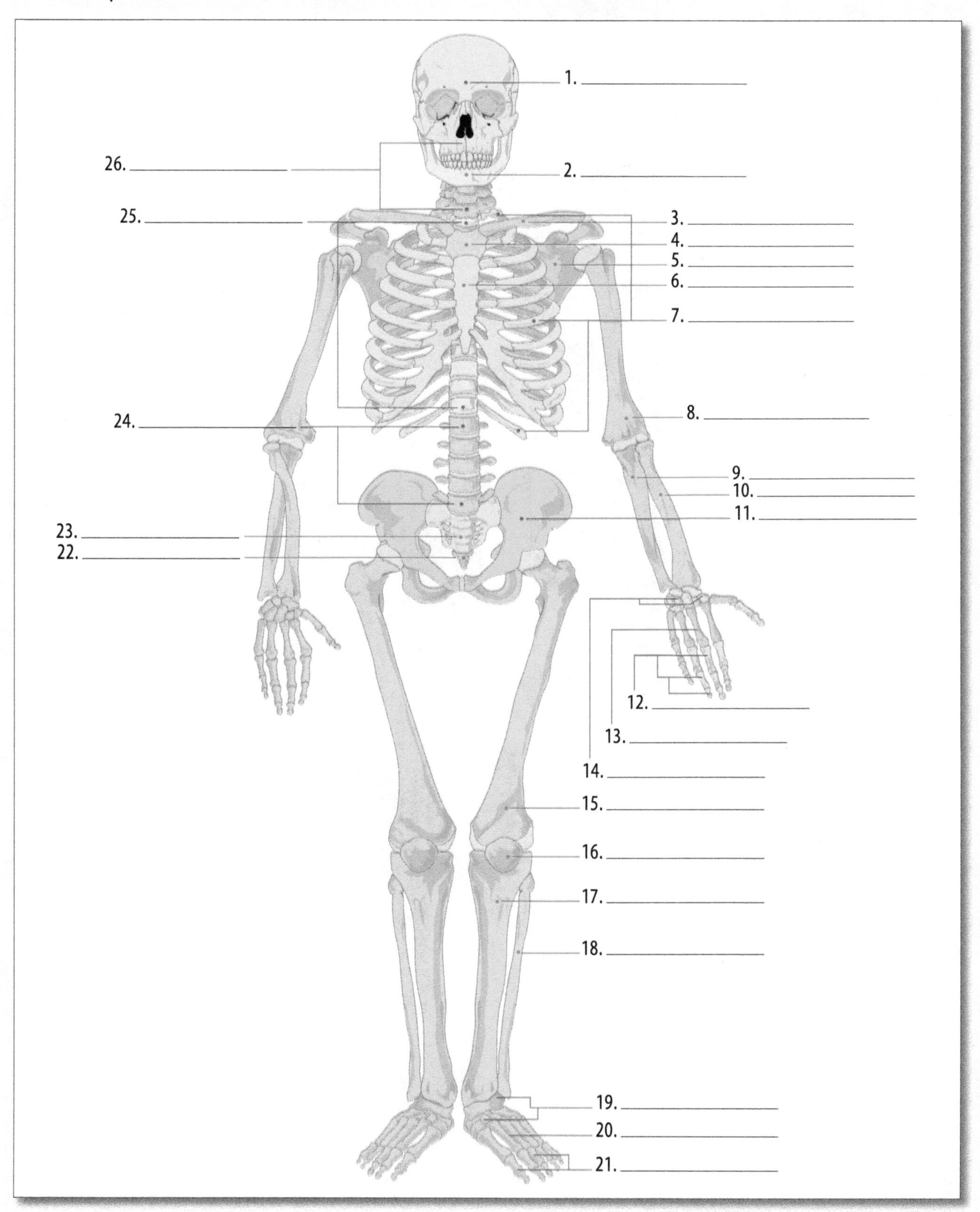

2. Identify the major muscle groups that are numbered below.

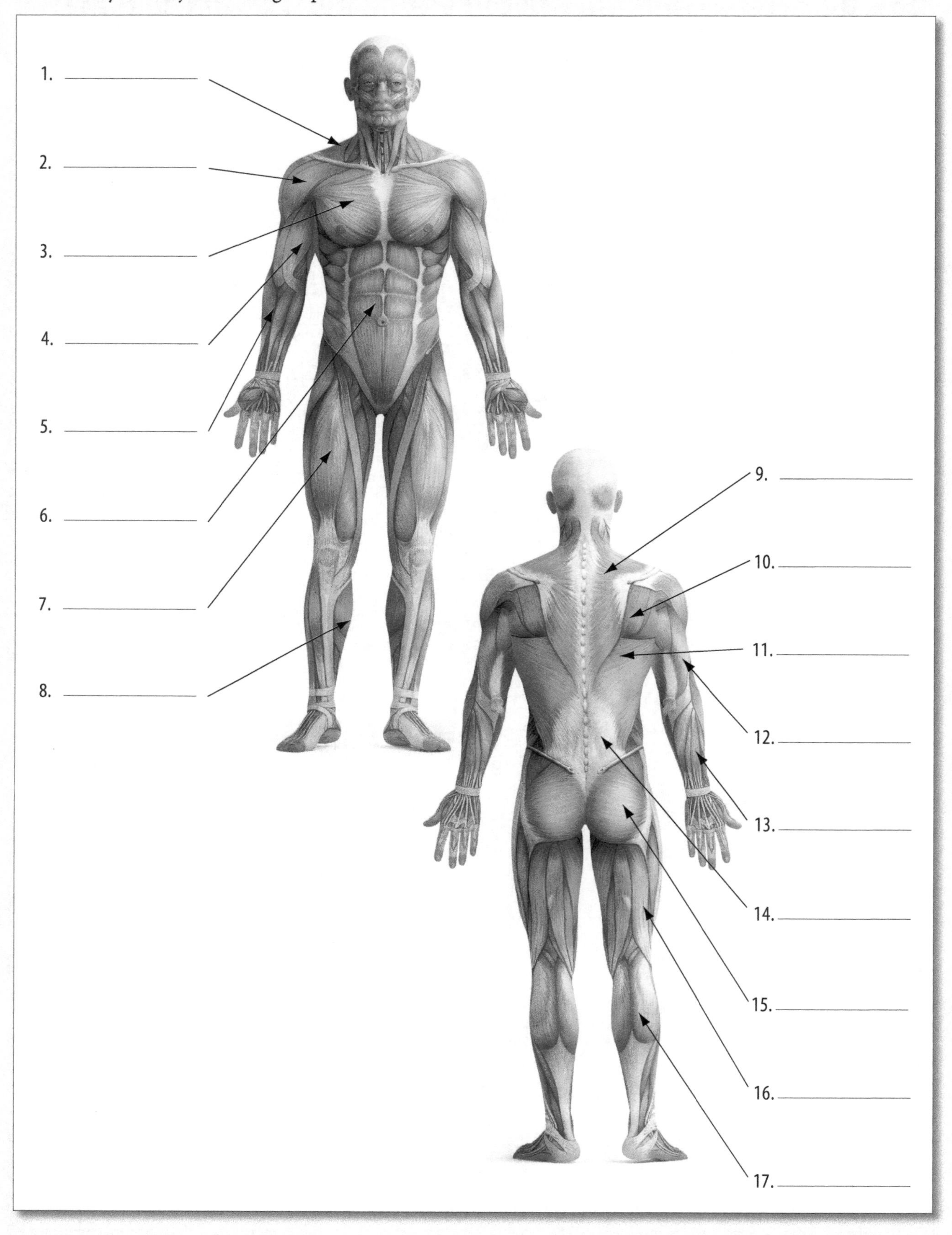

ASSIGNMENT 4.2 Health Benefits of Physical Activity

1. Drawing on the information presented in Chapter 4 and on your own knowledge, list eight health benefits of physical activity. How might they have an impact on your life? Your career? Place a star by the three most important.

	BENEFIT	IMPACT ON MY LIFE	IMPACT ON MY CAREER
1.			
2.			
3.			
4.			
5.			
6.			
7.			
8.			

2. After you have read this chapter, comment on the health benefits you believe are most important in law enforcement. What areas do you need to pay attention to in order to stay healthy throughout your career? Be specific.

ASSIGNMENT 4.3

Physical and Psychological Benefits of Physical Activity

Determine whether you are meeting the Canadian Physical Activity Guidelines.

Go to Canadian Physical Activity Guidelines (available at http://www.csep.ca/english/view.asp?x=804) and click on the Canadian Physical Activity Guideline for your age. Write out the guidelines that are recommended for your age group.

Your age: __________ years

Guidelines recommended for __________ – __________ years:

Comment on how close you are to those guidelines (i.e., what you do well; where you could improve; what issues you must face to achieve these standards):

Based on the above information and your personal values, list five physical benefits of physical activity that are important to you and that you would like to set as fitness training goals. Comment on why they are important to you.

	PHYSICAL BENEFIT	IMPORTANCE TO ME
1.		
2.		
3.		
4.		
5.		

Now do the same for five psychological benefits of physical activity.

	PSYCHOLOGICAL BENEFIT	IMPORTANCE TO ME
1.		
2.		
3.		
4.		
5.		

ASSIGNMENT 4.4 Reviewing Your Fitness Training Goals

Review the fitness training goals that you set for yourself in **assignment 4.3**. Do they address some of the principles that we have just examined? If you need to adjust your fitness training goals, go ahead. Be aware that these are short-term goals and therefore a reflection of your long-term goals. Accordingly, they should be continually reassessed and, if necessary, modified. Set a review date three to four months away. Once you pick your goals, use the information that you have learned from Chapter 4 to pick training techniques that you could use to accomplish these goals.

	GOAL	PHYSICAL TRAINING TECHNIQUES
SHORT-TERM GOALS *Think in terms of this semester.*	**1.**	
	2.	
	3.	
LONG-TERM GOALS *Think in terms of the next 2 to 5 years.*	**1.**	
	2.	
	3.	

Signature:	Date:
Witness signature:	Date:
Review date (When do I want to check on these?):	

ASSIGNMENT 4.5 Designing a Stretching Program

1. Determine how flexible you are.

   a. **Trunk Forward Flexion (Sit and Reach)**

   One of the tests in the fitness pin assessment done by the Police Fitness Personnel of Ontario (PFPO) is the sit and reach. It is a measure of posterior hip flexibility. Short hip flexors can lead to a higher risk of back problems and injuries.

   Before you attempt the test, warm up your hamstring and back muscles with a light aerobic activity for a few minutes. Add static stretching. When you are ready, take off your shoes and sit in front of the sit-and-reach apparatus with your feet flat against it. With your arms reaching forward, put one hand on top of the other. Reach as far forward as you can along the measurements. Hold the position for at least three seconds. *Do not bounce*. Repeat the test twice.

   From your first attempt during class assessment, record how you did and how it compares with the scores in Chapter 15 (see Table 15.3) If you have good flexibility, you should be able to touch your toes (a distance of about 26 cm).

TRUNK FORWARD FLEXION (SIT AND REACH) RESULT AND SCORE		
ATTEMPT	RESULT	SCORE (FROM TABLE 15.3)
1		
2		

   b. **Shoulder Flexibility**

   Move your right arm behind your back with your elbow bent. At the same time, bring your left arm over your shoulder and reach down your back as far as you can. Try to cross your left-hand fingers over your right hand. Repeat on the other side.

SHOULDER FLEXIBILITY RATING (✓ check one for each shoulder)			
SHOULDER	*Fail to touch fingers* BELOW AVERAGE	*Touch fingers* AVERAGE	*Overlap fingers* ABOVE AVERAGE
Right			
Left			

   c. **Lower Back Stretch**

   Lie on your back. While bending your knees, grasp the backs of your thighs and pull your knees toward your chest. If you have good flexibility, your upper legs should touch your chest.

LOW-BACK STRETCH RESULT (✓ check one)	
Upper legs touched chest	
PASS	ROOM FOR IMPROVEMENT

d. **Hip Flexor Stretch**

Lie on your back. With your left leg straight on the floor, try to pull your right knee to your chest by grasping the back of your right thigh. To pass, your right upper thigh must touch your chest while your straight left leg remains in contact with the floor. Then repeat the exercise, pulling your left knee to your chest while your right leg remains straight on the floor.

HIP FLEXOR STRETCH (✓ check one for each hip)		
	Upper thigh touched chest while other leg remained straight on floor	
HIP	**PASS**	**ROOM FOR IMPROVEMENT**
Right		
Left		

e. **Quadriceps Stretch**

Lie on your stomach with your knees together. Keeping your left leg straight, pull your right heel toward your buttocks by grasping your ankle. To pass, you should be able to touch your heel to your buttocks. Then repeat the exercise, keeping your right leg straight and pulling your left heel toward your buttocks.

QUADRICEPS STRETCH (✓ check one for each quadriceps)		
	Touched heel to buttocks	
QUADRICEPS	**PASS**	**ROOM FOR IMPROVEMENT**
Right		
Left		

2. Comment on how you did in these tests and how flexible you are in general. Describe your strengths and weaknesses:

____
____
____
____
____
____
____
____

3. Based on your assessment and comments, set some specific goals regarding a stretching program.

Goal 1: ____

Goal 2: ____

Goal 3: ____

4. Based on the information provided in Chapter 8 and on the FITT formula, design a stretching program that will fit your needs. Record your exercises in the chart below.

FLEXIBILITY LOG				
Date:		WORKOUT RESULTS		
EXERCISE		DURATION OF STRETCH	LENGTH OF REACH	CHANGE IN MOTION RANGE
Legs				
Chest				
Back				
Arms				

Comment on how your workout went (what went well, what you need to work on, which muscle groups you need to address):

ASSIGNMENT 5.1 Assessing Your Cardiorespiratory Fitness Level

Before you begin training, you should assess your cardiorespiratory fitness level, even if aerobic exercise is already a part of your routine. The following questions are designed to assist you.

1. What, if anything, are you doing to train your cardiorespiratory system?

____

____

____

____

____

____

2. Do your workouts follow the FITT formula? How many times a week do you participate in aerobic activities (frequency)? How strenuous is your workout (intensity)? How long is each session (time)? What kinds of activities do you participate in (type)?

Frequency: __________ times per week

Intensity: ____________________

Time: __________ minutes per workout

Type: ____________________

3. What do you think are the benefits of a regular aerobic training program?

____

____

____

____

____

____

4. If you do not regularly participate in aerobic activities, what strategies do you think you need to begin participating in a regular program?

____

____

____

____

____

____

5. What types of aerobic activities do you think will help you train to be successful in the 1.5-mile (2.4-km) run, shuttle run, and Bona Fide Occupational Requirements (PREP, PARE)?

____

____

____

____

____

____

6. What types of interval aerobic and anaerobic training do you think you have to incorporate to assist you to easily complete jumping the 4-foot (1.2-m) wall, going over the vault rail, completing the 4 and 12 sets of stairs in the PREP and PARE test, and completing the running involved in the PARE circuit and in the shuttle run in the PREP test?

____

____

____

____

____

____

ASSIGNMENT 5.2

Determining Your Resting Heart Rate and Target Heart Rate

To determine your true resting heart rate, you should test yourself first thing in the morning, before getting out of bed. Test yourself again later in the day.

Resting heart rate = ____________ bpm

Heart rate later in the day = ____________ bpm

Is there a large difference between your resting heart rate and your heart rate later in the day? If so, can you account for it? Be aware that caffeine, smoking, physical activity, stress, and even eating, including supplementation, can affect your heart rate. Is your heart rate later in the day at a healthy level (lower than 100 bpm)?

Comment:

____

____

____

____

____

Determine Your Target Heart Rate

Your target heart rate should be between 70 and 85 percent of your maximal heart rate. First, subtract your age from 220 to determine your maximal heart rate (MHR). Then, use your MHR to determine your target heart rate.

MHR = 220 − your age: ________ = ____________ bpm

YOUR TARGET HEART RATE:

BETWEEN

70% MHR = ____________ bpm × 0.70 = ____________ bpm

AND

85% MHR = ____________ bpm × 0.85 = ____________ bpm

Attempt a few aerobic activities to determine whether you are exercising within your target heart rate. If you are below 70 percent MHR, what can you do to get up to your target range? If you are above 85 percent MHR and not fit, what considerations should you be aware of?

ASSIGNMENT 5.3

Setting Up Your Cardiorespiratory Fitness Program

Drawing on the material in Chapter 5 and other sources, set up a cardiorespiratory fitness program for the semester. Include the cardiorespiratory exercises you most enjoy and create a program that follows the FITT formula.

Goals (for one semester):

Cardiorespiratory activities you want to engage in (remember to include aerobic and anaerobic activities):

Cardiorespiratory program (based on the FITT formula):

Date to check benchmarks for goals:

Success markers (based on semester goals):

Strategies for potential barriers (how you can overcome specific difficulties you might face in implementing your aerobic plan):

Maintaining a Cardiorespiratory Fitness Log

For each semester you may be required to maintain a fitness profile, including a log of the cardiorespiratory activities you engage in. You are encouraged to record all cardiorespiratory activities, including activities outside class. The pages that follow contain a Daily Workout Log and a Running Log that you may photocopy for this purpose. (They are also in the *Fit for Duty, Fit for Life Training Guide* that accompanies this textbook.) The logs include sections for noting the weather (which can affect outdoor activities) and recording your comments on how the workouts went. Your instructor will advise you on the specific requirements for your fitness profile and logs.

DAILY WORKOUT LOG

Dater: Week: Day:

MUSCLE GROUP	EXERCISE	SET 1		SET 2		SET 3		SET 4		SET 5	
		WEIGHT	REPS	WEIGHT	REPS	WEIGHT	REPS	WEIGHT	REPS	WEIGHT	REPS
1.											
2.											
3.											
4.											
5.											
6.											
7.											
8.											
MUSCLE GROUP	EXERCISE	WEIGHT	REPS	WEIGHT	REPS	WEIGHT	REPS	WEIGHT	REPS	WEIGHT	REPS
1.											
2.											
3.											
4.											
5.											
6.											
7.											
8.											

CARDIOVASCULAR WORKOUT /INTERVAL TRAINING

DATE	DISTANCE mi/km/laps	TIME h:mm:ss	PACE	HR	REST HR	TEMP °C/°F	SHOES	RUN TYPE	ROUTE NAME, DESCRIPTION	FEEDBACK
/										
/										
/										
/										

Comments on Workouts:

RUNNING LOG

Semester: Month: Name/Student ID:

WK	DATE	DISTANCE mi or km	TIME h:mm:ss	PACE	HR	REST HR	TEMP °C/°F	SHOES	RUN TYPE	ROUTE NAME, DESCRIPTION	FEEDBACK
1	/										
	/										
	/										
	/										
	/										
	/										
	/										
2	/										
	/										
	/										
	/										
	/										
	/										
	/										
3	/										
	/										
	/										
	/										
	/										
	/										
	/										
4	/										
	/										
	/										
	/										
	/										
	/										
	/										

ASSIGNMENT 6.1 Determining Your One-Repetition Maximum (1RM) for Bench Press

Muscular strength plays a vital role throughout an individual's lifespan. Your strength develops quite rapidly in your growing years, but as you get older, strength levels begin to decrease significantly. When assessing your muscular strength, most of the time you will use a hand-held dynamometer, which measures grip strength. There is a direct correlation between grip strength and overall body strength. There are established norms for gender and age. Chapter 15 lists the standards that are used by Peel Regional Police Service. (These are also reproduced in the *Fit for Duty, Fit for Life Training Guide* that accompanies this textbook.)

There are one-repetition maximum formulas for various lifts (such as bench press, leg press, or squats) that are also used to determine relative strength norms.

The following is the formula for determining a **one-repetition maximum (1RM)** from a submaximal test (for 2–20 repetitions):

1RM = [weight lifted] ÷ [1.0 – ([number of repetitions] × 0.02)]

For example, if an individual bench-presses 225 pounds 10 times, the formula would read:

1RM = 225 ÷ [1.0 – (10 × 0.02)] or 225 ÷ 0.8 = 281.25 pounds

To determine **relative strength**, take the individual's 1RM and divide it by his or her body weight in pounds. For example, using the 1RM from the example above and a 195-pound body weight:

281.25 ÷ 195 = 1.44

This individual has an upper-body relative strength that is 1.44 times his body weight (or 144% of his body weight).

The following are **norms established for relative strength**, with each norm being a percentage of body weight (in pounds).

Norms Established for Relative Strength, as Percentage of Body Weight (BW)

	UPPER BODY	LOWER BODY	
	BENCH PRESS	SQUATS	LEG PRESS
EXCELLENT	Above BW × 1.50 = 150%	Above BW × 2.00 = 200%	Above BW × 3.00 = 300%
GOOD	BW × 1.25 = 125%	BW × 1.75 = 175%	BW × 2.75 = 275%
AVERAGE	BW × 1.00 = 100%	BW × 1.50 = 150%	BW × 2.50 = 250%
FAIR	BW × 0.85–0.99 = 85%–99%	BW × 1.35 = 135%	BW × 2.25 = 225%
POOR	Below BW × 0.85 = 85%	BW × 1.25 = 125%	Below BW × 2.25 = 225%

SOURCE: Kraemer, W.J., & Fry, A.C. (1995). Strength testing: Development and evaluation of methodology. In P. Maud & C. Foster (Eds.), *Physiological Assessment of human fitness* (pp. 115–138). Champaign, IL: Human Kinetics.

Determining Your 1 RM for Bench Press (for 2–20 repetitions)

1RM = [weight lifted] ÷ [1.0 – ([number of repetitions] × 0.02)]

↓ ↓

1RM = ______ pounds ÷ [1.0 – (________________ × 0.02)] = ______ pounds

To see your potential score, look up bench press standards under "Additional Fitness Standards" in the *Fit for Duty, Fit for Life Training Guide* that accompanies this textbook.

Determining Your Relative Strength

Relative strength = [1RM for bench press] ÷ [body weight]

↓ ↓

= ______ pounds ÷ ______ pounds = ______ pounds

Now, from the **Norms Established for Relative Strength** chart on the previous page, determine your level of relative strength:

____

Comment on your absolute (maximal repetition) strength and your relative strength. Are you where you want to be? Are you meeting the standards for bench press? Set a goal for where you want to be by the end of the year.

____

____

____

____

____

____

____

____

SOURCE: Mayhew, J.L., Ball, T.E., Arnold, M.D., & Bowen, J.C. (1992). Prediction of 1RM bench press from relative endurance performance in college males and females. *Journal of Applied Sports Science Research, 6*, 200–206.

ASSIGNMENT 6.2 Designing Your Strength, Power, and Endurance Training Program

Before designing a strength, power, and endurance training program, determine your training goal. Table 6.4 lists the possible goals.

1. List the goals of your training program and indicate what sort of workout is necessary for each one. Specify the number of exercises associated with each goal. Goals can be general, such as developing greater muscle definition, or specific, such as increasing power to withstand an altercation. If your goal is to develop a specific muscle group, note that as well.

GOAL	WORKOUT EXERCISES	MUSCLE(S) DEVELOPED

2. Based on your goals, choose 6–10 exercises to perform during each weight training session. Pick exercises for each muscle group. Record them on the chart on the next page.
3. Choose starting weights. Follow the guidelines in Chapter 6 to determine what you can easily lift for 10–12 repetitions.
4. Choose a starting number of sets and repetitions. The optimal pattern for a weight training workout includes 3 sets of 10–12 repetitions for each exercise. If your program is focusing on strength alone, your sets can contain fewer repetitions using a heavier load.
5. Choose the number of training sessions per week. Choose a frequency between two and four days per week (three days per week is recommended).
6. Monitor your progress using a workout card. An example that you can photocopy is provided on page 439.

Exercises for a Weight Training Program

EXERCISE	MUSCLE(S) DEVELOPED	WEIGHT (KG OR LB.)	REPETITIONS	SETS	FREQUENCY (CHECK ✓)						
					S	M	T	W	T	F	S

WORKOUT CARD FOR:

EXERCISE		DATE																							
	WT																								
	SET																								
	REPS																								
	WT																								
	SET																								
	REPS																								
	WT																								
	SET																								
	REPS																								
	WT																								
	SET																								
	REPS																								
	WT																								
	SET																								
	REPS																								
	WT																								
	SET																								
	REPS																								
	WT																								
	SET																								
	REPS																								
	WT																								
	SET																								
	REPS																								
	WT																								
	SET																								
	REPS																								

ASSIGNMENT 7.1 Determining Your Body Mass Index (BMI)

To determine your BMI, follow these steps:

1. Measure your height in metres (m) to the nearest 0.005 m (that is, to the nearest half-centimetre):

   Your height = ____________________ m

2. Convert your height to metres squared (that is, multiply the figure by itself—for example, 1.955 m × 1.955 m).

   Your height squared = ____________________ m^2

3. Measure your weight in kilograms (kg) to the nearest 0.1 kg.

   Your weight = ____________________ kg

4. Determine your BMI by dividing your weight in kilograms by your height in metres squared.

   BMI = ____________________ kg ÷ ________________ m^2 = ________________ kg/m^2

   Alternatively, you can use the chart on the next page.

5. Comment on your BMI. According to the number, should you be concerned? Why or why not? Based on your family demographics, should you be concerned about this in the future?

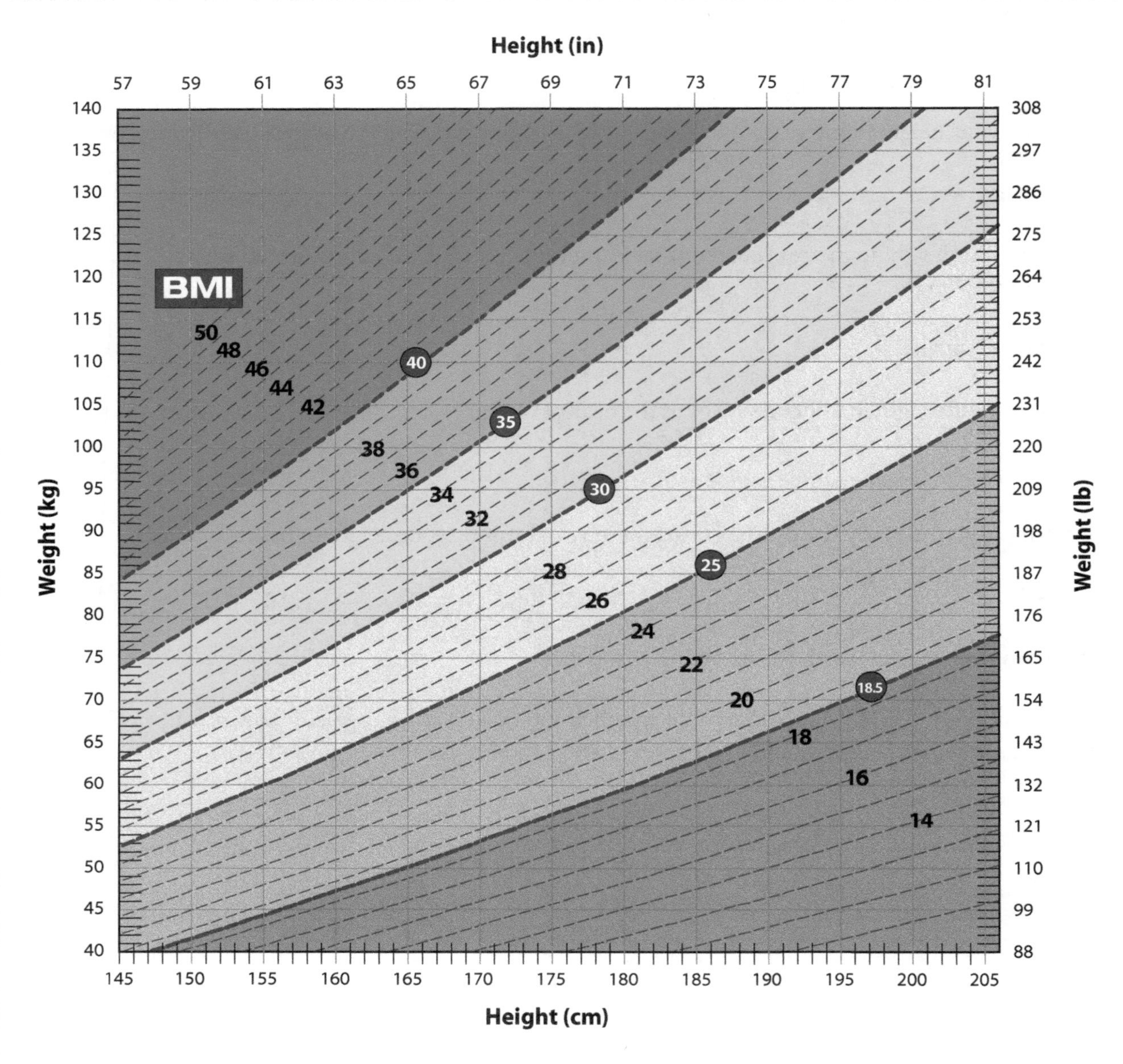

SOURCE: Health Canada. (2003). *Canadian guidelines for body weight classifications in adults*. Catalogue no. H49-179/2003-1E. http://www.hc-sc.gc.ca/fn-an/nutrition/weights-poids/guide-ld-adult/cg_quick_ref-ldc_rapide_ref_e.html. Reproduced with permission of the Minister of Public Works and Government Services Canada, 2007.

ASSIGNMENT 7.2 Determining Your Waist Circumference (WC)

Excess weight, as measured by BMI, is not the only risk to your health. The location of fat on your body is also a factor. If you carry fat mainly around your waist, you are more likely to develop health problems than if you carry fat mainly on your hips and thighs. This is true even if your BMI falls within the normal range.

To measure your WC, have someone place a tape measure at the part of the torso located midway between the lowest rib and the iliac crest (the top of the pelvic bone). Be sure that the tape is snug, but does not compress your skin and is parallel to the floor. Relax, exhale, and measure your waist. Repeat, to ensure that your WC has been measured accurately. The table below shows measurements that indicate increased risks to your health.

Measurement 1: __________ cm

Measurement 2: __________ cm

Waist Circumference and Risk for Type 2 Diabetes, Coronary Heart Disease, and Hypertension

	WAIST CIRCUMFERENCE	
	CUT-OFF POINT FOR RISK	**INCREASED RISK**
Males	102 cm (40 in)	Above 102 cm (40 in)
Females	88 cm (35 in)	Above 88 cm (35 in)

SOURCE: Adapted from WHO. (2000). *Obesity: Preventing and managing the global epidemic: Report on a WHO consultation on obesity*. Consultation Technical Report Series No. 894. Geneva: Author.

What does your score indicate? Are there any issues you should address? Comment:

____

____

____

____

____

____

____

____

____

____

____

____

____

____

____

ASSIGNMENT 7.3 Determining Your Waist-to-Hip Ratio

To determine your Waist-to-Hip Ratio (WHR), follow these steps:

1. Measure the girth of your waist by positioning a metric measuring tape horizontally at the place where the waist is noticeably narrowing, and take the measurement at the end of a normal exhale. Record the measurement to the nearest half-centimetre.

   Girth of waist = ________ cm

2. Measure the girth of your hips by positioning a metric measuring tape horizontally at the place where the circumference of the hips is the greatest. Record the measurement to the nearest half-centimetre.

   Girth of hips = ________ cm

3. Determine your WHR by dividing the girth of your waist by the girth of your hips.

   WHR = [girth of waist] ÷ [girth of hips]

   WHR = ________ cm ÷ ________ cm = ________ cm

4. What does your score indicate? Are there any issues you should address? Comment:

____

____

____

____

____

____

____

____

____

____

____

____

____

____

____

____

5. Based on the results you obtained above, what type of program do you need to develop or maintain in order to keep a healthy weight and waist measurement? What exercises would you include? Be specific:

ASSIGNMENT 8.1 Portion Distortion

Food portions in restaurants have have enlarged significantly since the 1950s and 1960s, when fast-food chains became mainstream. The "super-sizing" of portions to attract sales provides, in some cases, enough food for at least two people. Portion growth has resulted in increased waistlines and body weight.

Go to the National Heart, Lung, and Blood Institute (NHLBI) Portion Distortion Interactive Quizzes at http://hin.nhlbi.nih.gov/portion.

The two Portion Distortion quizzes compare current portion sizes with those that were available 20 years ago. The quizzes address caloric disparity and how much physical activity it would require to burn off the extra calories.

Comment on your results. How well did you do in determining caloric content and the amount of physical activity required to burn off the extra calories provided by today's portions? Do you need to look more closely at how much and what you are consuming?

ASSIGNMENT 8.2 Water Consumption

Water is a vital nutrient that is needed for regular cellular function and prevention of dehydration when working, exercising, and performing daily activities.

Determine your minimal daily water requirement based on your body weight:

Body weight (in pounds) × 0.55 = ________ daily ounces H_2O

________ daily ounces H_2O ÷ 8 = ________ cups of H_2O

Do you believe that you are consuming this quantity of water? Do you need to consume more (based on any symptoms you might be experiencing, your activity level, etc.)? Comment on the amount and types of fluid you typically drink in a day:

ASSIGNMENT 8.3 Sodium Consumption

Recognizing how much sodium you consume is important in keeping blood pressure and blood sodium levels down. Go to www.healthycanadians.gc.ca/init/sodium/interactive-guide-interactif-eng.php to explore your sodium intake using the Sodium Detector.

1. List the typical sources of sodium in your diet:

____

____

____

____

____

____

____

2. List 5 processed foods that contain high levels of sodium:
   - ____
   - ____
   - ____
   - ____
   - ____

   Comment on the sodium values and your typical intake of these foods:

   ____

   ____

   ____

   ____

   ____

   ____

3. Where in your usual diet can you lower your intake of sodium? What changes can you make?

____

____

____

____

____

____

____

ASSIGNMENT 8.4 Nutritional Labelling

At the Health Canada website, go to Interactive Tools—Nutritional Labelling at www.hc-sc.gc.ca/fn-an/label-etiquet/nutrition/cons/dv-vq/interact-eng.php.

Then, go to the Interactive Nutrition Facts table at www.hc-sc.gc.ca/fn-an/label-etiquet/nutrition/cons/index-eng.php.

List the 6 components that are required to be shown on food product labels in Canada since 2007:

1. ______________________________
2. ______________________________
3. ______________________________
4. ______________________________
5. ______________________________
6. ______________________________

Comment on the importance of learning how to read a food label:

____

____

____

____

____

____

____

____

Next, go to the interactive Amount of Food tool at www.hc-sc.gc.ca/fn-an/label-etiquet/nutrition/cons/amount-quantite/interact-d-eng.php—it will show you how the amount you eat changes the quantity of calories and nutrients you get from a food. Comment on what you have learned:

____

____

____

____

____

____

____

____

____

Finally, turn to the How to Compare interactive tool at www.hc-sc.gc.ca/fn-an/label-etiquet/nutrition/cons/dv-vq/interact-c-eng.php and compare two types of foods to assess quantities of calories, fats (saturated and trans fats), and other listed nutrients. Comment on your observations:

ASSIGNMENT 9.1 Are You at Risk for Diabetes?

1. Go the Canadian Diabetes Association website at www.diabetes.ca.
2. Click on **Diabetes & You**.
3. Under **What Is Diabetes?**, click on **Are You at Risk?**
4. Answer the **Are You at Risk? Questionnaire** to determine your level of risk for diabetes.
5. Comment on your results:

____

____

____

____

6. Click on **Diabetes Facts** and read the information provided.
7. Summarize two points that you feel are the most important to someone who lacks any knowledge of diabetes and why:
   - ____

     ____
   - ____

     ____

     ____
8. Click on **Metabolic Syndrome**. Define "metabolic syndrome."

____

____

____

Do you have three or more of the risk factors that contribute to a diagnosis of metabolic syndrome?

____

Comment on the risk factors that you need to be concerned about now or in the future based on family history or lifestyle:

____

____

____

____

____

____

____

ASSIGNMENT 10.1

Understanding Your Risks for Cardiovascular Disease

1. Go to www.heartandstroke.ca and complete the **Heart & Stroke Risk Assessment** to see if you are at risk for heart disease and/or stroke. This risk assessment will give you the opportunity to take an inventory of many facets of your health. The assessment looks at:
   - factors you cannot change or control, such as age, gender, ethnicity, and family medical history
   - risk factors for poor health and chronic disease that you can change or control, such as physical activity, diet, smoking, and stress
   - conditions that increase your risk of heart disease and stroke, such as high blood pressure or high cholesterol
   - any chronic conditions or diseases, such as asthma or arthritis, where you primarily access health care

   After completing the **Heart & Stroke Risk Assessment**, you will receive a comprehensive Health Assessment Report outlining your health strengths or advantages, as well as places where you might make improvements. If you have any chronic conditions, the Health Assessment Report will also provide links to disease-specific information.
2. Print a copy of the report provided for you.
3. After reading the report, comment on the risk factors that are putting you at risk or potentially could put you at risk, and what you can do to reduce or eliminate those risks.

ASSIGNMENT 10.2 First Aid for Heart Attack and Stroke Victims

1. Investigate and describe the first aid procedures for suspected victims of heart attacks and strokes, noting differences and similarities. Why are they important to know?

2. What is CPR? What is the purpose of CPR? How do you perform it?

3. Research what an AED is and what it does. Why do law enforcement officers need to know how to use it?

ASSIGNMENT 11.1 Healthy Back Assessment

1. Go to Chapter 15: Preparing to Meet Law Enforcement Fitness Standards and complete the following two assessments relating to back and core health. Then answer the questions that follow.
   a. Modified Biering-Sorensen Back Assessment (the Ontario Police Fitness Award (OPFA) Core Endurance Assessment)
   b. Sit-and-Reach Flexibility Test (the Trunk Forward Flexion in the OPFA Standards)
2. Record your results in the chart below.

TEST	RESULTS	SCORE
CORE ENDURANCE	sec	
SIT-AND-REACH	cm	

GET SCORES FROM CHAPTER 15
Get core endurance score from Table 15.2
Get sit-and-reach score from Table 15.3

3. Comment on your results. Did you meet the 75 percent standard, which is required to earn your fitness pin? What do you need to improve on?

4. What activities have either caused you back pain or made you feel your back was strained, tender, or sore when doing a certain activity: standing, sitting, bending to pick something up, going up/down stairs, driving, twisting, computer work, playing a specific sport, other? How long have you had/did you have these issues?

5. On a scale of 1 to 10 (with 10 being high), how intense is/was your back pain with each of the activities you identified? For each activity, in what area did you identify the pain? (neck, mid-back, low-back…) What made the pain better? Worse? Did you apply ice/heat or see a professional (physiotherapist, massage therapist, physician)? How long did the pain take to go away?

6. What body core and back issues do you need to address in your workouts to improve your performance (refer to what you have read in Chapter 11) to help keep your back strong? What precautions do you need to remind yourself about when exercising?

7. List 8 exercises you can incorporate into your fitness program that will improve your back health and core endurance based on what you answered above and what you should work on based on the workouts you have been doing and the test standards that exist.

EXERCISE	DESCRIPTION OR DIAGRAM OF EXERCISE
1.	
2.	
3.	
4.	
5.	
6.	
7.	
8.	

ASSIGNMENT 12.1 The Life Experience Survey

Listed on the following pages are a number of events that sometimes bring about change in the lives of those who experience them and necessitate social readjustment. Check those events that you have experienced in the past year and indicate how long ago the event occurred (0–6 months or 7–12 months).

For each item checked, assign a whole number between −3 and +3 to indicate the extent to which you viewed the event as having either a positive or a negative impact on your life at the time it occurred. A rating of −3 indicates an extremely negative impact, a rating of 0 indicates an impact that is neither positive nor negative, and a rating of +3 indicates an extremely positive impact.

Section I of the test is for everyone. It provides three blanks (items 45, 46, and 47) for you to list any recent experiences that have had an impact on your life but are not covered in items 1–44.

Section II of the test is designed for students only. If there are school-related experiences that have had a noticeable impact on your life but are not listed, you may list them in one or more of the three blanks in section I.

Some items apply only to males and some only to females; these are indicated in the survey.

After you complete the survey, consider the following questions:

1. Was your level of stress close to what you predicted it would be? Why or why not?

____

____

____

2. Can you highlight a few stressors that are affecting you, or are you experiencing overall stress? Is it good or bad stress?

____

____

____

3. Recognizing your stressors, are there any that you could work on to relieve your stress level?

____

____

____

4. What can you do to improve your positive stress?

____

____

____

5. Comment on any other observations you have made regarding your initial stress assessment.

____

____

____

The Life Experience Survey

SECTION I			0–6 months ✓	7–12 months ✓	Extremely negative	Moderately negative	Somewhat negative	No impact	Somewhat positive	Moderately positive	Extremely positive
1.	Marriage				−3	−2	−1	0	+1	+2	+3
2.	Detention in jail or comparable institution				−3	−2	−1	0	+1	+2	+3
3.	Death of spouse				−3	−2	−1	0	+1	+2	+3
4.	Major change in sleeping habits (much more or less sleep)				−3	−2	−1	0	+1	+2	+3
5.	Death of close family member	a. mother			−3	−2	−1	0	+1	+2	+3
		b. father			−3	−2	−1	0	+1	+2	+3
		c. brother			−3	−2	−1	0	+1	+2	+3
		d. sister			−3	−2	−1	0	+1	+2	+3
		e. child			−3	−2	−1	0	+1	+2	+3
		f. grandmother			−3	−2	−1	0	+1	+2	+3
		g. grandfather			−3	−2	−1	0	+1	+2	+3
		h. other (specify):			−3	−2	−1	0	+1	+2	+3
6.	Major change in eating habits (eating much more or much less)				−3	−2	−1	0	+1	+2	+3
7.	Foreclosure on mortgage or loan				−3	−2	−1	0	+1	+2	+3
8.	Death of a close friend				−3	−2	−1	0	+1	+2	+3
9.	Outstanding personal achievement				−3	−2	−1	0	+1	+2	+3
10.	Minor law violations (traffic ticket, disturbing the peace, etc.)				−3	−2	−1	0	+1	+2	+3
11.	Your or your partner's pregnancy				−3	−2	−1	0	+1	+2	+3
12.	Changed work situation (working conditions, working hours, etc.)				−3	−2	−1	0	+1	+2	+3
13.	New job				−3	−2	−1	0	+1	+2	+3
14.	Serious illness or injury of close family member	a. father			−3	−2	−1	0	+1	+2	+3
		b. mother			−3	−2	−1	0	+1	+2	+3
		c. sister			−3	−2	−1	0	+1	+2	+3
		d. brother			−3	−2	−1	0	+1	+2	+3
		e. grandfather			−3	−2	−1	0	+1	+2	+3
		f. grandmother			−3	−2	−1	0	+1	+2	+3
		g. spouse			−3	−2	−1	0	+1	+2	+3
		h. child			−3	−2	−1	0	+1	+2	+3
		i. other (specify):			−3	−2	−1	0	+1	+2	+3
15.	Sexual difficulties				−3	−2	−1	0	+1	+2	+3
16.	Trouble with employer (in danger of losing job, being suspended, demoted, etc.)				−3	−2	−1	0	+1	+2	+3
17.	Trouble with in-laws				−3	−2	−1	0	+1	+2	+3

SECTION I		0–6 months ✓	7–12 months ✓	Extremely negative	Moderately negative	Somewhat negative	No impact	Somewhat positive	Moderately positive	Extremely positive
18.	Major change in financial status (much better off or much worse off)			−3	−2	−1	0	+1	+2	+3
19.	Major change in closeness of family members (decreased or increased closeness)			−3	−2	−1	0	+1	+2	+3
20.	Gaining a new family member (through birth, adoption, family member moving in, etc.)			−3	−2	−1	0	+1	+2	+3
21.	Change of residence			−3	−2	−1	0	+1	+2	+3
22.	Marital separation from mate (due to conflict)			−3	−2	−1	0	+1	+2	+3
23.	Major change in church activities (increased or decreased attendance)			−3	−2	−1	0	+1	+2	+3
24.	Marital reconciliation with mate			−3	−2	−1	0	+1	+2	+3
25.	Major change in number of arguments with partner (many more or many fewer arguments)			−3	−2	−1	0	+1	+2	+3
26.	Change in partner's work outside the home			−3	−2	−1	0	+1	+2	+3
27.	Major change in usual type and/or amount of recreation			−3	−2	−1	0	+1	+2	+3
28.	Borrowing more than $10 000 (buying home, business, etc.)			−3	−2	−1	0	+1	+2	+3
29.	Borrowing less than $10 000 (buying car or TV, getting school loan, etc.)			−3	−2	−1	0	+1	+2	+3
30.	Being fired from job			−3	−2	−1	0	+1	+2	+3
31.	You or your partner having an abortion			−3	−2	−1	0	+1	+2	+3
32.	Major personal illness or injury			−3	−2	−1	0	+1	+2	+3
33.	Major change in social activities—e.g., parties, movies, visiting (increased or decreased participation)			−3	−2	−1	0	+1	+2	+3
34.	Major change in living conditions of family (building new home, remodeling, deterioration of home, neighbourhood, etc.)			−3	−2	−1	0	+1	+2	+3
35.	Divorce			−3	−2	−1	0	+1	+2	+3
36.	Serious injury or illness of close friend			−3	−2	−1	0	+1	+2	+3
37.	Retirement from work			−3	−2	−1	0	+1	+2	+3
38.	Son or daughter leaving home (due to marriage, college, etc.)			−3	−2	−1	0	+1	+2	+3
39.	Ending of formal schooling			−3	−2	−1	0	+1	+2	+3
40.	Separation from spouse (due to work, travel, etc.)			−3	−2	−1	0	+1	+2	+3
41.	Engagement			−3	−2	−1	0	+1	+2	+3
42.	Breaking up with boyfriend/girlfriend			−3	−2	−1	0	+1	+2	+3
43.	Leaving home for the first time			−3	−2	−1	0	+1	+2	+3
44.	Reconciliation with boyfriend/girlfriend			−3	−2	−1	0	+1	+2	+3

		0–6 months	7–12 months	*Extremely negative*	*Moderately negative*	*Somewhat negative*	*No impact*	*Somewhat positive*	*Moderately positive*	*Extremely positive*
SECTION I		✓	✓							
Other recent experiences that have had an impact on your life:										
45.				−3	−2	−1	0	+1	+2	+3
46.				−3	−2	−1	0	+1	+2	+3
47.				−3	−2	−1	0	+1	+2	+3
SECTION II (STUDENTS ONLY)										
48.	Beginning new school experience at a higher academic level (college, graduate school, professional school, etc.)			−3	−2	−1	0	+1	+2	+3
49.	Changing to a new school at same academic level (undergraduate, graduate, etc.)			−3	−2	−1	0	+1	+2	+3
50.	Academic probation			−3	−2	−1	0	+1	+2	+3
51.	Being dismissed from dormitory or other residence			−3	−2	−1	0	+1	+2	+3
52.	Failing an important exam			−3	−2	−1	0	+1	+2	+3
53.	Changing a major			−3	−2	−1	0	+1	+2	+3
54.	Failing a course			−3	−2	−1	0	+1	+2	+3
55.	Dropping a course			−3	−2	−1	0	+1	+2	+3
56.	Joining a fraternity/sorority			−3	−2	−1	0	+1	+2	+3

Scoring the Life Experience Survey

Total of Negative Scores:	
Total of Positive Scores:	
Overall Score (add the two scores together):	

Rating scale for life experiences and stress

	SUM OF NEGATIVE SCORES (DISTRESS SCORE)	SUM OF POSITIVE SCORES (EUSTRESS SCORE)
May need counselling	14+	
Above average stress	9–13	
Average	6–9	9–10
Below average stress	<6	

SOURCE: Sarason, I.G., Johnson, J.H., & Siegel, J.M. (1978). Assessing the impact of life changes: Development of the life experiences survey. *Journal of Consulting and Clinical Psychology, 46*(5), 932–946.

ASSIGNMENT 12.2 Recognizing Stress in Your Life

It's important to identify the events in your life that trigger your stress symptoms. Your ability to manage and prevent stress is built on your awareness of your stress symptoms and the events that fuel those symptoms.

Over the next few days, take a closer look at the stressful activities in your life. Keep track of the symptoms that helped you identify a stressful situation and the trigger that caused it.

After you've monitored your stress for several days, review the situation. Think about the coping strategies you used. Were there techniques that could have helped you better manage or eliminate the stressful situation?

Try to be prepared for the next time you encounter these or other stress-causing situations.

IN A RECENT STRESSFUL SITUATION, HOW DID YOU REACT? ANSWER TRUE (T) OR FALSE (F)			
1.	I ignored the fact that something was bothering me and tried to carry on as usual.	**T**	**F**
2.	I made sure that I had information on how to manage this stressful situation.	**T**	**F**
3.	I refused to admit that anything was bothering me, and I tried not to notice that I was experiencing signs of stress, such as an increase in heart rate, muscle tightness, and hurried behaviour.	**T**	**F**
4.	I used alcohol, smoking, or other substances as a way of relieving my stress.	**T**	**F**
5.	I made a plan and followed it, one step at a time.	**T**	**F**
6.	Every so often I took time to relax and forget about my stress. I read, listened to music, watched a film, or rested.	**T**	**F**
7.	I looked at the humorous side of the situation, or I gave my support and understanding to people around me who were also under stress.	**T**	**F**
8.	I took time to remind myself of the important things in life. I received the goals for my personal life and the priorities of my work.	**T**	**F**
9.	I took out my anger and frustration on my friends and family.	**T**	**F**
10.	I kept thinking that I was helpless to deal with this situation.	**T**	**F**
11.	I didn't let anyone know what was really bothering me, even though there were people available who would have been supportive or helpful.	**T**	**F**
12.	I started exercising or doing a hobby, so that I could enjoy myself for a while.	**T**	**F**

Compare your answers to the following to find out if your coping strategies are "stress fit."

The Best Coping Strategies to Keep "Stress Fit"

If you've answered in the same manner as below, you're already practising some "stress fit" strategies. If not, you may want to review the situations and consider alternative strategies that may help you live a healthier, more enjoyable life.

Remember, there is no single stress-coping skill that will effectively help you manage your stress in all situations or all of the time. The best approach to stress management is developing a flexible set of techniques that works for you as an individual.

	THE BEST WAY TO REACT IN A STRESSFUL SITUATION	
1.	**F**	The first step to managing stress is acknowledging the need for change. Take some quiet time to try to identify the source of your stress.
2.	**T**	Once you've identified what causes stress in your life, it's important to find information on how to develop new skills or improve already existing ones. A certified professional can help.
3.	**F**	A number of problems—an increase in heart rate and blood pressure, muscle tension, poor concentration, irritability, and sleep problems—can all be symptoms of excessive stress in your life. Don't ignore these signs—they're your body's way of telling you something's wrong. See your doctor or stress management specialist.
4.	**F**	You may feel that alcohol, smoking, or other substances may numb your stress and help you deal with a difficult situation. But any relief is only temporary, and this behaviour can only lead to additional problems for your physical and emotional health.
5.	**T**	Setting some priorities and being flexible about things that aren't critical can help you adapt to a particularly stressful time. Learn to manage your time and set realistic deadlines. This should be part of your overall management plan.
6.	**T**	Realize that there are equally rewarding sources of satisfaction available to you. You may want to look for inspiration in art, literature, philosophy, or religion. Or simply spend time on the activities you enjoy.
7.	**T**	Stressful situations often present an opportunity for you to grow in your positive emotions and attitudes. These can include the ability to see the humour in your situation, to trust in your convictions, and to develop more confidence in the people close to you.
8.	**T**	Sometimes it may be necessary to re-examine your life goals to see if they still effectively reflect what you want out of your life or career. If they don't, maybe it's time to re-assess your goals and priorities.
9.	**F**	When you're under pressure or stress you may be more irritable with the people closest to you. There are more positive ways of letting out the emotional and physical tension contributing to stress. Try to avoid situations that are bound to be stressful, exercise to reduce tension, or temporarily remove yourself from a situation.
10.	**F**	At times stress can lead to feelings of anxiety or helplessness. It's important to break the cycle of negative throughts by looking for ways to reduce stress or cushion how much it disrupts your life.
11.	**F**	Talking to others can give you a fresh perspective on a stressful situation. Plus, friends and family can provide valuable moral support when you need to feel good about yourself.
12.	**T**	Sometimes it's important to get some emotional distance from your daily hassles. Take on an activity that lets you temporarily forget what's going on. Enjoy yourself.

SOURCE: Adapted from Heart & Stroke Foundation. (n.d.). Heart & stroke stress test: How fit are you when it comes to managing stress? Ottawa: Author.

ASSIGNMENT 12.3 What Is Your Behaviour Type?

1. Based on the information you have read in Chapter 12, which environments (social, work, school, family, and so on) tend to bring out type A behaviour in you? What is it about these environments that you believe elicits this behaviour?

2. Answer the questions above as they apply to type B behaviour.

3. Answer the questions above as they apply to type C behaviour.

4. Which personality traits do you think cause stress in your life?

5. Which personality traits do you think will positively assist you in a career in law enforcement? Why?

6. Which of your personality traits would you like to change? Why? Which coping skills do you require to do this?

ASSIGNMENT 13.1 Handling Shiftwork Based on Understanding Your Sleeping Patterns and Chronotype

Part A

An individual's tolerance toward shiftwork has been found to be related to his or her *chronotype*, which is the scientific name given to an individual's particular circadian rhythm. Humans can be categorized as falling into three chronotypes, using such measures as the Horne-Ostberg Morningness–Eveningness Scale. The three types are "morning" (Larks), "evening" (Owls), and "indifferent" (sometimes known as "Hummingbirds").

Morning and evening types each represent approximately 15 to 20 percent of the human population, while the remaining 60 to 70 percent of the population fall into the "indifferent" category.

- Morning-type individuals (Larks) can be described as those persons who naturally waken about 2 hours earlier than the majority of the population and are ready for sleep between 8 p.m. and 10 p.m. To them, midnight is the middle of the night. Larks cope more easily with early shifts.
- Evening-type individuals (Owls) can be described as those persons who naturally waken about 2 hours later than the majority of the population and don't feel sleepy until between 12 midnight and 2 a.m. Owls cope more easily with late shifts.

If you don't readily identify yourself as a Lark or an Owl, then you most likely fall into the "indifferent" category. If you have any doubts, then you can take the Morningness–Eveningness Self-Assessment found at http://www.fileden.com/files/2008/10/6/2131219/ModifiedMEQ-SA-Terman.pdf.

- Studies show that in the short term, Larks have greater difficulty coping with night shifts than Owls, as their natural tendency to wake early reduces their daytime sleep after a night shift.
- If you identify yourself as a Lark, then napping in the evening is one strategy to help boost mental alertness on a night shift, although this does not replace good-quality sleep time.
- At the end of the survey, there is a table that recommends light therapy as an antidepressant means of coping with shiftwork.

SOURCE: Horne, J.A., & Östberg, O. (1976). A self-assessment questionnaire to determine morningness—eveningness in human circadian rhythms. *International Journal of Chronobiology*, 4, 97–100.)

Part B

1. What chronotype are you? Comment on the information obtained in the survey.

___

___

___

2. Do you have problems falling asleep or staying asleep? What situations make it most difficult?

___

___

___

3. Have you ever suffered from jet lag? If so, what were the symptoms?

4. When you wake up, do you feel rested, refreshed, and able to remain alert throughout the day without a nap? If you don't, how do you feel?

5. Have you lived in a household where someone was a shiftworker? If so, how did this affect you? What are the positive and negative aspects of living with a shiftworker?

6. Examine your sleeping environment and comment on the following.
   a. Is your bedroom a comfortable temperature (ideally, around 18 °C)?

   b. Do you have a humidifier for the winter and an air conditioner for the summer? (Humidity levels that are too high or too low can affect your sleep.) How does humidity affect your quality of sleep?

   c. Are your mattress and pillow in good condition, and are they comfortable?

   d. Does your bed partner disrupt your sleep?

   e. What do you need to address in order to make your sleeping environment more effective?

7. List what you think might be the benefits and drawbacks of shiftwork. What coping techniques can you develop to survive working shifts?

If you have negative responses to most of these questions, you may be one of those people who has difficulty with sleep, which could lead to a sleep disorder or difficulty working shifts.

ASSIGNMENT 13.2 How Will You Cope with Shiftwork?

1. What aspects of your life will you have to change in order to cope with shiftwork (sleeping habits, eating habits, etc.)?

2. What changes in your house or other dwelling might make it a better place to sleep?

3. What nutritional concerns do you need to address in order to adjust to shiftwork?

4. What habits will you have to change so that you will be able to sleep more effectively?

5. How do you think shiftwork will affect you socially? How can you moderate these effects?

6. How will you help your significant other and family members cope with your shiftwork?

7. What changes do you think you may have to make to ensure that you get the proper amount of fitness activity?

Glossary

1RM
one maximal repetition of weight; the maximal amount of weight that can be lifted through the full range of motion, for one repetition, with proper form

active living
a way of life in which individuals make meaningful and satisfying physical activities an integral part of daily living

aerobic conditioning
an exercise program that incorporates activities that are rhythmic in nature, using large muscle groups at moderate intensities for 4 to 7 days per week

agonist
a muscle that causes specific movement by contracting

amino acids
the fundamental constituents of proteins; amino acids can be divided into two types—complete (essential) and incomplete

anatomy
the study of the structure and parts of the body in relationship to one another

aneurysm
a weak or thin area in a blood vessel that causes it to expand and fill with blood; aneurysms may occur as a result of a disease, an injury, or a congenital abnormality in the vessel

angina pectoris
severe chest pains associated with advanced cases of coronary heart disease

anorexia nervosa
an eating disorder in which individuals do not eat enough to maintain a healthy body weight

antagonist
a muscle that acts in opposition to the movement caused by the agonist, returning a limb to its initial position

arteriosclerosis
blanket term for a group of ischemic cardiovascular diseases characterized by a narrowing or hardening of the arteries

arteriovenous malformation (AVM)
a malformation of the blood vessels of the brain, usually present at birth; an arteriovenous malformation can increase the risk of stroke

arthritis
a group of conditions in which there is a degeneration of a joint following trauma to the joint (as a result of an infection or aging)

atherosclerosis
a common type of arteriosclerosis; a slow, progressive disease in which arterial blockage results from fatty deposits collecting in the arteries

attitude
value added to one's beliefs

ballistic stretching
a stretching technique that promotes the stretch reflex but increases the risk of injury to muscles and tendons; it requires quick, well-coordinated action–reaction movements that stretch the muscles beyond their normal range of motion

basal metabolic rate (BMR)
the speed at which energy is used by the body

basal metabolism
the amount of energy a body at rest needs to maintain essential functions

belief
acceptance of an idea on the basis of knowledge and conviction

binge eating disorder (BED)
an eating disorder associated with obesity, where the person alternately eats obsessively and then diets and restricts eating; the disorder is diagnosed if the person does not follow the binge eating with compensatory behaviours such as vomiting, excessive exercise, or laxative abuse

blood cholesterol
the cholesterol produced by the liver

body composition
the proportion of lean tissue to fat in the body

body mass index (BMI)
a method for assessing body composition, based on weight and height

Borg scale
a method for determining the intensity of exercise, used as an alternative to heart rate monitoring

bulimia nervosa
an eating disorder in which individuals have an intense fear of overweight and overfat that causes binge eating followed by self-induced vomiting

bursitis
inflammation of a bursa (a sac of fluid near a joint)

cardiac arrest
cessation of the heart's pumping action

cardiorespiratory endurance
heart and respiratory system endurance; the ability to perform prolonged large-muscle activities at moderate to high intensity

cardiovascular fitness
the ability to transport and use oxygen during prolonged, strenuous exercise or work; it reflects the combined efficiency of the lungs, heart, vascular system, and exercising muscles in the transport and use of oxygen

cerebrovascular disease
interruption of circulation to the brain due either to clotting or hemorrhage

cholesterol
a waxy, fat-like substance important for normal body function that travels through the blood and is linked to atherosclerosis

chronic time urgency
a constant state of stress due to putting pressure on yourself to do too much in too little time

chronotype
a person's individual circadian rhythms, including body temperature, cognitive faculties, and eating and sleeping patterns

circadian rhythm
the 24-hour cycle on which the human biological clock is based

concurrent training
training for either strength or power at the same time as training for endurance

congenital heart disease
problems with the structure of the heart resulting from a birth defect

coronary heart disease
a type of ischemic heart disease in which fatty deposits block one or more coronary arteries (arteries supplying the heart)

critical incident
a situation faced by police and other emergency service personnel that causes them to experience unusually strong emotional reactions that have the potential to interfere with their ability to function at the scene (current stress) or later (residual stress)

DASH diet
a diet that follows Canada's Food Guide in order to reduce sodium, cholesterol, and fat in Canadians' diet

degenerative disc disease (DDD)
degeneration of the intervertebral disc

delayed-onset muscle soreness (DOMS)
soreness of muscles 12 hours or more after exercise

diabetes
a chronic disease in which your body cannot properly use glucose for energy

dietary cholesterol
the cholesterol in food

dietary fibre
food components that cannot be digested, found exclusively in plants; the two types of dietary fibre are insoluble and soluble

dynamic stretching
a stretching technique that involves performing movements within the full range of motion of the joint; it gradually increases reach and range of motion while the limbs are moving

exercise
a form of leisure-time physical activity that is planned, structured, and repetitive, with the goal of improving or maintaining physical fitness

exercising heart rate
your heart rate when your body is in motion during sustained exercise

extrinsic motivation
motivation to perform a task or goal based on external rewards

fartlek training
interval training of running distances at intense levels followed by recovery periods at predetermined intervals

fatty acids
the fundamental constituents of fats; fatty acids can be divided into two types—saturated and unsaturated

female athlete triad
an eating disorder among female athletes that is defined by three conditions: disordered eating, amenorrhea, and osteoporosis

fibromyalgia
chronic disorder characterized by widespread musculoskeletal pain, fatigue, and multiple "tender points," particularly in the neck, spine, shoulders, and hips

fixator
a muscle that provides support while movement occurs

flexibility
the ability to move the joints freely through their full range of motion

frostbite
severe condition where both the skin and the underlying tissue (fat, muscle, and bone) are frozen

frostnip
a mild form of frostbite, where only the top layer of skin freezes

general adaptation
the process of preparing your muscles, joints, tendons, and ligaments for intense training by educating the neuromuscular component so that gains can be seen; characterized by higher repetitions, lower intensities, and short rest periods

general adaptation syndrome (GAS)
the body's reaction to stress

gestational diabetes
a temporary condition in which hormonal changes associated with pregnancy and the growth demands of the fetus increase insulin needs to two to three times the normal level; generally occurs after the 24th week of pregnancy and resolves after delivery

glucose
a simple form of sugar that acts as fuel for the body

glycemic index
the amount of blood glucose (sugar) levels of certain foods within two hours of digestion

glycemic load (GL)
a measure of how quickly a food is converted into sugar in relation to how much sugar it contains

health
the ability of an individual to function independently in a constantly changing environment

health benefits
improvements to physical, mental, and psychological health

health-related fitness
the components of physical fitness that are related to health status, including cardiovascular fitness, musculoskeletal fitness, body composition, and metabolism

healthy living
the practice of health-enhancing behaviours; the physical, mental, and spiritual capacity to make healthy choices including healthy eating and physical activity, and an understanding of their relationship to maintaining a healthy weight

heart failure
inability of the heart to pump enough blood to the body

heat cramps
illness caused by a water and sodium deficiency; heat cramps feel like severe muscle pulls

heat exhaustion
illness caused by extreme body heat; excessive heat and dehydration can raise body temperature to 38–40 °C (100–104 °F)

heat stroke
illness caused by failure of the body's heat-regulating mechanism; may lead to permanent disability or death

high-density lipoprotein (HDL) cholesterol
"good" cholesterol; it helps clean out undesirable LDL deposits

high-intensity interval training (HIIT)
a form of training designed to increase aerobic performance

hyperhydration
water "intoxication," characterized by an abnormal increase in the body's water content

hypertension
high blood pressure—the term "essential hypertension" is used for cases in which the cause is unknown

hypertrophy
the process characterized by high training volume with moderate training intensity in order to build muscle mass

hypothermia
condition occurring when the body's control mechanism can no longer maintain a normal body temperature, and the body's temperature drops to an abnormally low level

impingement syndrome
squeezing of the rotator cuff (the group of muscles that surrounds the shoulder)

intention
a determination to achieve an aim

interval training
training that is based on the concept that the body's energy systems can make both aerobic and anaerobic gains by training with relatively intense exercises followed by a period of recovery

intervertebral discs
flexible, gelatinous, shock-absorbing pads that separate the vertebrae

intracerebral hemorrhage
bleeding in the brain resulting from the rupture of a blood vessel

intrinsic motivation
motivation to perform a task or goal based on enjoyment of doing the task itself

ischemic heart disease
blockage of the coronary arteries resulting in lack of oxygen, angina, and dyspnea

isokinetic contraction
occurs when muscle length changes, contracting maximally throughout the full range of movement

isometric contraction
occurs when muscle length remains constant, or when contractile force equals resistive force

isotonic contraction
contraction of a muscle in response to a load applied to it; includes concentric and eccentric contractions

kilocalorie (kcal)
a measure of the amount of energy in food; also referred to as a calorie. An individual's energy needs are the number of calories he or she must consume to maintain health based on age, sex, weight, height, and activity level.

ligament
fibrous tissue that connects bones to other bones

low-density lipoprotein (LDL) cholesterol
"bad" cholesterol; it can build up in the arteries and cause health problems

maximum aerobic capacity (VO_2 max or MVO_2)
a measure of cardiorespiratory fitness; estimated as the point at which oxygen uptake plateaus and does not increase with further increases in workload

maximal heart rate (MHR)
your heart rate when your heart beats at maximal effort during a sustained aerobic activity

metabolic syndrome
a cluster of risk factors including abdominal obesity, hypertension, high blood triglycerides, insulin resistance, low HDL (good) and high LDL (bad) cholesterol, and vascular inflammatory markers

mission statement
a concise statement of major values and goals that is meant to give direction to the decisions a person will make throughout his or her life

moderate-intensity physical activity
on an absolute scale, moderate intensity refers to activity that is performed 3.0–5.9 times the intensity of rest; on a scale relative to an individual's personal capacity, moderate-intensity physical activity is usually about 10–12 on the Borg scale of 0–20

morbidity
number of ill people in a population, usually expressed as an annual rate

mortality
number of deaths in a population, usually expressed as an annual rate

muscular endurance
the ability of a muscle to sustain a prolonged contraction or to contract over and over again

muscular strength
the amount of force a muscle can produce with a single maximum effort

musculoskeletal fitness
a combined measure of muscular strength, flexibility, and muscular endurance to provide a measure of health

myocardial infarction
a heart attack

narcolepsy
a disorder that causes brain malfunction, leading to one's falling asleep without warning

osteoporosis
a condition common in older people, in whom bones become increasingly soft and porous, thinner, and more brittle, making them susceptible to risk of fracture, particularly of the hip, spine, and wrist

overload principle
the principle that muscle mass can be built up only if the muscle is subjected to a greater than normal load

performance/skill-related fitness
the degree of fitness required to perform a particular job or sport

periodization
overall training plan where an individual maximizes performances at peak times; an organized approach to training that involves progressive cycling of various aspects of a training program during a specific period of time

peripheral vascular disease
reduced circulation to the extremities due to hardening of the arteries

personal goals
goals that reflect personality—who we are, how we think, and how we look

physical activity
all leisure and non-leisure body movement that results in an expenditure of energy

physical fitness
a person's health and performance, specifically in the areas of cardiorespiratory fitness, body composition, muscular strength and endurance, and flexibility

physiology
the study of function of the human body, or how the parts work and carry out their life-sustaining activities

plyometric training
a form of resistance training that works on developing strength and power

plyometrics
a method of training that enhances an individual's "explosive" reaction through rapid and powerful muscular contractions through stretch-shortening cycles; a concentric action immediately preceded by an eccentric action

post-traumatic stress disorder (PTSD)
disorder that changes the way the body responds to stress, probably as a result of chemical imbalances that increase the levels of stress hormones and alter the reaction of the nervous system

power training
the process where an athlete works to build overall body explosiveness and reactive ability by taking the strength gained in the strength phase and converting it to activity-specific power

prediabetes
impaired fasting glucose or impaired glucose tolerance; refers to blood glucose levels that are consistently higher than normal but not over 7.0 mmol/L

principle of progressive overload
refers to training and overloading the muscles that help the body to adapt to more and more stress

principle of recovery
refers to the recuperation time or amount of rest required after a workout

principle of reversibility
refers to all the benefits of exercise that are lost if you stop training

principle of specificity
refers to the ability of the body to adapt to a particular type and amount of stress placed on it

procrastination
the postponement of unpleasant or burdensome tasks

professional goals
goals that reflect career aspirations

proprioceptive neuromuscular facilitation (PNF)
a stretching technique that involves contracting and relaxing the muscles before stretching a measure of cardiorespiratory fitness; estimated as the point at which oxygen uptake plateaus and does not increase with further increases in workload

psychosomatic symptoms
physical symptoms resulting from mental conflict

pyramid training
a system that combines the light to heavy and heavy to light approaches for weight training

range of motion
the distance and direction a joint can move to its full potential

rapid-eye movement (REM) sleep
a stage of sleep that allows your body to recover from mental fatigue and helps to store memories and consolidate learning

repetition (rep)
one complete movement of an exercise

repetition maximum loading
progressive resistance training using a load that is heavy enough to result in "task failure" (muscular exhaustion on the tenth repetition)

repetitive strain injury (RSI)
an injury that arises when soft tissue is subjected to repeated trauma (such as may be caused by typing or using a computer mouse) without the chance to recover from each trauma

resistance training
the most common form of weight training which incorporates exercises that result in gains to muscle mass and strength as well as the potential for improved flexibility and range of motion; an exercise program that uses repeated, progressive contractions of specific muscle groups to increase muscle strength, endurance, or power

resting heart rate
your heart rate when you are in a resting state such as sleep

restless legs syndrome (RLS)
a condition characterized by an overwhelming urge to move the legs when they are at rest

rheumatic heart disease
defects in heart valve function resulting from an infection by *Streptococcus* bacteria

sciatica
pain anywhere along the sciatic nerve as the result of compression, inflammation, or irritation; generally, the pain travels from the back of the thigh to the back of the calf, and also may extend upwards, to the hip

self-efficacy
one's ability to take action and perform a specific behaviour

self-esteem
how one feels about oneself and one's characteristics

self-management behavioural strategies
having the ability to shift your attention from barriers and toward ideas, feelings, and actions that support change

set
a group of repetitions

six basic nutrients
the basic nutrients that the body requires to function efficiently: water, carbohydrates, protein, fats, vitamins, and minerals.

skinfold measurement
measurement of fat just below the skin surface at five points on the body to determine the percentage of body fat

sleep apnea
a breathing-related sleep disorder in which inappropriate brain signals do not tell the breathing muscles to initiate respiration

social involvement
the support of other people to assist you in achieving your goals

somatotype
there are three somatotypes (body types): ectomorphic, mesomorphic, and endomorphic

sprain
a stretching or tearing injury to a ligament

static stretching
a stretching technique that involves bringing a muscle to a maximum or near-maximum stretch by contracting the opposing muscle and holding the stretch for 20–30 seconds without pain

strain
a twisting or pulling injury to a muscle or tendon

stress
a "non-specific response of the body to any demands made upon it" (Selye, 1974)

stressor
any physical, psychological, or environmental event or condition that initiates the stress response

stroke
paralysis and a sudden loss of consciousness caused by an interruption of blood flow to the brain; a thrombotic or thromboembolic stroke occurs when blood flow is interrupted by a blood clot that travels to the brain; a hemorrhagic stroke occurs when very high blood pressure causes a weakened blood vessel near the brain to break

subarachnoid hemorrhage
hemorrhage that occurs when a blood vessel on the surface of the brain bleeds into the space between the brain and the skull

superset training
a system that involves performing two exercises in succession, without rest; often used to exercise opposing muscle groups, it results in increased strength and muscle mass of the targeted muscle group

synergist
a muscle that assist an agonist indirectly in producing a joint's movement

talk test
a method for determining the intensity of exercise, used as an alternative to heart rate monitoring; if a person is breathless and cannot carry on a conversation while exercising, he or she is working too hard

target heart rate (THR) zone
the zone that a person's heart rate must reach during exercise to improve or maintain aerobic fitness

tendinitis
inflammation of a tendon

tendon
fibrous tissue that connects muscles to bones

trans fats
unsaturated fatty acids that have been hydrogenated to give them a longer shelf life; diets high in trans fats increase the risk of atherosclerosis and coronary heart disease

transient ischemic attack (TIA)
a temporary interference with the blood supply to the brain

trisets
combining three exercises with little rest in between; can involve working the same muscle group from three different angles, working three different muscle groups, or working different areas of the same muscle from three different angles

type 1 diabetes
diabetes that occurs when the pancreas no longer produces insulin or produces very little

type 2 diabetes
diabetes that occurs when the pancreas cannot produce enough insulin or the body is unable to use the insulin effectively

values
the things that matter most to us and guide our daily behaviour, activities, and decisions

vertebrae
the bones of the spine (singular: vertebra)

vigorous-intensity physical activity
on an absolute scale, vigorous intensity refers to activity that is performed at 6.0 or more times the intensity of rest for adults and typically 7.0 or more times for children and youth; on a scale relative to an individual's personal capacity, vigorous-intensity physical activity is usually about 14–16 on the Borg scale of 0–20

waist circumference (WC)
an indicator of health risk associated with abdominal fat

waist-to-hip ratio (WHR) measurement
a method for assessing body composition, based on the relationship between the girth of the waist and the girth of the hips

wellness
a way of life in which you make decisions and choices to enjoy the highest level of health and well-being possible

wind chill index (WCI)
measure representing how the temperature would feel on your skin if the wind were reduced to a walking pace of 4.8 km/h

Workplace Hazardous Materials Information System (WHMIS)
a system that familiarizes workers with safety information about potentially hazardous products in their workplace

Index

Credits

Images

1, 3, 27, 43 © Image Source/Corbis; **57, 59, 95, 117** © Roy Morsch/Corbis; **62, 403** Wikipedia; **63** Luka Veselinovic/Shutterstock; **64** Universal Image Group/Visuals Unlimited, Inc.; **65, 404** malinx/Shutterstock; **66** Alila Medical Images/Shutterstock; **143, 145, 161** © F. Hammond/photocuisine/Corbis; **203, 205, 223, 253, 275, 303, 317** © Henglein and Steets/cultura/Corbis; **232** Nucleus Medical Media/Visuals Unlimited, Inc.; **327 top, 329** Peter Gardiner/Science Photo Library; **327 bottom** © Nucleus Medical Art, Inc./Alamy; **341, 343** Shaun Lowe/iStockphoto. All other medical illustrations: LifeArt. Exercise photos: Nancy Wagner Wisotzki.

Text

10 Adapted from Statistics Canada, Leading causes of death, by sex, CANSIM Table 102-0561 and Catalogue no. 84-215-X, 2008. This does not constitute an endorsement by Statistics Canada of this product; **15** Adapted from R.V. Hockey, *Physical fitness: The pathway to healthful living* (7th ed.) (Boston: Mosby-Year Book, 1993), p. 18. Reproduced with permission of The McGraw-Hill Companies; **29** Tabular adaptation of "The five stages of change" [pp. 36–50] from CHANGING FOR GOOD by JAMES O. PROCHASKA and JOHN C. NORCROSS AND CARLO C. DICLEMENTE. COPYRIGHT © 1994 BY JAMES O. PROCHASKA, JOHN C. NORCROSS AND CARLO C. DICLEMENTE. Reprinted by permission of HarperCollins Publishers; **30–31** Prochaska, J.O., & Vilicer, W.F. (1997). The transtheoretical model of health behavior change. *American Journal of Health Promotion, 12*(1), 39–40. AJHP Copyright 2012 by AMERICAN JOURNAL OF HEALTH PROMOTION. Reproduced with permission of AMERICAN JOURNAL OF HEALTH PROMOTION in the format republish in a textbook via Copyright Clearance Center; **75** Adapted from Statistics Canada, Leisure-time physical activity by sex, household population aged 12 and over, Canada, provinces and territories, occasional, CANSIM Table 105-0433, 2006. This does not constitute an endorsement by Statistics Canada of this product; **102** Adapted from Borg, G. (1982). Psychological bases of perceived exertion—Perceived rate of exertion. *Medicine & Science in Sports & Exercise, 14*, 344–386. Borg RPE Scale ®. Scales with instructions can be obtained from Borg Perception; **150** Adapted from World Health Organization (WHO). (2000). *Obesity: Preventing and managing the global epidemic: Report of a WHO consultation on obesity.* Geneva; **151** Adapted from National Heart, Lung, and Blood Institute; National Institutes of Health; U.S. Department of Health and Human Services. (1998). *Clinical guidelines on the identification, evaluation and treatment of overweight and obesity in adults: The evidence report*. Bethesda, MD; **167** Adapted from Foster-Powell, K., Holt, S.H., & Brand-Miller, J.C. (2002). International table of glycemic index and glycemic load values: 2002. *American Journal of Clinical Nutrition, 76*, 5–56. AJCN by American Society for Nutrition. Reproduced with permission of American Society for Nutrition in the format republish in a book/textbook via Copyright Clearance Center; **176–177** National Heart, Lung, and Blood Institute; National Institutes of Health; U.S. Department of Health and Human Services (n.d.). Low-calorie, lower-fat alternative foods. Department of Health and Human Services, National Heart, Lung, and Blood Institute. *Obesity Education*; **179** Adapted from Sizer, F., & Whitney, E. (1997). *Nutrition: Concepts and controversies* (7th ed.). Belmont, CA: Wadsworth; **180** Adapted from Sizer, F., & Whitney, E. (1997). *Nutrition: Concepts and controversies* (7th ed.). Belmont, CA: Wadsworth; National Heart, Lung, and Blood Institute; National Institutes of Health; U.S. Department of Health and Human Services, Office of Dietary Supplements (n.d.). Nutrient recommendations: Dietary reference intakes (DRI*)*; **182** Interactive nutrition label: Get the facts! Health Canada, 2011. Adapted and reproduced from the Minister of Health, 2013; **183** Nutrient content claims and what they mean. Health Canada, 2011. Adapted and reproduced from the Minister of Health, 2013; **184** Nutrition labelling: Get the facts! Health Canada, 2012. Adapted and reproduced with permission of the Minister of Health, 2013; **186 Table 8.7 and Table 8.8** *Eating well with Canada's Food Guide*. © Her Majesty the Queen in Right of Canada, represented by the Minister of Health Canada, 2011. This publication may be reproduced without permission. No changes permitted. HC Pub.: 4651 Cat.: H164-38/1-2011E-PDF ISBN: 978-1-100-19255-0; **187 Table 8.10** *Eating well with Canada's Food Guide*.

© Her Majesty the Queen in Right of Canada, represented by the Minister of Health Canada, 2011. This publication may be reproduced without permission. No changes permitted. HC Pub.: 4651 Cat.: H164-38/1-2011E-PDF ISBN: 978-1-100-19255-0; **222** Adapted from World Health Organization (WHO). (2008). *The global burden of disease: 2004 update*. Figure 4: Distribution of deaths by leading cause groups, males and females, world, 2004 (p. 10). http://www.who.int/healthinfo/global_burden_disease/GBD_report_2004update_full.pdf; **242** 7th WHO-ISH Meeting on Hypertension, Fukuoka, Japan, 29 September to October, 1998: 1999 World Health Organization—International Society of Hypertension Guidelines for the Management of Hypertension, *Journal of Hypertension*. International Society of Hypertension. Chalmers J. et al. Hpertens 1999; 17: 151.85. Table 11.1, Classification of hypertension. Journal of Hypertension by EUROPEAN SOCIETY OF HYPERTENSION; INTERNATIONAL SOCIETY OF HYPERTENSION. Reproduced with permission of LIPPINCOTT WILLIAMS & WILKINS, LTD. in the format reprint in a book/textbook via Copyright Clearance Center; **269** The DRIs for calcium, Health Canada, 2012. Adapted and reproduced from the Minister of Health, 2013; **284–285** American Psychiatric Association, 2000, pp. 429–484; **334** U.S. Search and Research Task Force; **348** *FITCO: Fitness text for Ontario correctional officer applicants*, Ministry of Community Safety and Correctional Services, 2015; **349** *Physical abilities requirement evaluation (PARE)*, http://www.rcmp-grc.gc.ca/recruiting-recrutement/rec/pare-tape-requirement-exigences-eng.htm, RCMP 2012. Reproduced with the permission of the Minister of Public Works and Government Services Canada, 2013; **350–355, 351, 352, 354, 355** Reprinted with permission of the RCMP; **359, 361–364** Ontario Police Fitness Award, Police Fitness Personnel of Ontario, *Fitness appraisal protocol and standards*, 2012; **369–370** Fantastic lifestyle checklist, Douglas M.C. Wilson and Donna Ciliska, *Canadian Family Physician*, July 1984, Vol. 30, pp. 1529–1530; **371–372** *Physical activity readiness questionnaire (PAR-Q)* © 2002. Used with permission from the Canadian Society for Exercise Physiology www.csep.ca; **373–376** *Physical activity readiness medical examination (PARmed-X)* © 2002. Used with permission from the Canadian Society for Exercise Physiology www.csep.ca; **386** *Canadian physical activity, fitness & lifestyle approach: CSEP health & fitness program's appraisal & counselling strategy* (3rd ed.) © 2003. Adapted with permission from the Canadian Society for Exercise Physiology www.csep.ca; **423** Kraemer, W.J., & Fry, A.C. (1995). Strength testing: Development and evaluation of methodology. In P. Maud & C. Foster (Eds.), *Physiological assessment of human fitness* (pp. 115–138). Champaign, IL: Human Kinetics; **430** Body Mass Index (BMI) nomogram. Health Canada, 2008. Reproduced with permission from the Minister of Health, 2013; **431** Adapted from WHO (2000). *Obesity: Preventing and managing the global epidemic: Report on a WHO consultation on obesity.* Consultation Technical Report Series No. 894. Geneva; **452–454** Copyright © 1978 by the American Psychological Association. Reproduced with permission. The official citation that should be used in referencing this material is *Journal of Consulting and Clinical Psychology*, Sarason, I.G., Johnson, J.H., and Siegle, J.M., Assessing the impact of life changes: Development of the life experiences survey, 1978, 46(5), 932–946; **455–456** © 2011 Heart and Stroke Foundation of Canada. Reproduced with permission of the Heart and Stroke Foundation of Canada. www.heartandstroke.ca.